Nanotechnology in Tissue Engineering and Regenerative Medicine

Nanotechnology in Tissue Engineering and Regenerative Medicine

Edited by Ketul Popat

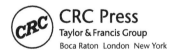

CRC Press
Taylor & Francis Group
Boca Raton   London   New York

CRC Press is an imprint of the
Taylor & Francis Group, an **informa** business

CRC Press
Taylor & Francis Group
6000 Broken Sound Parkway NW, Suite 300
Boca Raton, FL 33487-2742

First issued in paperback 2019

© 2011 by Taylor & Francis Group, LLC
CRC Press is an imprint of Taylor & Francis Group, an Informa business

No claim to original U.S. Government works

ISBN-13: 978-1-4398-0141-3 (hbk)
ISBN-13: 978-0-367-38332-9 (pbk)

Library of Congress Cataloging-in-Publication Data

Nanotechnology in tissue engineering and regenerative medicine / edited by Ketul Popat.
    p. ; cm.
    Includes bibliographical references and index.
    Summary: "Referred to as "nanomedicine" or "nanobiomedicine," the application of nanotechnology to medicine can impact diagnosis, monitoring, and treatment of diseases as well as control and understanding of biological systems. Bringing together an unparalleled field of experts, this volume explores various aspects of nanotechnology and its applications in biomedical fields. The book uses an application-based approach to relate laboratory-based research to the development of technologies that can be readily adaptable to an industrial environment, focusing chiefly on drug delivery, tissue engineering, and regenerative medicine"--Provided by publisher.
    ISBN 978-1-4398-0141-3 (hardcover : alk. paper)
    1. Nanomedicine. 2. Tissue engineering. 3. Regenerative medicine. I. Popat, Ketul. II. Title.
    [DNLM: 1. Tissue Engineering. 2. Biocompatible Materials. 3. Nanostructures. 4. Nanotechnology. 5. Regenerative Medicine--methods. QT 37 N1875 2011]

R857.N34N362 2010
610.28'4--dc22
    2010018864

Visit the Taylor & Francis Web site at
http://www.taylorandfrancis.com

and the CRC Press Web site at
http://www.crcpress.com

Contents

Preface

Nanotechnology has become a rapidly growing field with potential applications ranging from electronics to cosmetics. The term "nanotechnology" varies greatly based on the specific definition that is used. The National Science Foundation and the National Nanotechnology Initiative define nanotechnology as understanding and control of matter at dimensions of 1–100 nm where unique phenomena enable novel applications. Nanomaterials and devices provide unique opportunities to advance medicine. The application of nanotechnology to medicine is referred to as "nanomedicine" or "nanobiomedicine" and could impact diagnosis, monitoring, and treatment of diseases as well as control and understanding of biological systems. This multicontributed book discusses the use of nanotechnology for medical applications with focus on its use for drug delivery and tissue engineering.

Nanotechnology for Regenerative Medicine

Controlled drug-delivery strategies have made a dramatic impact in medicine. In general, controlled-release polymer systems deliver drugs in the optimum dosage for long periods, thus increasing the efficacy of the drug, maximizing patient compliance and enhancing the ability to use highly toxic, poorly soluble or relatively unstable drugs. Nanoscale materials can be used as drug delivery vehicles to develop highly selective and effective therapeutic and diagnostic modalities. There are a number of advantages with nanoparticles in comparison to microparticles. For example, nanoscale particles can travel through the blood stream without sedimentation or blockage of the microvasculature. Small nanoparticles can circulate in the body and penetrate tissues such as tumors. In addition, nanoparticles can be taken up by the cells through natural means such as endocytosis. Nanoparticles have already been used to deliver drugs to target sites for cancer therapeutics and deliver imaging agents for cancer diagnostics. These vehicles can be engineered to recognize biophysical characteristics that are unique to the target cells and therefore minimize drug loss and toxicity associated with delivery to nondesired tissues.

Nanotechnology in Tissue Engineering

Tissue engineering combines biology, medicine, engineering, and materials science to develop tissues that restore, maintain, or enhance tissue function. To recapitulate proper function and organization of native tissues in tissue engineering approaches, it is important to mimic tissue properties at the nanoscale. For example, in the body, the extracellular matrix (ECM) provides a natural web of tissue-specific and organized nanofibers that supports and maintains the cell microenvironment. In addition, cells in the body reside in a unique environment that is regulated by cell–cell, cell–ECM, and cell-soluble factors presented in a spatially and temporally dependent manner. Thus, engineering approaches and methods that aim to use tissue engineering principles must have the same level of complexity. Nanotechnologies and microtechnologies can be merged with biomaterials to generate scaffolds for tissue engineering that can maintain and regulate cell behavior. Also, such technologies can be used to regulate *in vitro* cellular microenvironment to direct stem cell differentiation.

Nanotechnology is an emerging field that is potentially changing the way we treat diseases through drug delivery and tissue engineering. However, significant challenges remain in pushing this field into clinically viable therapies. For drug delivery, the design and testing of novel methods of controlling the interaction of nanomaterials with the body are some of the current barriers to translating these technologies to therapies. Methods of targeting nanomaterials to specific sites of the body while avoiding capture by organs, such as the liver and spleen, are major challenges that need to be addressed. With respect to tissue engineering, it is envisioned that new nanomaterials that provide proper signals and environmental cues to cells as well as generate three-dimensional microenvironments may be advantageous over today's polymers. This book brings insight into these issues and discusses cutting edge research in these areas.

Editor

Ketul Popat is an assistant professor in the Department of Mechanical Engineering and School of Biomedical Engineering at Colorado State University. His research is on developing nanoscale materials for tissue engineering regenerative medicine, with particular emphasis on understanding the structure–function relationship between nanomaterials and tissues. He has published over 30 peer-reviewed papers, 50 abstracts, and 3 pending patents. He received his PhD in bioengineering from University of Illinois at Chicago, MS in chemical engineering from Illinois Institute of Technology, and BE in chemical engineering from Maharaja Sayajirao University, India.

Contributors

Kristy M. Ainslie
Department of Bioengineering and Therapeutic Sciences
University of California, San Francisco
San Francisco, California

Jorge L. Almodóvar
Department of Chemical and Biological Engineering
Colorado State University
Fort Collins, Colorado

Treena Livingston Arinzeh
Department of Biomedical Engineering
New Jersey Institute of Technology
Newark, New Jersey

Harinder K. Bawa
Department of Chemistry, Chemical Biology, and Biomedical Engineering
Stevens Institute of Technology
Hoboken, New Jersey

Daniel A. Bernards
Department of Bioengineering and Therapeutic Sciences
University of California, San Francisco
San Francisco, California

Zarna Ashwin Bhavsar
Department of Bioengineering
University of Texas at Arlington
Arlington, Texas

Sandra Whaley Bishnoi
Department of Biological, Chemical, and Physical Sciences
Illinois Institute of Technology
Chicago, Illinois

Walter Bonani
Department of Mechanical Engineering
University of Colorado at Boulder
Boulder, Colorado

Karla S. Brammer
Materials Science and Engineering
University of California, San Diego
La Jolla, California

Philip J. Chuang
Department of Biomedical Engineering
Columbia University
New York, New York

Nicole Clarke
Department of Chemical Engineering
University of Florida
Gainesville, Florida

Christine J. Cobb
Materials Science and Engineering
University of California, San Diego
La Jolla, California

Tejal A. Desai
Department of Bioengineering and
    Therapeutic Sciences
University of California, San Francisco
San Francisco, California

Cevat Erisken
Department of Biomedical Engineering
Columbia University
New York, New York

Anirban Sen Gupta
Department of Biomedical Engineering
Case Western Reserve University
Cleveland, Ohio

Albena Ivanisevic
Department of Chemistry
Purdue University
West Lafayette, Indiana

Sungho Jin
Materials Science and Engineering
University of California, San Diego
La Jolla, California

Radoslaw Junka
Department of Chemistry, Chemical Biology,
    and Biomedical Engineering
Stevens Institute of Technology
Hoboken, New Jersey

Matt J. Kipper
Department of Chemical and Biological
    Engineering
Colorado State University
Fort Collins, Colorado

Soujanya Kona
Department of Biomedical Engineering
University of Texas
Arlington, Texas

Bhanu Prasanth Koppolu
Department of Biomedical Engineering
University of Texas at Arlington
Arlington, Texas

Marcus Kramer
Weldon School of Biomedical
    Engineering
Purdue University
West Lafayette, Indiana

Jiyeon Lee
Department of Chemical
    Engineering
University of Florida
Gainesville, Florida

Yee-Shuan Lee
Department of Biomedical
    Engineering
New Jersey Institute of Technology
Newark, New Jersey

Tanmay P. Lele
Department of Chemical Engineering
University of Florida
Gainesville, Florida

Helen H. Lu
Department of Biomedical Engineering
Columbia University
New York, New York

Krishna Madhavan
Department of Mechanical Engineering
University of Colorado at Boulder
Boulder, Colorado

Kytai Truong Nguyen
Department of Bioengineering
University of Texas
Arlington, Texas

Seunghan Oh
Department of Dental Biomaterials
Wonkwang University
Iksan, South Korea

Parth N. Shah
Department of Chemical and Biomolecular
    Engineering
The University of Akron
Akron, Ohio

John Shapiro
Department of Molecular Virology,
    Immunology, and Medical
    Genetics
The Ohio State University
Columbus, Ohio

Sadhana Sharma
College of Engineering
The Ohio State University
Columbus, Ohio

Piyush M. Sinha
Intel Corporation
Hillsboro, Oregon

Justin A. Smolen
Department of Biomedical Engineering
The University of Akron
Akron, Ohio

Siddarth D. Subramony
Department of Biomedical Engineering
Columbia University
New York, New York

Wei Tan
Department of Mechanical Engineering
University of Colorado at Boulder
Boulder, Colorado

Sarah L. Tao
The Charles Stark Draper Laboratory
Cambridge, Massachusetts

Rahul G. Thakar
Department of Bioengineering and
    Therapeutic Sciences
University of California, San Francisco
San Francisco, California

Chandra M. Valmikinathan
Department of Chemistry, Chemical Biology
    and Biomedical Engineering
Stevens Institute of Technology
Hoboken, New Jersey

Robbie J. Walczak
Thermo Fisher Scientific
Indianapolis, Indiana

Hao Xu
Department of Bioengineering
University of Texas at Arlington
Arlington, Texas

Xiaojun Yu
Department of Chemistry, Chemical Biology,
    and Biomedical Engineering
Stevens Institute of Technology
Hoboken, New Jersey

Yang H. Yun
Department of Biomedical Engineering
The University of Akron
Akron, Ohio

1

Atomic Force Microscope Lithography on Biomimetic Surfaces

Marcus Kramer
Purdue University

Albena Ivanisevic
Purdue University

1.1 Introduction to Patterning of Substrates

As our scientific comprehension advances, our search to understand the world requires scientists to investigate smaller and smaller features. In the field of tissue engineering this is no different. The constant endeavor for new knowledge drives the development of methods of study involving cells, and/or biomaterials to heal illness and improve longevity (Khademhosseini et al., 2006). However, it is necessary to fully understand the current applications to enable the development of future techniques. These applications focus on the combination of biological and engineering techniques to mimic the structures of the human body like the extracellular matrix (ECM) in order to rebuild tissue function (Khademhosseini et al., 2006; Nelson and Tien, 2006). This is a very difficult task. The ECM is a highly heterogeneous structure composed of many biomolecules with different chemical features that create different microenvironments (Nelson and Tien, 2006). Cells in these different environments respond, grow, and (in the case of stem cells) develop differently (Bettinger et al., 2009). These cells receive different migration, proliferation, and adhesion signals from the ECM microenvironment around them. It has been shown *in vitro* that micro and nanoscale patterned substrates can be used to produce structural and chemical cues to cause changes in cell behavior (Khademhosseini et al., 2006; Nelson and Tien, 2006; Bettinger et al., 2009). Still, researchers lack the ability to recreate these unique matrices synthetically and can only recreate chemical or structural microenvironments mimicking a few natural cues (Nelson and Tien, 2006). This chapter will focus on two-dimensional micro and nanopatterning of biomimetic substrates. The heterogeneity of the microenvironment is important in regulating cellular function (Nelson and Tien, 2006; Bettinger et al., 2009). Modification of natural and synthetic biomimetic substrates is necessary to tailor them to the specific application of interest (i.e., cell study, treatment, etc.).

There are many techniques capable of patterning on nanometer length scales and they are generally characterized as contact and noncontact printing (Barbulovic-Nad et al., 2006). Examples of these techniques range from micro/nanocontact printing (μCP/nCP) (being more general) to electrospray depositions (ESD) (being more selective). All of these techniques offer advantages and disadvantages ranging from the inexpensive, high throughput of single ink μCP (Zhao et al., 1997) to the high registry, inherently serial scanning probe techniques (Tseng et al., 2005). Since tissue engineering inheritably involves tissue and cell experiments the primary inks of interest are biomolecule inks (Mendes et al., 2007). Biomolecule inks are solutions of biological molecules used for patterning including peptides, proteins, DNA, viruses, and cells, which are primarily used in the study of fundamental cell/molecular biology, and nanoarray production for biosensors and biochips (Mendes et al., 2007; Salaita et al., 2007). The ideal patterning technique for tissue engineering should pattern variable biomolecular inks on the biomimetic substrate. It should also be generally useable and scalable for mass replication. (I.e., it should be capable of patterning in a parallel fashion so it could be scaled for mass production or mass parallel experimentation). However, patterning biomimetic substrates in parallel becomes more difficult while considering the soft, sometimes uneven nature of the substrates on the nanometer scale. Dip-pen nano-lithography (DPN) is an atomic force microscope (AFM) lithographic technique which uses an AFM probe to pattern a highly confluent self-assembled monolayer (SAM) to various substrates. Further this technique is capable of patterning bimolecular and soft substrates without damaging them. Therefore, the remainder of this chapter will explore patterning of biomimetic substrates with AFM lithography primarily focusing on DPN.

1.2 Atomic Force Microscopy and Applications

1.2.1 Atomic Force Microscopy

The AFM is an instrument capable of imaging various substrates all the way down to the level of atoms. Some of its greatest strengths are its ease of use, fast image acquisition, and reproducibility. Image collection works by bringing a solid tip with a nanometer radius in contact with the substrate. The tip is controlled by a laser which is bounced off the cantilever that bends when in contact with the substrate. The bending of the cantilever changes the signal to the AFM. This signal is processed and returns as a change in the height of the substrate. By moving the tip across the substrate in a raster pattern (scanned back and forth) a constant change in the substrate height is recorded as an image (Figure 1.1). The most common AFM operation modes are contact mode and tapping mode. In contact mode the tip is kept

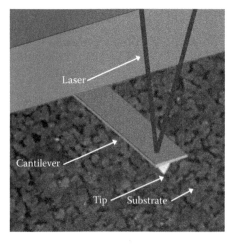

FIGURE 1.1   (See color insert following page 10-24.) Representation of AFM imaging of a gold substrate.

in constant contact with the substrate during scanning. Tapping mode operates by tapping the tip on the substrate during imaging this tapping produces an image through feedback. However, because the imaging is performed by tapping the substrate it is a softer method of imaging and can be used to image soft substrates. One problem with imaging is that under ambient conditions a water meniscus forms around the tip–substrate interface. Understanding this characteristic of AFM, Piner et al. realized a new method of patterning molecules, with micro and nanometer control, to substrates called DPN, a form of AFM lithography (Piner et al., 1999). Other methods of AFM lithography include nanoshaving/nanografting which will be covered here in brief; however, the remainder of this chapter will focus on DPN.

1.2.2 Nanoshaving/Nanografting

Nanoshaving and nanograftting are very similar techniques and can be covered together (Avseenko et al., 2002; Barbulovic-Nad et al., 2006; Mendes et al., 2007). These techniques use an AFM tip which is placed in contact with an SAM covered substrate. Under high forces, the tip scraps away a line of the SAM exposing the substrate underneath (Figure 1.2a–c). In nanoshaving, the substrate can be repatterned with a new functional molecule after shaving or left with empty trenches (Figure 1.2c and f) (Banerjee et al., 2004). In nanografting the only difference is that the SAM removal is done in the presence of the new functional molecule which is coated on the AFM tip. In this way the new molecule replaces the removed one immediately (Figure 1.2d–f) (Wadu-Mesthrige et al., 1999). Both methods have been used to immobilize biomolecules and show good nanometer resolution (Wadu-Mesthrige et al., 1999; Liu et al., 2002; Banerjee et al., 2004; Tinazli et al., 2007). However, these techniques are inherently serial because they use a scanning probe method (Barbulovic-Nad et al., 2006). Also the SAM must be readily removable and the replacement molecule quickly binding to facilitate patterning (Leggett, 2006). Further the technique has been limited to hard substrates (Mendes et al., 2007), due to the increased forces, used during patterning.

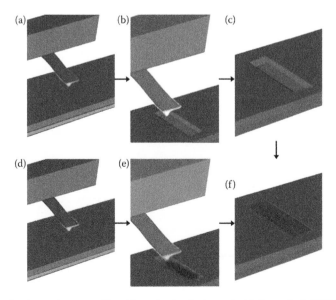

FIGURE 1.2 Nanoshaving and nanografting. Nanoshaving is shown in (a) tip contact, (b) SAM removal, and (c) removed SAM (trench). Nanografting is shown in (d) tip contact, (e) SAM removal and replacement, and (f) new functional molecule patterned to substrate.

1.2.3 Dip-Pen Nanolithography

DPN is unique in its ability to both image and pattern various molecules on the micro and nanoscales (Piner et al., 1999). DPN has shown versatility using DNA (Zhang et al., 2002), proteins (Agarwal et al., 2003a), peptides (Cho and Ivanisevic, 2004), viruses (Cheung et al., 2003), and cells (Hsiao et al., 2008) as inks for patterning to various substrates. It works by delivering molecular inks to the substrate through diffusion. First, the AFM tip is inked with the desired ink (in this case biologic) then the tip is brought into contact with the substrate of interest (Figure 1.3a). Upon contact a meniscus forms between the tip and the substrate. This water meniscus facilitates primary diffusion of the inks that are on the surface of the tip to the substrate (Figure 1.3b) (Piner et al., 1999). The tip can then be scanned across the substrate (usually in contact mode) (Piner et al., 1999; Zhang et al., 2002; Agarwal et al., 2003a) but also shown to work in tapping mode (Agarwal et al., 2003b) to produce SAM patterns on a substrate (Piner et al., 1999; Ginger et al., 2004) (Figure 1.3c). Using the AFMs imaging capabilities it is possible to view patterns produced on substrates immediately after production. These patterns can be of various shapes (Piner et al., 1999; Ginger et al., 2004) and composed of a range of molecular inks (Piner et al., 1999; Zhang et al., 2002; Agarwal et al., 2003a). DPN has shown versatility using DNA (Zhang et al., 2002), proteins (Agarwal et al., 2003a), peptides (Cho and Ivanisevic, 2004), viruses (Cheung et al., 2003), and cells (Hsiao et al., 2008) as inks for patterning to various substrates including the natural ECM of the Bruch's membrane (Sistiabudi and Ivanisevic, 2007, 2008). These SAMs are highly confluent and multiple inks can be patterned side by side, with multiple runs, at a high spatial resolution due to the techniques read and write ability (Hong et al., 1999). Therefore, DPN has many advantages toward biological patterning of biomimetic substrates. However, by nature DPN is a serial process (Piner et al., 1999; Barbulovic-Nad et al., 2006; Christman et al., 2006; Salaita et al., 2007). To overcome this, two main ideologies have been developed (Ginger et al., 2004). The first is a passive array DPN, in which a multiple probe array is brought into contact with the substrate simultaneously for patterning with only one probe being controlled by the AFM feedback loop (Mirkin, 2001; Ginger et al., 2004). This is by far the simpler of the two techniques (Ginger et al., 2004). However, this method has difficulties contacting all of the probes, to the substrate, at the same time, though techniques have been developed to overcome this inefficiency to produce passive parallel DPN (Mirkin, 2001). The second technique is active array DPN in which each of the cantilevers in the array is bent by thermal or electrical signals to make substrate contact (Ginger et al., 2004; del Campo and Bruce, 2005). Using this method individual probe(s) may be bent into and out of contact (Bullen et al., 2004; del Campo and Bruce, 2005) with the substrate. Using this technique many molecular patterns have been produced. However, it severely detracts from the ease of use of DPN for patterning. Also, heat is a primary method for bending the probes which

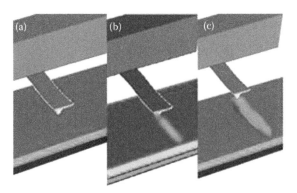

FIGURE 1.3 Patterning of a substrate with DPN from (a) contact to, (b) deposition, and (c) withdrawal of the probe.

poses a risk of denaturing and poor patterning of bioinks (Salaita et al., 2007). Even with the drawbacks of these techniques both have shown the capability of patterning in parallel onto various substrates with multiple inks (Mirkin, 2001; Bullen et al., 2004; Lee et al., 2006). In review, this technique produces highly confluent SAMs whose patterns are easily controlled and has the potential for multiple ink patterning simultaneously (Ginger et al., 2004; Salaita et al., 2007). Further this technique can easily be repeated in the same area with good alignment and multiple inks facilitating complex pattern production (Hong et al., 1999). The remainder of the chapter will focus on an in-depth look at DPN as a biomolecule patterning technique on biomimetic substrates followed by an analysis of its current state and future directions.

1.3 Serial DPN of Biological Inks and Applicable Substrates

The topic of patterning biologically active molecules to various biomimetic substrates with DPN has been reviewed in literature (Zhang et al., 2002; Agarwal et al., 2003b; Sistiabudi and Ivanisevic, 2008). The importance of this work lies with the variety of inks accessible to DPN including those composed of proteins (Lee et al., 2002; Lim et al., 2003; Nam et al., 2004), peptides (Cho and Ivanisevic, 2004; Onyeneho and Ivanisevic, 2004; Sistiabudi and Ivanisevic, 2007, 2008), viruses (Cheung et al., 2003; Smith et al., 2003; Vega et al., 2005), cells (Hsiao et al., 2008), and oligonucleotides (Jiang and Stupp, 2005; Baserga et al., 2008). These have been patterned on various substrates from SAMs (Cho and Ivanisevic, 2004) to inorganic substrates (Nam et al., 2004) and basement membrane (Sistiabudi and Ivanisevic, 2008). There are a variety of techniques which have been employed to both deposit and link the various types of biomolecules to their substrates. However all of the technique's variations can be divided into two general methods indirect and direct (Mendes et al., 2007). Direct patterning to the substrate relies on strong chemical attachment (Lim et al., 2003), and indirect patterning relies on a linker, which is patterned to the substrate, prior to attachment (Smith et al., 2003) of the biomolecules (Mendes et al., 2007). Each of these methods of patterning is reviewed in Table 1.1 which follows the general order of this section.

1.3.1 Indirect Patterning

Indirect DPN is very important as it allows the patterning of substrates and inks not normally accessible to direct DPN (Smith et al., 2003; Valiokas et al., 2006). This capability has captured the attention of researchers in biosenors (Pena et al., 2003) and biomaterials (Nelson and Tien, 2006). There is a great body of work to expand into the nanoworld, using DPN (for instance, the use of these protein arrays, for sensors, produces almost 1000 times reduction in dot size thereby increasing its sensing capacity (Taha et al., 2003)). The first step in patterning is to directly pattern commonly used inks (Vega et al., 2005) (must contain secondary binding group, amine-terminated thiols are common (Smith et al., 2003; Valiokas et al., 2006)) on an acceptable substrate (usually gold). Various protein structures can then be attached to these linker molecules (including cell membrane proteins (Valiokas et al., 2006), IgG (Zhang et al., 2003), lysozyme (Lee et al., 2002), biotin (Hyun et al., 2002), deoxyribonucleic acid (DNA) (Baserga et al., 2008), viruses (Vega et al., 2005), and cells (Lee et al., 2002)). However, this method has some major drawbacks. First, it is very difficult to pattern more than one biomolecule at a time with this technique primarily due to substrate passivation after patterning (Hyun et al., 2002; Demers et al., 2002). Further even with methods (primarily nanografting/shaving (Lim et al., 2003)) to overcome this weakness it would require multiple time-consuming steps to pattern each biomolecule which can lead to nonspecific binding and contamination (Demers et al., 2002; Hyun et al., 2002). Therefore the ideal method for patterning multiple biological functionalities to the substrate is a direct method allowing the production of multicomponent patterns for biosensors, cell scaffolds, and cell experiments (Demers et al., 2002; Lee et al., 2003; Hsiao et al., 2008).

TABLE 1.1 Overview of Current Serial DPN with Various Biomolecules on Every Substrate from Inorganic to Biologic

Method	Biomolecule	Surface Patterning Technique	Reference
Indirect	Proteins	Patterned cell membrane proteins to gold through amine-terminated linkers placed by DPN	Valiokas et al. (2006)
		Biotin–BSA was patterned to gold through DPN pattern of MHA bound by biotin and then streptavidin	Hyun et al. (2002)
		Rabbit IgG placed on gold nanofeatures made via DPN of MHA and etching	Zhang et al. (2003)
	Proteins/Cells	Placed lysozyme rabbit IgG and retronectin for the attachment of cells to gold as proof of concept for cell studies	Lee et al. (2002)
	DNA	DNA patterned to MHA rafts made via DPN on ODT passivated gold	Demers et al. (2001)
		DNA patterned to gold nanofeatures made via DPN and wet etching	Zhang et al. (2002)
		DNA arrays were indirectly patterned to gold through a thiol to show feasibility of combo gold–silver substrate for DPN experiments	Baserga et al. (2008)
	Viruses	Cow pea mosaic virus was attached to maleimide linker patterned on a gold substrate	Smith et al. (2003)
		Tobacco mosaic virus was placed at the single particle level on gold through Zn^{2+} an MHA scaffold generated via DPN	Vega et al. (2005)
		Cow pea mosaic virus indirectly immobilized using thiol linker that was patterned to a gold substrate	Cheung et al. (2003)
Direct	Proteins	Tween-20 surfactant facilitates DPN of maleimide linked biotin onto hydrophobic 3-mercaptopropyltrimethoxysilane (MPTMS) SAM on silicon	Jung et al. (2004)
		Peptide patterned via DPN using tapping mode AFM on gold	Agarwal et al. (2003b)
		Synthetic peptide and T1pA protein patterned using electrochemical DPN in tapping mode	Agarwal et al. (2003a)
		Streptavidin was patterned, using combined dynamic mode DPN, to DNA wires on gold	Li et al. (2004)
		Nanofountain pen to directly pattern yeast protein G to an aldehyde and GFP to an BSA-coated glass	Taha et al. (2003)
		Use nanopen to directly deliver IgG to gold nanowells on glass	Bruckbauer et al. (2004)
		Biotin patterned to polyethyleneimine functionalized silicon oxide	Pena et al. (2003)
		Lysozyme and rabbit IgG dot arrays produced on gold	Lee, 2003)
		Various IgG antibodies modified and unmodified were written to negatively charge silicon oxide and a SAM of aldehyde on silicon oxide	Lim et al. (2003)
		Histidine-tagged ubiquitin and thioredoxin were patterned to nickle oxide	Nam et al. (2004)
		Patterned silicon oxide surface with TAT peptide through an amine SAM	Cho and Ivanisevic (2004)
		Patterned gold with TAT peptide SAM using DPN, μCP, and from solution for comparison	Cho and Ivanisevic (2005)
		Patterned peptide sequence to the retina of harvested eyes	Onyeneho and Ivanisevic (2004)
		Patterned polyarginine and poly(glutamic acid) to SAMs on silicon oxide and the inner collagenous zone of the Bruchs membrane	Sistiabudi and Ivanisevic (2007)
		Patterning of biotin using collagen binding peptide as a linker to the Bruch's membrane	Sistiabudi and Ivanisevic (2008)

TABLE 1.1 (continued) Overview of Current Serial DPN with Various Biomolecules on Every Substrate from Inorganic to Biologic

Method	Biomolecule	Surface Patterning Technique	Reference
	DNA/ Proteins	Patterned DNA and proteins using an argarose carrier to facilitate equal deposition rates of various biomolecules for future use in parallel patterning	Senesi et al. (2009)
	DNA	Oligonucleotide SAM was selectively patterned (degraded) on gold with DNase DPN	Hyun et al. (2004)
		DNA patterned onto a gold and mercaptopropyltrimethoxysilane	Demers et al. (2002)
	Cells	Cells were patterned using complementary DNA linkages on the cells, probe, and substrate	Hsiao et al. (2008)
	Other	Only dynamic patterning observed of PAMAM dendrimers to NHS and NHS-PS-b-PtBA SAM	Salazar et al. (2006)
		Patterned various dendrimers to silicon and silicon oxide to explore interactions and DPN patterning	McKendry et al. (2002)
		Patterning of peptide amphiphiles to silicon	Jiang and Stupp (2005)
		Thiolated collagen patterned onto gold substrate via DPN	Wilson et al. (2001)

1.3.2 Direct Patterning

Direct patterning of proteins and peptides has produced a number of profound discoveries which make patterning to biologically derived substrates more feasible (Jung et al., 2004; Onyeneho and Ivanisevic, 2004; Cho and Ivanisevic, 2005; Sistiabudi and Ivanisevic, 2007, 2008). For example, it is possible to pattern biomolecules to hydrophobic substrates through activation with a surfactant (Jung et al., 2004). From this work Tween-20 (surfactant) has been used to enable the direct patterning of hydrophobic substrates which were previously unusable (Jung et al., 2004; Sistiabudi and Ivanisevic, 2007). However, patterning is still usually performed on hard, hydrophilic conductive substrates (Agarwal et al., 2003a; Lim et al., 2003; Nam et al., 2004). Tapping mode has also been found to be DPN compatible (Agarwal et al., 2003b), but the forces applied to the substrate had to be increased to near contact mode forces. Additionally, the proteins were not strongly bound to the substrate (Agarwal et al., 2003b). This makes tapping mode an interesting but not commonly used mode of DPN. To improve patterning in tapping mode electrochemical deposition was used during which a current between the tip and substrate drives the proteins to deposit (Agarwal et al., 2003a). This technique facilitates patterning but requires a conductive substrate (Nam et al., 2004). Another study used dynamic mode patterning in which the probe was switched between contact and tapping mode for writing and imaging on the substrate. This method has the advantages of imaging in tapping mode and writing in contact mode (Li et al., 2004). There are also a number of studies which modify the substrate to facilitate patterning. Included in these is the production of etched wells which contain the biomolecules in a localized spot (Bruckbauer et al., 2004). This would be a viable method to trap cells in a localized spot for study, inside each well the cell could have its own microenvironment. Some of the more interesting progress in patterning biomimetic substrates involves biomolecules patterned to SAMs. For example, the yeast protein G (Taha et al., 2003), biotin (Pena et al., 2003), and the TAT peptide (Cho and Ivanisevic, 2004) were patterned to SAM-covered substrates. The SAMs serve as a good biomimetic substrate for patterning. However they are homogeneous and are not indicative of the complex microenvironments in biologically derived substrates. Through multiple biomolecule patterning it may be possible to renew some of the complex microenvironment for study. All of these studies merely mimic the biologically derived substrate which was directly patterned (retina (Onyeneho and Ivanisevic, 2004), and Bruch's membrane (Sistiabudi and Ivanisevic, 2007, 2008)) by peptides (Onyeneho and Ivanisevic, 2004; Sistiabudi and Ivanisevic, 2007)

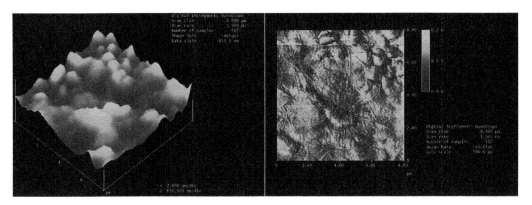

FIGURE 1.4 (Left) Topographical image of the Bruch's membrane of the retina, (right) friction image of polypeptide patterned to the same Bruch's membrane substrate.

and proteins (Sistiabudi and Ivanisevic, 2008) (example of patterning peptides to Bruch's membrane shown in the left image of Figure 1.4). This is the only work which presented studies of the patterning of a biologically derived collagen scaffold (essentially a heterogeneous uneven substrate). During this work Tween-20 (Jung et al., 2004) was used for the patterning process as the substrate (dried Bruch's membrane) was hydrophobic (Sistiabudi and Ivanisevic, 2008). There are two main areas for enhancement in this work. First, the patterning is performed using DPN and is therefore carried out in a serial manner (Piner et al., 1999; Barbulovic-Nad et al., 2006; Christman et al., 2006; Salaita et al., 2007). Second, parallelization of this technique becomes even more complex when considering the uneven nature of the substrate (on micrometer scales) as shown in the left image of Figure 1.4. Patterning with the standard array of silicon nitride tips would have the tendency to either damage the substrate with some tips or not contact the substrate with others.

Patterning of biologically derived substrates is extremely important for the study of cell interactions with the substrate and other cells. Combined with the patterning of cells (Hsiao et al., 2008) and DNA (Hsiao et al., 2008) scientists would be enabled to study cellular responses to specific environmental stimuli. In patterning of cells complementary DNA tethers were attached to the probe and to the substrate to facilitate cell attachment (Hsiao et al., 2008). This sort of work in combination with virus immobilization (Cheung et al., 2003; Smith et al., 2003; Vega et al., 2005) would allow for multifaceted cell infection studies to be carried out with different cells and different viruses on the micron scale. Further, DNA has been explored for direct patterning partly due to its ability to complementary base pair (Demers et al., 2001, 2002). This theoretically allows for the immobilization of any particle that can be functionalized to the DNA. DNA has been selectively patterned onto insulators (Demers et al., 2002; Senesi et al., 2009) and conductors (Demers et al., 2002; Hyun et al., 2004) (enzymatically depatterned (Hyun et al., 2004)) to create various scaffolds. Recently, an argarose accelerant was used as a method of depositing different inks (DNA and proteins) which normally have varying deposition rates (Hyun et al., 2004) at near the same rate. Finally, exploration into the patterning of other biomolecules including dendrimers (McKendry et al., 2002; Salazar et al., 2006), peptide amphiphiles (Jiang and Stupp, 2005), and collagens (Wilson et al., 2001) has been performed. These studies primarily looked at the patterning capabilities of DPN, including research on DPN control (McKendry et al., 2002) and substrate bioactivity after patterning (Wilson et al., 2001). These experiments expanded the technical understanding of the deposition process of bioinks during DPN. In the end these kinds of studies helped to show that DPN on biologically derived substrates with biomolecules was possible (Sistiabudi and Ivanisevic, 2007, 2008). However, parallelization is an important step to making this an accessible technique to multiple research fields (McKendry et al., 2002).

1.4 Parallel DPN of Biological Inks and Applicable Substrates

A substantial drawback of the DPN process is its inherently serial nature (del Campo and Bruce, 2005). There have been numerous efforts to develop parallel DPN too turn it into a production scale technique. There are two main methods used to produce parallel DPN active and passive (Ginger et al., 2004) (Figure 1.5). The ideal generalized parallel DPN technique should be compatible with many substrates (including soft uneven heterogeneous substrates), instruments, inks, and users. In addition to these characteristics, the system should be simple enough to use so that its complexity does not inhibit adoption. Under these confinements, passive pen DPN emerges as a stronger methodology (Salaita et al., 2007). Active pen DPN is a complex method which requires special setup, cantilevers, and instruments to actuate each pen (Bullen et al., 2004). Further, certain well explored methods of actuation (heat) can denature the bioinks or interfere with patterning (Salaita et al., 2007). There has been considerable research and development in the passive probe DPN arena and the remainder of this section will review the use of parallel DPN for the patterning biomolecules (a synopsis is shown in Table 1.2).

Parallel DPN was originally used to pattern biomolecules indirectly. Indirect patterning was used because the proteins (Lee et al., 2006) and virus (Vega et al., 2007) particles did not possess a binding modality that allowed them to adhere to the substrates. The substrates patterned are generally extremely flat and can be positioned (i.e., angled) to bring all of the probes into contact simultaneously (Mirkin, 2001). One of the first studies employed a DPN-patterned thiol layer on gold. The remainder of the gold substrate was passivated with PEG and proteins A/G were then selectively immobilized on the $NHSC_{11}SH$ pattern. This allowed the human antibody IgG to be selectively bound to these locations thereby patterning a bioactive antibody to the substrate (Lee et al., 2006). In a similar experiment, active virus particles were immobilized onto a gold substrate through a series of linkers attached to a 16-mercaptohexadecanoic acid (MHA) pattern. These virus particles were shown to be active through the selective infection of cells placed onto the array (Vega et al., 2007). The use of this scaffold could allow new studies into virus function and infectivity with different cells types on a massively parallel scale. This technique for immobilizing biomolecules is extremely useful in the production of bioarrays and scaffolds. However, it is limited to the patterning of one ink at a time (different inks have varying diffusion times, making it difficult to use a different ink with each probe (Senesi et al., 2009)). Even if multiple patterns could be placed with good spatial registry, this process is both laborious and difficult as it is hard to place the biomolecules without contamination.

The direct patterning of the biomolecules is preferred for patterning multiple biomolecules quickly. It has been shown that many biomolecules can be patterned directly using passive parallel DPN (and variations). For example, multilayers of 1,2-dioleoyl-*sn*-glycero-3-phosphocholine (DOPC) were directly patterned to a glass slide in a high humidity environment. This system eventually reorganized into bilayers after patterning (Lenhert et al., 2007). These systems would be extremely useful for studying cell-to-cell adhesion and cell-to-cell signaling processes as DPN allows for multiple functionalities to be patterned in close spatial arrangements without contamination. Further, these systems could be used to study bilayer mobility and perfusion *in vitro*. Proteins have also been patterned in parallel directly onto

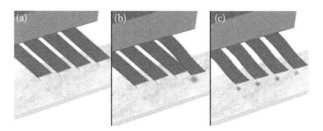

FIGURE 1.5   (a) Parallel probes for (b) active and (c) passive DPN.

TABLE 1.2   Overview of Applicable Parallel DPN of Biomolecules with None on Soft Heterogeneous Uneven Substrates

Probe Type	Patterned Biomolecule(s)	Substrate Patterned	Patterning Technique
Passive parallel AFM	Proteins A/G and human antibody IgG	Gold patterned with NHSC11SH by DPN	Indirectly immobilized the human antibody IgG onto proteins A/G on patterned NHSC11SH Lee et al. (2006)
Passive parallel AFM	Antibody and rSV5-EGFP virus particles	Gold patterned with MHA	Indirectly imobilized rSV5-EGFP virus particles onto rabit antibodies held by a zinc layer on patterned MHA Vega et al. (2007)
Passive parallel AFM	DOPC	Glass slide patterned with DOPC bilayer	Directly immobilized phospholipid (DOPC) bilayer onto glass slide (Showed multilayer formation which changed with high humidity and time) Lenhert et al. (2007)
Passive parallel aluminum electrode tips	DNA and antirabit IgG	Glass slide patterned with DNA and antigoat IgG	Directly immobilized DNA and antigoat IgG onto glass slides coated with dendrimer crosslinkers Belaubre et al. (2003)
Passive parrallel NFP	DNA	Gold patterned with DNA	Directly immobilized DNA onto a gold surface through microchannels in the AFM probes Kim et al. (2008)
Passive parrallel NFP	IgG and BSA	IgG and BSA patterned to MHA SAM on gold	Directly immobilized IgG (rabbit) and biotin-BSA on SAM of MHA and confirmed activity Loh et al. (2008)

substrates (SAMs). These SAMs provide an evenly functionalized substrate for the proteins to bind to. This was initially performed using a DPN variant technique in which an electric current was used to pattern DNA and antirabbit IgG to a dendrimer-coated glass slide. The current was applied through a specially designed aluminum electrode probe (Belaubre et al., 2003). This is a commonly used technique for patterning proteins which have a low or uncontrollable diffusion (Agarwal et al., 2003a). Though this works well with an SAM it may not be feasible with a biologically derived substrate. To pattern to a soft uneven substrate, there would be a constant balancing act between making good contact with all tips and avoiding substrate damage because of excess tip pressure in some areas.

Another variant of DPN is the nanofountain pen (NFP) which shows great promise to overcome the throughput limitations of DPN. By using microchannels to supply ink directly to the tips, from wells in the base of the probe, it delivers a constant flow of ink to the substrate in a passive parallel manner (Moldovan et al., 2006). Through this technique, proteins (Loh et al., 2008) and DNA (Kim et al., 2008) have been patterned to gold (Loh et al., 2008) and glass (Kim et al., 2008) respectively. First, DNA was patterned directly to glass by using the built-in microchannels to wet the tip. This transport mechanism was shown to be efficient in both the patterning of the DNA and in maintaining its functionality (Kim et al., 2008). It was later shown that both IgG and BSA proteins could be patterned to an MHA SAM on gold. Using the NFP system and an electric current, they demonstrated that a current-induced deposition of proteins occurred instead of a diffusion process. Additionally, these proteins maintained their bioactivity after patterning (Loh et al., 2008). This advancement of the DPN method allows for the high throughput parallel passive fabrication of bioarrays. The MHA multilayer was both flat and homogenous. Switching to the patterning of uneven heterogeneous substrates will introduce additional complications for this technique. It will be extremely difficult to bring the tips into contact with a soft uneven substrate and not apply forces which could cause substrate damage or clog the volcano tips with debris from the substrate. Also, the heterogeneity and limited conduction of the substrate are poor attributes for this process. Although much work has been done in the field of passively patterning biomolecules, there is still no technique which has shown all of the suitable qualities necessary for the reliable parallel patterning of biologically derived substrates. A major extension of DPN would be probe modifications which allow for the patterning of an assortment of inks under varying conditions. Although research on optimizing the technique, to the unique challenges of patterning biomolecules, has not occurred.

1.5 Future Directions for AFM Lithography

DPN is a highly versatile patterning technique which has been used in serial to pattern many substrates with a variety of inks. None so important as the patterning of biomimetic substrates which includes a vast array of substrates such as silicon, SAMs, or any others which may be used in biological experimentation. The primary focus of patterning these substrates inherently involves biological inks. These serial techniques are important in developing patterning techniques for various inks and substrates. However, this inherently slow patterning process involves patterning with one tip at a time and therefore to advance DPN into a commonly used technique, it must be made parallel. To advance the technique many groups have developed different variations which allow patterning in parallel for a number of reasons including tilting the substrate and active pens. To make this technique a manufacturing and commercially common technique it is necessary to advance parallel patterning techniques. This technique must be capable of overcoming throughput limitations and be simple enough as to not exclude use. Further, it must be compatible with a wide variety of inks and substrates.

Mirkins group has explored probe modifications (reviewed Table 1.3) which have not been tested with biological inks but may provide a viable option for parallel patterning. The first-probe modifications for DPN involved combining the advantages of the polydimethylsiloxane (PDMS) soft tip from μCP with DPN. In 2003, scanning probe contact printing (SC-CP) was developed (Wang et al., 2003). Then, later in 2004 the DPN stamp tip was developed (Zhang et al., 2004). These are the only prevalent examples in literature of soft tip DPN. The SP-CP tip has displayed the potential to overcome the simultaneous multiink and alignment limitations of μCP. This was shown with the printing of 1-octadecanethiol (ODT) dot patterns. This model compound showed reliable pattern formation when printed. By combining a row of dots this technique offered the production of lines and patterns (Wang et al., 2003). However, the tip is composed of sharpened PDMS on a polyimide cantilever with a PDMS base and the fabrication process produced cantilevers that were not reflective. This lead to a lack of AFM feedback control which made it difficult to produce proper alignment and patterning (Zhang et al., 2004). To further develop this work it was shown that SP-CP can be used in parallel using active pens. This was done using an array of DPN, reader, and SP-CP pens which could be individually actuated (Wang and Liu, 2005). However, the use of active pens makes the technique less diversifiable, more complex, and more time consuming. To address the limitations of SP-CP the DPN stamp tip was developed and it showed considerable improvements (Zhang et al., 2004). This method employs a normal silicon nitride AFM probe which is modified by polymerizing PDMS directly and selectively only to the tip. This is done by dipping the tip into an inkwell filled with the monomer solution. The tip is then removed from solution and the coating is cured. Using this tip multiple inks were printed on gold (MHA, ODT, and

TABLE 1.3   Probe Modifications Applicable to and Used in DPN of Soft Substrates

Probe Modification	Probe Type	Serial/Parallel	Specification	Application
Polymer coat	Tipped	Serial	Fabricated PDMS tip	Contact printing with soft tip Wang et al. (2003)
			PDMS-coated AFM probe	DPN with soft coated tip Zhang et al. (2004)
		Parallel	SC-CP, DPN and reader tips in parallel	Simultaneous reading and writing with both DPN and SP-CP (Wang and Liu (2005)

cystamine) and Si/SiOx (dendrimer G6-OH) in dot, line, and hollow line patterns. This tip modification is relatively simple, inexpensive, and effective. It also allows for a high level of reproducibility (Zhang et al., 2004). This technique is unique in its ability to easily produce hollow nanostructures quickly. Further it provides a soft tip substrate interaction which could be useful in patterning soft substrates which would otherwise be damaged by a regular tip in contact mode. These are viable techniques which could lead to the future of biomimetic patterning with biomolecules on varying substrates.

In conclusion, AFM-lithographic techniques have the potential to greatly expand our ability to pattern and control molecular microenvironments. The ability to control the patterning of biomolecules with high registry and confluence, sets up the future of biological studies. Using varying lithographic features it is possible to study cell–substrate interactions. Ultimately current parallel patterning techniques are not sufficient to pattern soft uneven substrates though they may work with even homogenous substrates. However, a substrate such as a biologically derived substrate would prove a difficult to impossible balancing act between maintaining contact with the probes and not damaging the substrate. Therefore, it is necessary to develop new techniques which must be capable of overcoming throughput limitations, simple enough as to not exclude use and compatible with a wide variety of inks and substrates. Finally, this chapter has reviewed the advancements in the field of AFM lithography mainly involving DPN which has allowed the patterning of various biomimetic substrates with diverse bioinks.

References

Agarwal, G., R. R. Naik, and M. O. Stone. 2003a. Immobilization of histidine-tagged proteins on nickel by electrochemical dip pen nanolithography. *Journal of the American Chemical Society* 125 (24):7408–7412.

Agarwal, G., L. A. Sowards, R. R. Naik, and M. O. Stone. 2003b. Dip-pen nanolithography in tapping mode. *Journal of the American Chemical Society* 125 (2):580–583.

Avseenko, N. V., T. Y. Morozova, F. I. Ataullakhanov, and V. N. Morozov. 2002. Immunoassay with multicomponent protein microarrays fabricated by electrospray deposition. *Analytical Chemistry* 74 (5):927–933.

Banerjee, I. A., L. T. Yu, R. I. MacCuspie, and H. Matsui. 2004. Thiolated peptide nanotube assembly as arrays on patterned Au substrates. *Nano Letters* 4 (12):2437–2440.

Barbulovic-Nad, I., M. Lucente, Y. Sun, M. J. Zhang, A. R. Wheeler, and M. Bussmann. 2006. Bio-microarray fabrication techniques—A review. *Critical Reviews in Biotechnology* 26 (4):237–259.

Baserga, A., M. Vigano, C. S. Casari, S. Turri, A. L. Bassi, M. Levi, and C. E. Bottani. 2008. Au–Ag template stripped pattern for scanning probe investigations of DNA arrays produced by dip pen nanolithography. *Langmuir* 24 (22):13212–13217.

Belaubre, P., M. Guirardel, G. Garcia, J. B. Pourciel, V. Leberre, A. Dagkessamanskaia, E. Trevisiol, J. M. Francois, and C. Bergaud. 2003. Fabrication of biological microarrays using microcantilevers. *Applied Physics Letters* 82 (18):3122–3124.

Bettinger, C. J., R. Langer, and J. T. Borenstein. 2009. Engineering substrate topography at the micro- and nanoscale to control cell function. *Angewandte Chemie—International Edition* 48:2–12.

Bruckbauer, A., D. J. Zhou, D. J. Kang, Y. E. Korchev, C. Abell, and D. Klenerman. 2004. An addressable antibody nanoarray produced on a nanostructured surface. *Journal of the American Chemical Society* 126 (21):6508–6509.

Bullen, D., S. W. Chung, X. F. Wang, J. Zou, C. A. Mirkin, and C. Liu. 2004. Parallel dip-pen nanolithography with arrays of individually addressable cantilevers. *Applied Physics Letters* 84 (5):789–791.

Cheung, C. L., J. A. Camarero, B. W. Woods, T. W. Lin, J. E. Johnson, and J. J. De Yoreo. 2003. Fabrication of assembled virus nanostructures on templates of chemoselective linkers formed by scanning probe nanolithography. *Journal of the American Chemical Society* 125 (23):6848–6849.

Cho, Y. and A. Ivanisevic. 2004. SiOx surfaces with lithographic features composed of a TAT peptide. *Journal of Physical Chemistry B* 108 (39):15223–15228.

Cho, Y. and A. Ivanisevic. 2005. TAT peptide immobilization on gold surfaces: A comparison study with a thiolated peptide and alkylthiols using AFM, XPS, and FT-IRRAS. *Journal of Physical Chemistry B* 109 (13):6225–6232.

Christman, K. L., V. D. Enriquez-Rios, and H. D. Maynard. 2006. Nanopatterning proteins and peptides. *Soft Matter* 2 (11):928–939.

del Campo, A. and I. J. Bruce. 2005. Substrate patterning and activation strategies for DNA chip fabrication. In *Immobilisation of DNA on Chips I*. Berlin: Springer-Verlag.

Demers, L. M., D. S. Ginger, S. J. Park, Z. Li, S. W. Chung, and C. A. Mirkin. 2002. Direct patterning of modified oligonucleotides on metals and insulators by dip-pen nanolithography. *Science* 296 (5574):1836–1838.

Demers, L. M., S. J. Park, T. A. Taton, Z. Li, and C. A. Mirkin. 2001. Orthogonal assembly of nanoparticle building blocks on dip-pen nanolithographically generated templates of DNA. *Angewandte Chemie—International Edition* 40 (16):3071–3073.

Ginger, D. S., H. Zhang, and C. A. Mirkin. 2004. The evolution of dip-pen nanolithography. *Angewandte Chemie—International Edition* 43 (1):30–45.

Hong, S. H., J. Zhu, and C. A. Mirkin. 1999. Multiple ink nanolithography: Toward a multiple-pen nano-plotter. *Science* 286 (5439):523–525.

Hsiao, S. C., A. K. Crow, W. A. Lam, C. R. Bertozzi, D. A. Fletcher, and M. B. Francis. 2008. DNA-coated AFM cantilevers for the investigation of cell adhesion and the patterning of live cells. *Angewandte Chemie—International Edition* 47 (44):8473–8477.

Hyun, J., S. J. Ahn, W. K. Lee, A. Chilkoti, and S. Zauscher. 2002. Molecular recognition-mediated fabrication of protein nanostructures by dip-pen lithography. *Nano Letters* 2 (11):1203–1207.

Hyun, J., J. Kim, S. L. Craig, and A. Chilkoti. 2004. Enzymatic nanolithography of a self-assembled oligonucleotide monolayer on gold. *Journal of the American Chemical Society* 126 (15):4770–4771.

Jiang, H. Z. and S. I. Stupp. 2005. Dip-pen patterning and surface assembly of peptide amphiphiles. *Langmuir* 21 (12):5242–5246.

Jung, H., C. K. Dalal, S. Kuntz, R. Shah, and C. P. Collier. 2004. Surfactant activated dip-pen nanolithography. *Nano Letters* 4 (11):2171–2177.

Khademhosseini, A., R. Langer, J. Borenstein, and J. P. Vacanti. 2006. Microscale technologies for tissue engineering and biology. *Proceedings of the National Academy of Sciences of the United States of America* 103 (8):2480–2487.

Kim, K. H., R. G. Sanedrin, A. M. Ho, S. W. Lee, N. Moldovan, C. A. Mirkin, and H. D. Espinosa. 2008. Direct delivery and submicrometer Patterning of DNA by a nanofountain probe. *Advanced Materials* 20 (2):330–+.

Lee, K. B., J. H. Lim, and C. A. Mirkin. 2003. Protein nanostructures formed via direct-write dip-pen nanolithography. *Journal of the American Chemical Society* 125 (19):5588–5589.

Lee, K. B., S. J. Park, and C. A. Mirkin. 2002. Protein nanoarrays generated by dip-pen nanolithography. *Abstracts of Papers of the American Chemical Society* 223:506-PHYS.

Lee, S. W., B. K. Oh, R. G. Sanedrin, K. Salaita, T. Fujigaya, and C. A. Mirkin. 2006. Biologically active protein nanoarrays generated using parallel dip-pen nanolithography. *Advanced Materials* 18 (9):1133–+.

Leggett, G. J. 2006. Scanning near-field photolithography—surface photochemistry with nanoscale spatial resolution. *Chemical Society Reviews* 35:1150–1161.

Lenhert, S., P. Sun, Y. H. Wang, H. Fuchs, and C. A. Mirkin. 2007. Massively parallel dip-pen nanolithography of heterogeneous supported phospholipid multilayer patterns. *Small* 3 (1):71–75.

Li, B., Y. Wang, H. P. Wu, Y. Zhang, Z. X. Zhang, X. F. Zhou, M. Q. Li, and J. Hu. 2004. Combined-dynamic mode "dip-pen" nanolithography and physically nanopatterning along single DNA molecules. *Chinese Science Bulletin* 49 (7):665–667.

Lim, J. H., D. S. Ginger, K. B. Lee, J. Heo, J. M. Nam, and C. A. Mirkin. 2003. Direct-write dip-pen nano-lithography of proteins on modified silicon oxide surfaces. *Angewandte Chemie—International Edition* 42 (20):2309–2312.

Liu, M. Z., N. A. Amro, C. S. Chow, and G. Y. Liu. 2002. Production of nanostructures of DNA on surfaces. *Nano Letters* 2 (8):863–867.

Loh, O. Y., A. M. Ho, J. E. Rim, P. Kohli, N. A. Patankar, and H. D. Espinosa. 2008. Electric field-induced direct delivery of proteins by a nanofountain probe. *Proceedings of the National Academy of Sciences of the United States of America* 105 (43):16438–16443.

McKendry, R., W. T. S. Huck, B. Weeks, M. Florini, C. Abell, and T. Rayment. 2002. Creating nanoscale patterns of dendrimers on silicon surfaces with dip-pen nanolithography. *Nano Letters* 2 (7):713–716.

Mendes, P. M., C. L. Yeung, and J. A. Preece. 2007. Bio-nanopatterning of surfaces. *Nanoscale Research Letters* 2 (8):373–384.

Mirkin, C. A. 2001. Dip-pen nanolithography: Automated fabrication of custom multicomponent, sub-100-nanometer surface architectures. *Mrs Bulletin* 26 (7):535–538.

Moldovan, N., K. H. Kim, and H. D. Espinosa. 2006. A multi-ink linear array of nanofountain probes. *Journal of Micromechanics and Microengineering* 16:1935–1942.

Nam, J. M., S. W. Han, K. B. Lee, X. G. Liu, M. A. Ratner, and C. A. Mirkin. 2004. Bioactive protein nanoarrays on nickel oxide surfaces formed by dip-pen nanolithography. *Angewandte Chemie—International Edition* 43 (10):1246–1249.

Nelson, C. M. and J. Tien. 2006. Microstructured extracellular matrices in tissue engineering and development. *Current Opinions in Biotechnology* 17 (5):518–523.

Onyeneho, N. A. and A. Ivanisevic. 2004. Tissue and cell-based biomimetic templates generated via dip-pen nanolithography. Paper read at *Conference on Imaging, Manipulation and Analysis of Biomolecules, Cells and Tissues II*, Jan. 27–28, San Jose, CA.

Pena, D. J., M. P. Raphael, and J. M. Byers. 2003. "Dip-pen" nanolithography in registry with photolithography for biosensor development. *Langmuir* 19 (21):9028–9032.

Piner, R. D., J. Zhu, F. Xu, S. H. Hong, and C. A. Mirkin. 1999. "Dip-pen" nanolithography. *Science* 283 (5402):661–663.

Salaita, K., Y. H. Wang, and C. A. Mirkin. 2007. Applications of dip-pen nanolithography. *Nature Nanotechnology* 2 (3):145–155.

Salazar, R. B., A. Shovsky, H. Schonherr, and G. J. Vancso. 2006. Dip-pen nanolithography on (bio)reactive monolayer and block-copolymer platforms: Deposition of lines of single macromolecules. *Small* 2 (11):1274–1282.

Senesi, A. J., D. I. Rozkiewicz, D. N. Reinhoudt, and C. A. Mirkin. 2009. Agarose-assisted dip-pen nanolithography of oligonucleotides and proteins. *ACS Nano ASAP* 3 (8):2394–2402.

Sistiabudi, R. and A. Ivanisevic. 2007. Patterning of polypeptides on a collagen-terminated tissue surface. *Journal of Physical Chemistry C* 111 (31):11676–11681.

Sistiabudi, R. and A. Ivanisevic. 2008. Dip-pen nanolithography of bioactive peptides on collagen-terminated retinal membrane. *Advanced Materials* 20 (19):3678–+.

Smith, J. C., K. B. Lee, Q. Wang, M. G. Finn, J. E. Johnson, M. Mrksich, and C. A. Mirkin. 2003. Nanopatterning the chemospecific immobilization of cowpea mosaic virus capsid. *Nano Letters* 3 (7):883–886.

Taha, H., R. S. Marks, L. A. Gheber, I. Rousso, J. Newman, C. Sukenik, and A. Lewis. 2003. Protein printing with an atomic force sensing nanofountainpen. *Applied Physics Letters* 83 (5):1041–1043.

Tinazli, A., J. Piehler, M. Beuttler, R. Guckenberger, and R. Tampe. 2007. Native protein nanolithography that can write, read and erase. *Nature Nanotechnology* 2 (4):220–225.

Tseng, A. A., A. Notargiacomo, and T. P. Chen. 2005. Nanofabrication by scanning probe microscope lithography: A review. *Journal of Vacuum Science & Technology B* 23 (3):877–894.

Valiokas, R., A. Vaitekonis, G. Klenkar, G. Trinkunas, and B. Liedberg. 2006. Selective recruitment of membrane protein complexes onto gold substrates patterned by dip-pen nanolithography. *Langmuir* 22 (8):3456–3460.

Vega, R. A., D. Maspoch, K. Salaita, and C. A. Mirkin. 2005. Nanoarrays of single virus particles. *Angewandte Chemie—International Edition* 44 (37):6013–6015.

Vega, R. A., C. K. F. Shen, D. Maspoch, J. G. Robach, R. A. Lamb, and C. A. Mirkin. 2007. Monitoring single-cell infectivity from virus-particle nanoarrays fabricated by parallel dip-pen nanotithography. *Small* 3 (9):1482–1485.

Wadu-Mesthrige, K., S. Xu, N. A. Amro, and G. Y. Liu. 1999. Fabrication and imaging of nanometer-sized protein patterns. *Langmuir* 15 (25):8580–8583.

Wang, X. F. and C. Liu. 2005. Multifunctional probe array for nano patterning and imaging. *Nano Letters* 5 (10):1867–1872.

Wang, X. F., K. S. Ryu, D. A. Bullen, J. Zou, H. Zhang, C. A. Mirkin, and C. Liu. 2003. Scanning probe contact printing. *Langmuir* 19 (21):8951–8955.

Wilson, D. L., R. Martin, S. Hong, M. Cronin-Golomb, C. A. Mirkin, and D. L. Kaplan. 2001. Surface organization and nanopatterning of collagen by dip-pen nanolithography. *Proceedings of the National Academy of Sciences of the United States of America* 98 (24):13660–13664.

Zhang, H., R. Elghanian, N. A. Amro, S. Disawal, and R. Eby. 2004. Dip pen nanolithography stamp tip. *Nano Letters* 4 (9):1649–1655.

Zhang, H., K. B. Lee, Z. Li, and C. A. Mirkin. 2003. Biofunctionalized nanoarrays of inorganic structures prepared by dip-pen nanolithography. *Nanotechnology* 14 (10):1113–1117.

Zhang, H., Z. Li, and C. A. Mirkin. 2002. Dip-pen nanolithography-based methodology for preparing arrays of nanostructures functionalized with oligonucleotides. *Advanced Materials* 14 (20):1472–+.

Zhao, X. M., Y. N. Xia, and G. M. Whitesides. 1997. Soft lithographic methods for nano-fabrication. *Journal of Materials Chemistry* 7 (7):1069–1074.

2

Nanofiber-Based Integrative Repair of Orthopedic Soft Tissues

Siddarth D.
Subramony
Columbia University

Cevat Erisken
Columbia University

Philip J. Chuang
Columbia University

Helen H. Lu
Columbia University

2.1 Introduction

Trauma and degeneration of orthopedic tissues are commonly associated with injuries to soft tissues such as ligaments and tendon, which connect bone to bone, and muscle to bone, respectively. Given their inherent nanoscale structural organization (Figure 2.1), nanotechnology-based treatment modalities are actively being researched for the repair of these connective tissues. This chapter will highlight the current nanotechnology-based approaches in the treatment of injuries to tendons and ligaments, with an emphasis on the integrative repair, or biological fixation, of these complex soft tissues.

In the musculoskeletal system, the integration of ligament or tendon to bone is facilitated by an intricate multitissue interface or insertion site, which exhibits a gradient of structure–function properties that enables it to minimize the formation of stress concentrations as well as mediating load transfer between soft and hard tissues. Given its functional significance and as injuries often occur at the soft tissue–bone junction, its regeneration will be critical for functional graft integration. To this end, design considerations for the new paradigm of integrative soft-tissue repair must include, in addition to the formation of the constitutive soft tissue and bone, also the regeneration of the interface which connects these distinct tissue types, resulting in a *multitissue* grafting unit consisting of distinct yet contiguous soft tissue, interface, and bone regions, that is both functional and integrative with the host environment (e.g., osteointegrative or soft-tissue integrative).

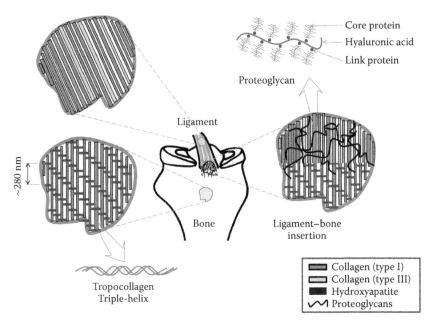

FIGURE 2.1   (See color insert following page 10-24.) Overview of the nanoscale structural organization of bone, ligament/tendon, and direct ligament/tendon-to-bone insertion site.

Focusing on these design considerations, the objective of this chapter is to provide an overview of current approaches to integrative soft tissue repair, beginning with a brief description of the application of nanotechnology in bone repair, with an emphasis on osteointegration. This section is followed by a review of nanofiber-based approaches to tendon and ligament repair, while the final section of this chapter highlights the exciting research into interface regeneration or interface tissue engineering, with an emphasis on the concurrent formation of multitissue systems for integrative soft-tissue repair. Each of these sections will begin with a summary of the structure–function relationship of the tissue at the nanoscale, which provides the biomimetic design inspiration for the scaffold systems intended for the regeneration of each tissue type. The chapter will conclude with a summary and future direction section which will outline the challenges in this exciting field.

2.2 Bone

2.2.1 Structure–Function Relationships of Bone

Bone serves as the main structural unit of the human body and is the most commonly replaced organ with over 800,000 grafting procedures performed annually in the United States alone (Langer and Vacanti, 1993). It is composed of approximately 25% extracellular matrix (ECM), 50% mineral, and 25% water (Ozawa et al., 2008) and is populated largely by three cell types: osteoblasts, osteocytes, and osteoclasts. Osteoblasts, which form new bone, and osteoclasts, which resorb bone, serve to continuously remodel and rebuild the skeleton. This cycle is mediated by osteocytes, the most abundant cell type present in bone that acts as mechanosensors.

The organic component of bone ECM consists predominantly of type-I collagen fibrils. The collagen molecule is typically built on the repetition of the sequence glycine-proline-4-hydroxyproline with slight variations (Mann, 2001). Individual collagen filaments are composed of three molecules of this sequence wrapped around each other, resulting in a superhelical structure called tropocollagen. For type-I collagen, the tropocollagen fibrils are organized at the nanoscale into the revised quarter stagger model (Figure 2.1). The adjacent parallel fiber rows are spaced by 64 nm longitudinally, with each tropo-collagen strand being about 280 nm long, and 1.5 nm in width (Mann, 2001). This arrangement allows for maximum crosslinking of hydroxylysine and lysine residues for maximum stability of the matrix (Knott and Bailey, 1998). The natural spacing formed between the ends of the collagen fibers are 40×5 nm in size (Mann, 2001). It is proposed that these vacancies between the collagen fibers serve as nucleation sites for the mineral component of bone (Landis and Silver, 2008).

Hydroxyapatite crystals constitute the inorganic phase of bone, with the mineralized collagen fibers exhibiting greater mechanical properties than unmineralized collagen fibers (Buehler, 2007). Buehler et al. investigated the difference in tensile mechanical properties between mineralized and unmineralized collagen fibers and found that uncalcified collagen behaves mechanically like an elastic polymer with a Young's modulus of 4.59 GPa and a maximum stress of 0.3 GPa, while the mineralized collagen fibers were reported to have a Young's modulus of 6.23 GPa and a maximum stress of 0.6 GPa. This observed increase in mechanical properties is attributed to the hydroxyapatite crystals, which act as strengthening precipitates that impart resistance to plastic deformation and fracture. Interestingly, the weak adhesion between collagen and hydroxyapatite also allows for slip deformation to occur at these interfaces, which prevents the presence of mineral from making the overall fiber too brittle. Furthermore, the nanoscale organization of the collagen fibrils and hydroxyapatite crystals is theorized to increase the strength of the overall fiber by maximizing intermolecular forces.

Given the complex nanoscale organization of bone, the ideal scaffold must be biomimetic with nanoscale organization, able to support bone growth (osteoconductive), induce bone formation (osteoinductive), and structurally integrate with the host bone tissue (osteointegrative). Many such biomimetic systems have been actively researched which combine collagenous or synthetic nanofibrils and hydroxyapatite nanoparticles, with the ultimate goal of engineering a bone grafting system that can meet all of these aforementioned design criteria. Examples discussed below include composite nanofiber scaffolds (Table 2.1) and hydroxyapatite coatings on biodegradable polymeric scaffolds for osteointegration (Table 2.2).

2.2.2 Composite Nanofiber Scaffolds for Bone Regeneration

The natural fibril morphology of the collagen in the ECM can be readily mimicked with nanofibers in order to optimize osteoblast response on polymeric biomaterials. The most common polymers used include polylactide-*co*-glycolide acid (PLGA) and polycaprolactone (PCL) which are selected for their favorable biodegradation profiles and mechanical properties (Agrawal and Ray, 2001).

In general, nanofibers are fabricated via the classical method of electrospinning (Reneker and Chun, 1996). For example, electrospinning was used to generate unaligned PLGA (Li et al., 2001) as well as PCL nanofiber scaffolds (Yoshimoto et al., 2003). In each case, the polymer is dissolved in a solvent and dispensed by a syringe pump, and drawn out into nanofibers under the application of high voltage, and a ground collector is used to capture the polymer fibers formed. It was reported that when mesenchymal stem cells (MSCs) were seeded on the PCL scaffolds (Yoshimoto et al., 2003), they differentiated into

TABLE 2.1 Nanofiber Scaffolds for Bone Formation

Study	Scaffold Design	Application	Study Model
Li et al., 2002	Poly(D,L-lactide-*co*-glycolide) nanofiber (500–800 nm)	Biocompatibility	*In vitro*/Mouse fibroblasts
Yoshimoto et al., 2003	Poly(ε-caprolactone) nanofibers (400 nm)	Bone	*In vitro*/Mouse MSCs
Venugopal et al., 2008	Poly(ε-caprolactone) nanofibers(411 nm), hydroxyapatite, gelatin (856 nm)	Bone	*In vitro*/Human fetal osteoblasts
Song et al., 2008	Collagen type-I nanofibers (70–170 nm), hydroxyapatite	Bone	*In vitro*/MC3T3-E1 osteoblastic cells

TABLE 2.2   Simulated Body Fluid Coating Methods to Improve Osteointegration

Study	Material	Immersion Time	Mineral	Function
Murphy et al., 2002	Poly(lactide-*co*-glycolide), SBF	16-day immersion	Carbonated apatite	Shown to improve bone regeneration in a rat cranial defect model
Yang et al., 2008	PCL, SBF, and 10× SBF	7 day immersion in 1× SBF; two 10 h immersion in 10× SBF	Brushite and apatite	Uses a plasma discharge treatment prior to SBF treatment; compared normal SBF with 10× SBF
Mavis et al., 2009	PCL, 10× SBF	6 h immersion	Brushite, monetite, and apatite	Evaluated response of osteoblasts on coated PCL scaffolds, and demonstrate superior osteoconductivity *in vitro* over uncoated scaffolds

osteoblasts under rotational culture in osteogenic differentiation medium, with abundant type-I collagen matrix formation and mineralization observed throughout the scaffold. In addition, aligned polymer scaffolds have been formed using the same technique with a rotating collecting target in order to not only replicate the fibrous structure of collagen but also the natural alignment of the native collagen matrix (Moffat et al., 2009). The versatility of the electrospinning process also enables the incorporation of other biomaterials, both organic (e.g., collagen, chitosan) and synthetic, into these nanofiber meshes (Reneker and Chun, 1996; Matthews et al., 2002; Shin et al., 2005) which will further promote bone formation.

Moreover, the fabrication of composite nanofibers or incorporation of organic–inorganic nanocomposite complexes into nanofiber scaffolds has been of significant interest. For example, Song et al. electrospun nanofiber scaffolds from hydroxyapatite–collagen nanocomposites, whereby a coprecipitation method was first used to form the nanocomposites, which involved the addition of two emulsions (hydroxyapatite and collagen) drop-wise into a reaction vessel while the pH is fixed with a reaction time on the order of 48 h (Song et al., 2008). The resulting nanocomposites were dried and dissolved in 1,1,1,3,3,3-hexafluoro-2-propanol and electrospun into unaligned nanofiber meshes. When MC3T3-E1 preosteoblasts were seeded onto these substrates, these cells measured a significant increase in alkaline phosphatase activity over time, demonstrating the osteoconductive potential of these novel nanofiber composites. Recently, using the same fabrication system, Venugopal et al. substituted gelatin for collagen in order to reduce cost and further enhance the osteoconductivity of these nanocomposite scaffolds (Venugopal et al., 2008). Specifically, hydroxyapatite, PCL, and gelatin were electrospun together to form composite nanofibers. While the mechanical properties of these composite nanofibers were several orders of magnitudes lower than those of bone in terms of both Young's modulus and ultimate tensile strength (UTS), the scaffolds supported osteoblast proliferation, higher ALP activity, and mineralization.

For composite nanofiber scaffolds, the primary challenge is in how to successfully match scaffold mechanical properties (such as Young's modulus, UTS) with those of native bone, as well as optimizing the induction of mineralization and addresses the need for osteointegration. Introduction of additional elements into the nanofiber systems, such as peptides and growth factors, as well as the incorporation of the other nanofibers into polymeric or titanium implants are examples of how these scaffolds can be further tailored to improve osteoconductivity and osteoinductivity (Khang et al., 2006; Horii et al., 2007; Sargeant et al., 2008).

2.2.3 Hydroxyapatite Coatings of Polymeric Scaffolds and Osteointegration

A common method that has been researched extensively for improving osteointegration involves the formation of a calcium phosphate layer directly onto the scaffold surface (Table 2.2), specifically by incubating the scaffolds in a simulated body fluid (SBF) with physiologic or supra-physiologic calcium and/or phosphate concentrations. These ions promote the nucleation of mineral crystals on the polymeric substrate, and it is anticipated that this newly formed calcium phosphate layer can thereby lead to improved osteointegration *in vivo*. Incubation in the SBF offers a relatively low temperature processing technique, ideal for substrates such as polymers that cannot sustain the high temperature treatments necessary for the well established plasma spraying of metallic or ceramic implants (Du et al., 2002). Another advantage of this method is the ability to form a relatively uniform coating on surfaces with complex topography and predesigned geometries.

Modification of the polymeric substrate has been reported to improve the efficiency of forming a calcium phosphate layer on polymer scaffolds. Murphy and Mooney showed that carbonate-apatite can be deposited onto PLGA surfaces after pretreating the polymer surface in a NaOH solution (Murphy and Mooney, 2002). In this study, polymeric films were immersed in a SBF solution for 16 days at 37°C, with the solution replaced daily. Moreover, it was observed that when the PLGA films were presoaked in 0.5 M NaOH, a hydrolyzed, carboxylic acid-rich surface was formed which resulted in improved mineral deposition. A follow-up study elegantly demonstrated that a macroporous PLGA scaffold coated with a layer of carbonate-apatite formed through this method reported a 53% increase in bone formation when evaluated in a rat cranial defect model (Murphy et al., 2005).

Working with PCL nanofibers, Yang et al. as well as Mavis et al. demonstrated that the SBF soaking method can be applied to form calcium phosphate coatings on these scaffolds (Yang et al., 2008; Mavis et al., 2009). In contrast to Murphy et al., a concentrated SBF solution was used to expedite the coating process, reducing week-long immersion times to just a couple of hours. Specifically, Yang et al. pre-exposed the PCL scaffold to a plasma discharge treatment and then immersed the nanofibers in two types of solution: a SBF solution with calcium and phosphate ion concentrations matching those found in human blood plasma and a 10× concentrated SBF solution, and the scaffolds were incubated in each for 7 days or up to 6 h, respectively. Both methods resulted in the deposition of a calcium phosphate layer on the PCL nanofibers. Interestingly, the scaffolds immersed in the physiologic SBF exhibited a crystalline structure more closely resembling natural apatite whereas the scaffolds immersed in the concentrated SBF solution had a mixture of apatite and dicalcium phosphate dihydrate. The coating resulting from scaffold immersion in the normal SBF solution was also found to be porous, which may be beneficial for cell migration and nutrient transport. Later using a 10× concentrated SBF, Mavis et al. immersed the PCL scaffolds for 6 h and subsequently evaluated murine osteoblast response on these coated scaffolds. It was observed that the cells exhibited elevated ALP activity and expressed osteocalcin, indicating that the coated scaffolds enhance osteoblastic differentiation over PCL controls.

Collectively, these studies and others demonstrate that surface calcium phosphate coatings have the potential to increase osteoconductivity of polymeric scaffolds and enable them to be osteointegrative *in vivo*. Challenges to be addressed include matching the degradation and mechanical properties to enable functional repair, as well as controlling the stability of the preformed calcium phosphate coating and establishing long term osteointegration *in vivo*.

2.3 Tendons and Ligaments

2.3.1 Structure–Function Relationships of Tendons and Ligaments

Tendons and ligaments are fibrous tissues that connect muscle to bone and bone to bone, respectively. Similar in structure, they are primarily composed of fibroblasts that secrete a dense collagenous ECM (Amiel et al., 1984). The primary constituent of tendons and ligaments is type-I collagen which is responsible for resisting tensile deformation and sustain physiological loading (Woo et al., 1993). Also present is type-III collagen, distributed within the ECM in the form of loosely packed thin fibrils, which plays a role in wound healing and tendon–bone/ligament–bone attachment. Additionally, type-V collagen functions to regulate the assembly of collagen fibrils and ultimately controls fiber diameter

(Liu et al., 1995). Small amounts of proteoglycans and elastin are also present. While this overall similarity between tendon and bone has resulted in the two tissue types being largely regarded as identical structures suited for different functions, biochemical analyses of tendons and ligaments have revealed certain differences. Specifically, Amiel et al. compared rabbit tendons and ligaments and found that the tendons contain more type-I collagen, fewer cells, more proteoglycans, and exhibit a different collagen crosslinking pattern from ligaments. These studies also detected variations between different types of tendon (e.g., the patellar tendon and Achilles tendon), indicating that the observed tissue heterogeneity is site-specific and may depend on the specific physiological function of the soft tissue in the body (Amiel et al., 1983).

The highly organized nano-level structure of tendons and ligaments is characterized by closely packed parallel collagen fiber bundles, varying in diameter and are composed of bundles of individual collagen fibrils approximately 1–2 nm in diameter (Woo et al., 1995). This structural arrangement is critical in allowing tendons and ligaments to perform their physiological functions, including the stabilization and guidance of joint motion, transmission of physiological loads, and the maintenance of the anatomical alignment of the skeleton. Furthermore, this arrangement of collagen fibers, parallel to the direction of applied loads, results in one of the strongest tissues in the body (Jung et al., 2009). For example, the Young's modulus of the human patellar tendon and anterior cruciate ligament (ACL) is approximately 650 and 350 MPa, respectively (Butler, 1989). The collagen fibers of tendons and ligaments typically exhibit a bimodal diameter distribution in the nanometer range (approximately 40–400 nm) that varies according to the specific tissue type, as well as between individuals and may also be altered during the formation of scar tissue post injury (Liang et al., 2006).

Tendon and ligament injuries are among the most common trauma afflicting the young and physically active population (Kumbar et al., 2008). For example, over 100,000 ACL reconstructions and more than 75,000 rotator cuff tendon repairs are performed annually in the United States, many of which are accompanied by injuries to the surrounding ligaments and other tissues (Griffin et al., 2000; Vitale et al., 2007). Soft tissue tears are often susceptible to incomplete healing and recurrent injury even after treatment has been administered, with failure rates in excess of 90% in some instances (Galatz et al., 2004). Furthermore, the limited healing potential of the injured tissue, relative scarcity of autografts, and the inherent risks associated with allografts leave current repair strategies largely unsatisfactory. While previously evaluated synthetic approaches, such as the Kennedy Ligament Augmentation Device and the Proflex poly(ethylene terephthalate) graft, have proven to be insufficient, tissue engineering has emerged as a promising approach by which to form functional tissue replacements with material properties similar to that of native tissue (Ventura et al., 2009). Several research groups have explored tissue engineering approaches to tendon and ligament repair (Dunn et al., 1995; Altman et al., 2002b; Lu et al., 2005; Cooper et al., 2007; Kimura et al., 2008). Synthetic as well as biologically derived grafts have shown favorable results during *in vitro* culture trials as well as in relevant *in vivo* models. One of the most common approaches is the use of scaffolds composed of fibers that are several tens of micrometers in diameter. These include the use of a variety of synthetic polymers, such as poly-L-lactic acid, polylactide-*co*-glycolide, and polyurethane (Lu et al., 2005; Cooper et al., 2007), as well as biological materials, such as collagen (Dunn et al., 1995) and silk (Altman et al., 2002a; Horan et al., 2009). While these approaches have shown promising results, the scaffold architecture differs significantly from that of the native nanoscale organization of tendons and ligaments. Given that scaffold fiber diameters have been shown to directly affect fibroblast phenotype and matrix production (Bashur et al., 2006), there is significant interest in enhancing physiologically relevant ligament or tendon regeneration utilizing scaffolds that more closely mimics the native tissue nanostructure and mechanics.

2.3.2 Nanofiber Scaffolds for Tendon and Ligament Repair

When aiming to regenerate tendons/ligaments, the ideal tissue engineering scaffold must be able to mimic the native structure–function relation of the tissue to be replaced, and promote neo-tissue formation. Specifically, it must be able to support the growth of relevant cell populations and enable the deposition of a tendon- or ligament-like ECM. In addition, it should be able to support physiological loads while degrading at a rate that coincides with neo-tissue formation (Lu et al., 2005). It is anticipated that these characteristics would result in the eventual regeneration of grafts with properties equaling those of native tendon or ligaments, accompanied by the complete elimination of implanted materials.

The nanoscale architecture of the underlying collagen matrix of tendons and ligaments may be readily recapitulated with nanofiber scaffolds, which exhibits high surface to volume ratio, low density, high porosity, variable pore size, and mechanical properties approaching those of the native tissues. Similar to the bone-tissue engineering applications described above, these nanofibers can be fabricated using a variety of methods, such as drawing, template synthesis, temperature-induced phase separation, molecular self-assembly, and, most frequently, electrospinning (Kumbar et al., 2008). Currently, a number of polymer-based and naturally derived nanofiber scaffolds (Table 2.3) have been evaluated for tendon and ligament repair, predominantly for rotator cuff and ACL reconstruction, and these studies are highlighted below.

Designed for rotator cuff repair, Moffat et al. recently reported on the fabrication of polylactide-*co*-glycolide (PLGA) nanofiber scaffolds with physiologically relevant structural and mechanical properties (Moffat et al., 2009). It was observed that human rotator cuff fibroblast morphology and growth on aligned (615 nm mean fiber diameter) and unaligned (568 nm mean fiber diameter) fiber matrices was dictated by the substrate fiber alignment, with distinct cell morphology (Figure 2.2a and b) and integrin expression profiles. Upregulation of the $\alpha2$ integrin, a key mediator of cellular attachment to collagenous matrices, was observed when the fibroblasts were cultured on aligned fibers, and upon which the cells deposited a collagen-rich matrix containing both type-I and type-III collagen. Bashur et al., also working with PLGA nanofiber scaffolds, subsequently reported that fibroblast morphology is modulated by increasing or decreasing fiber diameter below a specific threshold. These interesting findings indicate that cellular response on these biomimetic scaffolds can be modulated by varying nanofiber alignment and organization.

Additionally, Lee et al. evaluated polyurethane (PU) nanofibers for ACL tissue engineering and examined the impact of cyclic uniaxial tensile strain on human ligament fibroblasts seeded on these scaffolds (Lee et al., 2005). It was observed that these nanofiber scaffolds with physiologically relevant mechanical properties supported ligament fibroblast proliferation and matrix deposition. The study also found that uniaxial tensile strain applied parallel to the direction of fiber alignment increases the amount of collagen deposited by the ligament fibroblasts. Recently, using a high throughput bioreactor system, Subramony et al. evaluated the effect of mechanical strain on pluripotent MSCs seeded on PLGA nanofibers (Subramony et al., 2010). Stem cells have been shown to differentiate toward a fibroblastic

TABLE 2.3　Nanofiber Scaffolds for Ligament and Tendon Tissue Engineering

Study	Scaffold Design	Application	Study Model
Moffat et al., 2009	Aligned (615 nm) and unaligned (568 nm) electrospun PLGA (85:15) nanofibers	Rotator cuff repair	*In vitro*/Human tendon fibroblasts
Bashur et al., 2006	Aligned (140–760 nm) and unaligned (130–660 nm) PLGA (75:25) nanofibers	Ligament repair	*In vitro*/NIH 3T3 fibroblasts
Rho et al., 2006	Electrospun collagen (type-I) nanofibers (460 nm)	Wound healing	*In vivo*/Rat model
Lee et al., 2005	Aligned electrospun polyurethane nanofibers (657 nm)	Ligament repair	*In vitro*/Human ligament fibroblasts
Subramony et al., 2010	Aligned (615 nm) electrospun PLGA (85:15) nanofibers	Ligament repair	*In vitro*/Human MSCs
Sahoo et al., 2006	PLGA (10:90) knitted scaffold with electrospun PLGA (65:35) nanofibers (300–900 nm) on surface	Ligament repair	*In vitro*/Porcine bone marrow stromal cells

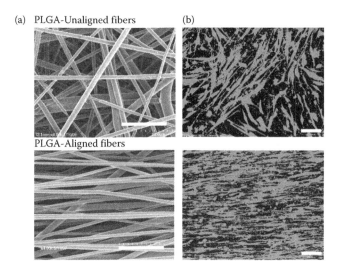

(a) PLGA-Unaligned fibers   (b)

PLGA-Aligned fibers

FIGURE 2.2   (See color insert following page 10-24.) (a) Aligned and unaligned nanofiber scaffolds evaluated with scanning electron microscopy (SEM) (4000×, bar = 10 μm); (b) Human rotator cuff tendon fibroblasts cultured on aligned and unaligned PLGA (85:15) nanofiber scaffolds (day 14, 20×, bar = 100 μm).

lineage when mechanically stimulated in a collagen hydrogel (Altman et al., 2002b). Subramony et al. observed that MSC attachment was guided by the nanofiber substrate, and the expression of ligament fibroblast markers and key integrins (e.g., $\alpha 2$, $\beta 1$, and $\alpha 5$) were significantly upregulated. These promising results suggest that nanofibers coupled with mechanical loading can be used to promote MSC-mediated ligament or tendon regeneration.

Biological response to polymeric nanofibers may also be enhanced by additional surface modifications. For example, when Rho et al. electrospun aligned type-I collagen nanofiber scaffolds with a mean fiber diameter of 460 nm and evaluated the response of human epidermal cells after coating the scaffolds with various adhesion proteins (Rho et al., 2006), it was found that proliferation was enhanced by coating the scaffolds with an additional layer of type-I collagen and laminin, two ECM proteins that modulate keratinocyte adhesion. It is likely that the polymeric scaffold described here may be similarly modified to promote tendon or ligament fibroblast attachment and biosynthesis.

Nanofibers have also been used to improve existing scaffold design, resulting in a graft with a more biomimetic surface for eliciting desired cell response. For example, Sahoo et al. electrospun PLGA nanofibers directly onto a woven microfiber PLGA scaffold in order to increase cell seeding efficiency while maintaining a scaffold that was mechanically competent for ACL reconstruction (Sahoo et al., 2006). The attachment, proliferation, and differentiation of porcine bone marrow stromal cells was evaluated on these scaffolds and when compared to scaffolds seeded using a fibrin gel delivery system, it was found that seeding the cells onto nanofiber-coated scaffolds enhanced proliferation, collagen production, and also increased the gene expression of several ligament/tendon-related markers, namely decorin, biglycan, and collagen I.

2.4 Soft Tissue-to-Bone Interface and Integrative Repair

2.4.1 Structure–Function Relationships of the Ligament/ Tendon-to-Bone Interface

Structural integration between soft and hard tissues is crucial for physiological function of the musculoskeletal system. Soft tissues, such as the ACL of the knee or the supraspinatus tendon (ST) of the rotator cuff connect to bone via the direct insertion site, a complex enthesis consisting of three distinct yet continuous regions of soft tissue, fibrocartilage, and bone (Cooper and Misol, 1970; Benjamin et al., 1986; Wang et al., 2006). The fibrocartilage region is further divided into noncalcified and calcified interface regions. The insertion site serves several functions, including enabling the transfer of loads between distinct tissues (Benjamin et al., 1986; Woo et al., 1988), minimizing the formation of stress concentrations (Woo et al., 1983; Benjamin et al., 1986; Moffat et al., 2008a) and supporting the communication between multiple cell types necessary for interface function and homeostasis (Lu and Jiang, 2006). Therefore, regeneration of this multi-tissue transition is a prerequisite for biological fixation. To this end, an in-depth understanding of interface structure–function relationship will be essential for developing effective strategies for integrative soft-tissue repair.

As noted above, direct insertion sites found at the ACL-bone or supraspinatus tendon–bone interface are anatomically divided into several distinct yet continuous tissue regions (Figure 2.3) with characteristic spatial variations in cell type and matrix composition (Cooper and Misol, 1970; Benjamin et al., 1986; Woo and Buckwalter, 1988; Kumagai et al., 1994; Niyibizi et al., 1995, 1996; Wei and Messner, 1996; Blevins et al., 1997; Messner, 1997; Petersen and Tillmann, 1999; Thomopoulos et al., 2003; Wang et al., 2006). The first region is the soft-tissue proper that contains tendon or ligament fibroblasts within a matrix rich in collagen types-I and III. Directly adjacent to this is the fibrocartilage interface region that is further divided into nonmineralized and mineralized regions. The nonmineralized fibrocartilage (NFC) region is populated by fibrochondrocytes in a matrix containing proteoglycans and types-I and II collagen fibrils. The mineralized fibrocartilage (MFC) region contains hypertrophic chondrocytes situated within a type-X collagen matrix with mineralized collagen fibrils containing hydroxyapatite nanoparticles. The MFC then connects directly to the bone in a parallel and oblique fashion (Woo and Buckwalter, 1988) whereby fibrils from the MFC blend with those of bone (Cooper and Misol, 1970; Raspanti et al., 1996; Oguma et al., 2001).

From a structure–function perspective, the matrix heterogeneity evident at the multiple-tissue interface is known to allow for a gradual increase in stiffness through the interface, thus minimizing stress concentrations and also enabling effective load transfer from soft tissue to bone (Woo and Buckwalter, 1988; Matyas et al., 1995; Moffat et al., 2008a). It has been reported that matrix organization at the tendon-to-bone transition is optimized to sustain both tensile and compressive stresses (Woo et al., 1988; Matyas et al., 1995; Benjamin and Ralphs, 1998). Using ultrasound elastography, Spalazzi et al. experimentally determined the strain distribution at the ACL-to-bone interface (Spalazzi et al., 2006a). The deformation across the insertion site is observed to be region-dependent, with the highest displacement found at the ACL and then decreasing in magnitude from the fibrocartilage interface to bone when the joint is loaded in tension. These regional differences suggest an increase in tissue stiffness from ligament to bone. Recently, Moffat et al. determined the compressive mechanical properties of the ACL-bone interface by combining microscopic mechanical testing with optimized digital image correlation methods (Moffat et al., 2008a). Similarly, it was observed that deformation decreased

	Tissue	Cell type	Major matrix composition
Ligament	Ligament/tendon	Fibrolasts	Collagen types I, III
	Non-mineralized fibrocartilage	Ovoid chondrocytes	Collagen types I, II proteoglycans
Fibrocartilage	Mineralized fibrocartilage	Hypertrophic chondrocytes	Collagen type X
Bone	Bone	Osteoblast, osteocytes, osteoclasts	Collagen type I

FIGURE 2.3 (See color insert following page 10-24.) Structure and composition of direct insertion site (ACL-to-bone interface, FTIR-I).

gradually from the fibrocartilage interface to bone. Moreover, these region-dependent changes in strain were accompanied by a gradual increase in compressive modulus. A significantly higher elastic modulus was found for the MFC (Moffat et al., 2008a), with the compressive modulus increasing more than 50% from the nonmineralized to the MFC region.

The presence of the noncalcified and calcified fibrocartilage regions at the interface is of functional significance, as higher matrix mineral content have been associated with greater mechanical properties in connective tissues (Currey, 1988; Ferguson et al., 2003; Radhakrishnan et al., 2004). Moffat et al. correlated the aforementioned increase in compressive modulus across the interface to the onset of mineral presence in the calcified fibrocartilage region (Moffat et al., 2008a). Characterization of the ACL-bone insertion site using Fourier Transform Infrared Imaging (FTIR-I, Figure 2.3) further revealed an exponential increase in calcium and phosphorous content progressing from ligament, interface, and then to bone (Spalazzi et al., 2007). Recently, Genin et al. carried out a Raman spectroscopic study of the rat tendon-to-bone transition and identified the presence of apatite crystals with increasing concentrations in regions approaching the bone (Genin et al., 2009).

On the basis of the analyses of the direct insertion site detailed above, any attempt to regenerate the soft tissue-to-bone interface must take into consideration the complex structure of the insertion and how to strategically mimic the native structure–function of the interface. The multi-tissue interface represents a significant challenge as several distinct types of tissue are observed. The ideal scaffold for interface tissue engineering should therefore exhibit a gradient of structural and mechanical properties mimicking those of the multi-tissue insertion. Compared to a homogenous structure, a stratified scaffold with predesigned tissue-specific matrix inhomogeneity can better sustain and transmit the distribution of complex loads inherent at the direct insertion site. A key criterion in stratified scaffold design is that the phases must be interconnected and preintegrated with each other, thereby supporting the formation of distinct yet continuous multi-tissue regions. In other words, the scaffold would exhibit a gradient of physical properties in order to allow for the recapitulation of interface-like heterogeneity throughout the scaffold. It should also support the growth and differentiation, as well as the interactions between heterotypic and homotypic cell populations, thereby promoting the formation and maintenance of multitissue interface. In addition, the scaffold phases should be biodegradable so it is gradually replaced by living tissue, and the degradation process must be balanced with respect to mechanical properties in order to permit physiological loading and neo-interface function. Finally, the interface scaffold must be compatible with existing ligament or tendon reconstruction grafts or preincorporated into tissue engineered graft design in order to achieve integrative and functional soft-tissue repair.

To this end, a scaffold recapturing the nanoscale interface organization, and particularly with preferentially aligned nanofiber organization would be highly advantageous, and current efforts in this exciting area are highlighted below.

2.4.2 Nanofiber Scaffolds for Ligament–Bone and Tendon–Bone Repair

Scaffolds with micro- and/or nano-scale structural features have been investigated for interface tissue engineering (Table 2.4). Modeled after the multi-tissue ACL-bone insertion, Spalazzi et al. designed a stratified scaffold consisting of three distinct yet continuous phases, with each engineered for a particular cell type and tissue region found at the interface (Spalazzi et al., 2006b): Phase I was designed with a PLGA (10:90) mesh for fibroblast culture and ligament formation, Phase II consists of PLGA (85:15) microspheres and is the interface region intended for fibrochondrocyte culture, and Phase III is comprised of sintered PLGA (85:15) and 45S5 bioactive glass composite microspheres for osteoblast culture and bone formation. To control the spatial distribution of the different cell types, a nanofiber-based barrier was incorporated between the three phases. This novel stratified design resulted in essence a "single" scaffold system with three *distinct yet continuous* phases mimicking the organization of the native insertion site.

TABLE 2.4 Nanofiber Scaffolds for Interface Tissue Engineering

Study	Scaffold Design	Application	Study Model
Spalazzi et al., 2008a	Triphasic Phase I: PLGA mesh Phase II: PLGA (85:15) microspheres Phase III: PLGA-45S5 composite	Ligament–bone	*In vivo*/Rat model with bovine *fibroblasts,* *chondrocytes, osteoblasts*
Spalazzi et al., 2008b	AlignedPLGA (85:15) nanofibers (900 nm) PLGA(85:15) microspheres	Ligament–bone	*In vitro*/Bovine patellar tendon graft
Moffat et al., 2008b	Biphasic Phase I: PLGA nanofibers (615 nm) Phase II: PLGA-HA composite nanofiber	Tendon–bone	*In vitro*/Human *fibroblasts,* *osteoblasts, chondrocytes*

Erisken et al., 2008a	Continuously graded
	PCL nanofibers (200–2000 nm)
	   incorporated with calcium
	   phosphate nanoparticles
		Cartilage–bone	*In vitro*/Mouse preosteoblasts

Li et al., 2009	Continuously graded Calcium phosphate on gelatin- coated PCL nanofibers	Tendon–bone	*In vitro*/Mouse preosteoblasts

Through *in vitro* (Spalazzi et al., 2006b) and *in vivo* (Spalazzi et al., 2008a) evaluations, it was reported that the triphasic scaffold supported multilineage interactions between interface-relevant cell populations, as well as tissue infiltration and abundant matrix production. In addition, controlled phase-specific matrix heterogeneity was established on the multiphased scaffold, with *distinct yet continuous* ligament-, fibrocartilage-, and bone-like tissue regions formed on the scaffold. In other words, the neo-fibrocartilage formed was continuous with the ligament-like tissue observed in Phase I as well as the bone-like tissue found in Phase III. In a related study, Spalazzi et al. designed a mechanoactive scaffold system for ligament-to-bone interface regeneration based on a composite of poly-α-hydroxyester nanofibers and sintered microspheres to be used as tendon graft collar (Spalazzi et al., 2008b). Taking advantage of the inherent contractile property of aligned PLGA nanofibers, compression was applied directly to tendon grafts using the novel graft collar. It was found that the nanofiber scaffold-mediated compression led to significant remodeling of the tendon matrix as well as the expression of fibrocartilage interface-related markers including type-II collagen, aggrecan, and transforming growth factor-β3. These promising results suggest that nanofiber scaffolds may be directly employed to induce the formation of fibrocartilage interface on biological grafts or incorporated into a tissue engineered scaffold system designed for interface regeneration.

These composite nano-/micro-scale structures have yielded promising results for ligament-to-bone applications, and scaffolds made entirely from nanofibrous structures could be advantageous for tendon-to-bone integration, especially when fabricated with aligned organization mimicking that of the native insertion. To this end, it is important that the fiber size, alignment, and the overall scaffold structure meet the requirements of the interface of interest. Building on the PLGA nanofiber scaffold described earlier, Moffat et al. subsequently designed a composite nanofiber system of PLGA and hydroxyapatite nanoparticles aimed at regenerating both the nonmineralized and mineralized fibrocartilage regions of the tendon-to-bone insertion site (Moffat et al., 2008b). The response of tendon fibroblasts, osteoblasts, and chondrocytes were evaluated on these nanocomposite scaffolds with promising results demonstrating the potential of a biodegradable nanofiber-based scaffold system for integrative tendon-to-bone repair.

Controlling scaffold mineral distribution may be another promising approach for repairing the soft tissue-to-bone insertion site. Working with PCL nanofibers and utilizing a novel extrusion system,

Erisken et al. incorporated calcium phosphate nanoparticles into nonwoven nanofiber meshes, resulting in a gradient of mineral distribution across the depth of the PCL scaffold (Erisken et al., 2008a,b). Within 4 weeks, culturing of MC3T3 cells on these nanofiber constructs led to the formation of a gradient of calcified matrix. Recently, using the SBF immersion method discussed earlier in this chapter, Li et al. formed a calcium phosphate coating on a nonwoven mat of gelatin-coated PCL nanofibers in a graded manner (Li et al., 2009). It was observed that the gradient in mineral content resulted in spatial variations in the stiffness and affected the number of mouse preosteoblast MC3T3 cells adhered to the substrate.

2.5 Summary and Future Directions

Nanotechnology-based approaches to connective tissue repair have several distinct advantages. Specifically, nanofibrous substrates are advantageous for tissue engineering due to their potential to directly mimic the native collagenous tendon/ligament matrix and ultimately direct cellular response. In addition, nanofibers can be fabricated from a variety of polymers, as well as natural materials, with relative ease and reproducibility. Furthermore, the versatility of the fabrication process allows for the construction of scaffolds that possesses tunable geometry, mechanical properties, porosity, permeability, degradation kinetics, and fiber diameter. The studies described in this chapter and many others collectively illustrate the promise and the excitement in the field regarding nanotechnology-based scaffolds for guided orthopedic tissue engineering and integrative repair, from nano-coatings for promoting osteointegration to nanofiber and composite nanofiber scaffolds for tissue engineering, be it for the regeneration of bone, ligaments, tendons, or the critical junction that connect soft and hard tissues together to enable musculoskeletal function and joint motion.

Several challenges remain to be overcome for the widespread clinical utilization of nanofiber scaffolds for orthopedic tissue engineering and integrative repair. One of the challenges is that the electrospinning process generally utilizes a variety of toxic solvents to dissolve polymers which may have undesired effects on biomolecules or cells. Additionally, high throughput fabrication and delivery processes need to be developed for nanofiber scaffolds in order to augment their commercial applicability. Furthermore, optimization of scaffold design strategies will be critical for effective clinical translation. To this end, biomimetic design of nanofiber-based scaffolds will be aided by continued elucidation of the structure–function relationship of the native tissue and increased understanding of the mechanisms governing its regeneration. Moreover, recent advances in nanotechnology and in the delivery of bioactive agents that are immobilized within the carriers would provide additional methods to control the formation of single or complex tissues. Finally, the establishment of physiologically relevant *in vivo* models to evaluate the clinical efficacy of these biomimetic scaffolds will validate their potential for regenerative medicine and advance these scaffold for integrative soft-tissue repair.

Acknowledgments

The authors gratefully acknowledge the National Institutes of Health (NIH/NIAMS AR052402; AR056459; and AR055280), the Wallace H. Coulter Foundation and the National Science Foundation Graduate Fellowship (SDS), and GK-12 Fellowship (GK-12 0338329, PJC) for funding support.

References

Agrawal, C. M. and R. B. Ray. 2001. Biodegradable polymeric scaffolds for musculoskeletal tissue engineering. *Journal of Biomedical Materials Research Part B: Applied Biomaterials* 55:141–150.

Altman, G. H., R. L. Horan, H. H. Lu, J. Moreau, I. Martin, J. C. Richmond, and D. L. Kaplan. 2002a. Silk matrix for tissue engineering anterior cruciate ligaments. *Biomaterials* 23(20):4131–4141.

Altman, G. H., R. L. Horan, I. Martin, J. Farhadi, P. R. Stark, V. Volloch, J. C. Richmond, G. Vunjak-Novakovic, and D. L. Kaplan. 2002b. Cell differentiation by mechanical stress. *The FASEB Journal* 16(2):270–272.

Amiel, D., C. Frank, F. Harwood, J. Fronek, and W. Akeson. 1984. Tendons and ligaments: A morphological and biomechanical comparison. *Journal of Orthopaedic Research* 1(3):257–365.

Bashur, C. A., L. A. Dahlgren, and A. S. Goldstein. 2006. Effect of fiber diameter and orientation on fibroblast morphology and proliferation on electrospun poly(D, L-lactic-*co*-glycolic acid) meshes. *Biomaterials* 27(33):5681–5688.

Benjamin, M. and J. R. Ralphs. 1998. Fibrocartilage in tendons and ligaments—an adaptation to compressive load. *Journal of Anatomy* 193:481–494.

Benjamin, M., E. J. Evans, and L. Copp. 1986. The histology of tendon attachments to bone in man. *Journal of Anatomy* 149:89–100.

Blevins, F. T., M. Djurasovic, E. L. Flatow, and K. G. Vogel. 1997. Biology of the rotator cuff tendon. *Orthopedic Clinics in North America* 28:1–16.

Buehler, M. J. 2007. Molecular nanomechanics of nascent bone: Fibrillar toughening by mineralization. *Nanotechnology* 18:1–9.

Butler, D. L. 1989. Anterior cruciate ligament: Its normal response and replacement. *Journal of Orthopaedic Research* 7:910–921.

Cooper Jr, J. A., J. S. Sahota, W. J. Gorum 2nd, J. Carter, S. B. Doty, and C. T. Laurencin. 2007. Biomimetic tissue-engineering anterior cruciate ligament replacement. *Proceedings of the National Academy of Sciences* 104(9):3049–3054.

Cooper, R. R., and S. Misol. 1970. Tendon and ligament insertion. A light and electron microscopic study. *Journal of Bone and Joint Surgery of America* 52:1–20.

Currey, J. D. 1988. The effect of porosity and mineral content on the Young's modulus of elasticity of compact bone. *Journal of Biomechanics* 21:131–139.

Du, C., P. Klasens, R. E. de Haan, et al. 2002. Biomimetic calcium phosphate coatings on PolyActive 1000/70/30. *Journal of Biomedical Materials Research* 59:535–546.

Dunn, M. G., J. B. Liesch, M. L. Tiku, and J. P. Zawadsky. 1995. Development of fibroblast-seeded ligament analogs for ACL reconstruction. *Journal of Biomedical Materials Research* 29(11):1363–1371.

Erisken, C., D. M. Kalyon, and H. Wang. 2008a. Functionally graded electrospun polycaprolactone and beta-tricalcium phosphate nanocomposites for tissue engineering applications. *Biomaterials* 29:4065–4073.

Erisken, C., D. M. Kalyon, and H. J. Wang. 2008b. A hybrid twin screw extrusion/electrospinning method to process nanoparticle-incorporated electrospun nanofibres. *Nanotechnology* 19 (16): 165–302.

Ferguson, V. L., A. J. Bushby, and A. Boyde. 2003. Nanomechanical properties and mineral concentration in articular calcified cartilage and subchondral bone. *Journal of Anatomy* 203:191–202.

Galatz, L. M., C. M. Ball, S. A. Teefey, W. D. Middleton, and K. Yamaguchi. 2004. The outcome and repair integrity of completely arthroscopically repaired large and massive rotator cuff repairs. *Journal of Bone and Joint Surgery* 86A:219–224.

Genin, G. M., A. Kent, V. Birman, B. Wopenka, J. D. Pasteris, P. J. Marquez, and S. Thomopoulos. 2009. Functional grading of mineral and collagen in the attachment of tendon to bone. *Biophysical Journal* 97:976–985.

Griffin, L. Y., J. Agel, M. J. Albohm, E. A. Arendt, R. W. Dick, W. E. Garrett, J. G. Garrick et al. 2000. Noncontact anterior cruciate ligament injuries: Risk factors and prevention strategies. *Journal of the American Academy of Orthopaedic Surgeons* 8:141–150.

Horan, R. L., I. Toponarski, H. E. Boepple, P. P. Weitzel, J. C. Richmond, and G. H. Altman. 2009. Design and characterization of a scaffold for anterior cruciate ligament engineering. *Journal of Knee Surgery* 22(1):82–92.

Horii, A., X. Wang, F. Gelain, and S. Zhang. 2007. Biological designer self-assembling peptide nanofiber scaffolds significantly enhance osteoblast proliferation, differentiation and 3-D migration. *PLoS ONE* 2:e190.

Jung, H-J., M. B. Fisher, and S. L-Y. Woo. 2009. Role of biomechanics in the understanding of normal, injured, and healing ligaments and tendons. *Sports Medicine, Arthroscopy, Rehabilitation Therapy & Technology* 1(1):9.

Kay, M. I., R. A. Young, and A. S. Posner. 1964. Crystal structure of hydroxyapatite. *Nature* 204:1050–1052.

Khang, D., M. Sato, R. L. Price, A. E. Ribbe, and T. J. Webster. 2006. Selective adhesion and mineral deposition by osteoblasts on carbon nanofiber patterns. *International Journal of Nanomedicine* 1:65–72.

Kimura, Y., A. Hokugo, T. Takamoto, Y. Tabata, and H. Kurosawa. 2008. Regeneration of anterior cruciate ligament by biodegradable scaffold combined with local controlled release of basic fibroblast growth factor and collagen wrapping. *Tissue Engineering Part C* 14(1):47–57.

Knott, L. and A. J. Bailey. 1998. Collagen cross-links in mineralizing tissues: A review of their chemistry, function, and clinical relevance. *Bone* 22:181–187.

Kumagai, J., K. Sarkar, H. K. Uhthoff, Y. Okawara, and A. Ooshima. 1994. Immunohistochemical distribution of type I, II and III collagens in the rabbit supraspinatus tendon insertion. *Journal of Anatomy* 185:279–284.

Kumbar, S. G., R. James, S. U. Nukavarapu, and C. T. Laurencin. 2008. Electrospun nanofiber scaffolds: Engineering soft tissues. *Biomedical Materials* 3(3):034002.

Landis, W. J. and F. H. Silver. 2008. Mineral deposition in the extracellular matrices of vertebrate tissues: Identification of possible apatite nucleation sites on type I collagen. *Cells Tissues Organs* 189:20–24.

Langer, R. and J. P. Vacanti. 1993. Tissue engineering. *Science* 260:920–926.

Lee, C. H., H. J. Shin, I. H. Cho, Y. M. Kang, I. A. Kim, K. D. Park, and J. W. Shin. 2005. Nanofiber alignment and direction of mechanical strain affect the ECM production of human ACL fibroblast. *Biomaterials* 26(11):1261–1270.

Li, W. J., C. T. Laurencin, E. J. Caterson, R. S. Tuan, and F. K. Ko. 2002. Electrospun nanofibrous structure: A novel scaffold for tissue engineering. *Journal of Biomedical Materials Research* 60:613–621.

Li, X. R., J. W. Xie, J. Lipner, X. Y. Yuan, S. Thomopoulos, and Y. N. Xia. 2009. Nanofiber scaffolds with gradations in mineral content for mimicking the tendon-to-bone insertion site. *Nano Letters* 9:2763–2768.

Liang, R., S. L-Y. Woo, Y. Takakura, D. K. Moon, F. Jia, and S. Abramowitch. 2006. Long-term effects of porcine small intestinal submucosa on the healing of the medial collateral ligament: A functional tissue engineering study. *Journal of Orthopaedic Research* 24(4):811–819.

Liu, S. H., R-S. Yang, R. Al-Shaikh, and J. M. Lane. 1995. Collagen in tendon, ligament, and bone healing. *Clinical Orthopaedics and Related Research* 318:265–278.

Lu, H. H. and J. Jiang. 2006. Interface tissue engineering and the formulation of multiple-tissue systems. *Advances in Biochemical Engineering and Biotechnology* 102:91–111.

Lu, H. H., J. A. Cooper Jr., S. Manuel, J. W. Freeman, M.A. Attawia, F. K. Ko, and C. T. Laurencin. 2005. Anterior cruciate ligament regeneration using braided biodegradable scaffolds: *In vitro* optimization studies. *Biomaterials* 26(23):4805–4816.

Mann, S. 2001. *Biomineralization: Principles and Concepts in Bioinorganic Materials Chemistry*. New York: Oxford University Press.

Matthews, J. A., G. E. Wnek, D. G. Simpson, and G. L. Bowlin. 2002. Electrospinning of collagen nanofibers. *Biomacromolecules* 3:232–238.

Matyas, J. R., M. G. Anton, N. G. Shrive, and C. B. Frank. 1995. Stress governs tissue phenotype at the femoral insertion of the rabbit MCL. *Journal of Biomechanics* 28:147–157.

Mavis, B., T. T. Demirtas, M. Gumusderelioglu, G. Gunduz, and U. Colak. 2009. Synthesis, characterization and osteoblastic activity of polycaprolactone nanofibers coated with biomimetic calcium phosphate. *Acta Biomaterialia* 5: 3098–3111.

Messner, K. 1997. Postnatal development of the cruciate ligament insertions in the rat knee. Morphological evaluation and immunohistochemical study of collagens types I and II. *Acta Anatomica* 160:261–268.

Moffat, K. L., W. H. Sun, P. E. Pena, N. O. Chahine, S. B. Doty, G. A. Ateshian, C. T. Hung, and H. H. Lu. 2008a. Characterization of the structure–function relationship at the ligament-to-bone interface. *Proceedings of the National Academy of Sciences USA* 105:7947–7952.

Moffat, K. L., W. N. Levine, and H. H. Lu. 2008b. *In vitro* evaluation of rotator cuff tendon fibroblasts on aligned composite scaffold of polymer nanofibers and hydroxyapatite nanoparticles. *Transactions of the 54th Annual Meeting of the Orthopaedic Research Society.*

Moffat, K. L., S. P. Kwei, J. P. Spalazzi, S. B. Doty, W. N. Levine, and H. H. Lu. 2009. Novel nanofiber-based scaffold for rotator cuff repair and augmentation. *Tissue Engineering Part A* 15:115–126.

Murphy, W. L., S. Hsiong, T. P. Richardson, C. A. Simmons, and D. J. Mooney. 2005. Effects of a bone-like mineral film on phenotype of adult human mesenchymal stem cells *in vitro. Biomaterials* 26:303–310.

Murphy, W. L. and D. J. Mooney. 2002. Bioinspired growth of crystalline carbonate apatite on biodegradable polymer substrata. *Journal of the American Chemical Society* 124:1910–1917.

Niyibizi, C., C. S. Visconti, K. Kavalkovich, and S. L. Woo. 1995. Collagens in an adult bovine medial collateral ligament: immunofluorescence localization by confocal microscopy reveals that type XIV collagen predominates at the ligament–bone junction. *Matrix Biology* 14:743–751.

Niyibizi, C., V. C. Sagarrigo, G. Gibson, and K. Kavalkovich. 1996. Identification and immunolocalization of type X collagen at the ligament-bone interface. *Biochemistry and Biophysics Research Communication* 222:584–589.

Oguma, H., G. Murakami, H. Takahashi-Iwanaga, M. Aoki, and S. Ishii. 2001. Early anchoring collagen fibers at the bone–tendon interface are conducted by woven bone formation: Light microscope and scanning electron microscope observation using a canine model. *Journal of Orthopedic Research* 19:873–880.

Ozawa, H., K. Hoshi, and N. Amizuka. 2008. Current concepts of bone biomineralization. *Journal of Oral Bioscience* 50:1–14.

Petersen, W. and B. Tillmann. 1999. Structure and vascularization of the cruciate ligaments of the human knee joint. *Anatomy and Embryology* 200:325–334.

Radhakrishnan, P., N. T. Lewis, and J. J. Mao. 2004. Zone-specific micromechanical properties of the extracellular matrices of growth plate cartilage. *Annales in Biomedical Engineering* 32:284–291.

Raspanti, M., R. Strocchi, V. De Pasquale, D. Martini, C. Montanari, and A. Ruggeri. 1996. Structure and ultrastructure of the bone/ligament junction. *Italian Journal of Anatomy and Embryology* 101:97–105.

Reneker, D. H., and I. Chun. 1996. Nanometre diameter fibres of polymer, produced by electrospinning. *Nanotechnology* 7:216–233.

Rho, K. S., L. Jeong, G. Lee, B. M. Seo, Y. J. Park, S. D. Hong, S. Roh, J. J. Cho, W. H. Park, and B. M. Min. 2006. Electrospinning of collagen nanofibers: Effects on the behavior of normal human keratinocytes and early-stage wound healing. *Biomaterials* 27(8):1452–1461.

Sahoo, S., H. Ouyang, J. C. Goh, T. E. Tay, and S. L. Toh. 2006. Characterization of a novel polymeric scaffold for potential application in tendon/ligament tissue engineering. *Tissue Engineering* 12(1):91–99.

Sargeant, T. D., M. O. Guler, S. M. Oppenheimer, et al. 2008. Hybrid bone implants: Self-assembly of peptide amphiphile nanofibers within porous titanium. *Biomaterials* 29:161–171.

Shin, S. Y., H. N. Park, K. H. Kim, et al. 2005. Biological evaluation of chitosan nanofiber membrane for guided bone regeneration. *Journal of Periodontology* 76:1778–1784.

Song, J., H. Kim, and H. Kim. 2008. Electrospun fibrous web of collagen-apatite precipitated nanocomposite for bone regeneration. *Journal of Material Science: Material and Medicine* 19:2925–2932.

Spalazzi, J. P., J. Gallina, S. D. Fung-Kee-Fung, E. E. Konofagou, and H. H. Lu. 2006a. Elastographic imaging of strain distribution in the anterior cruciate ligament and at the ligament-bone insertions. *Journal of Orthopedic Research* 24:2001–2010.

Spalazzi, J. P., S. B. Doty, K. L. Moffat, W. N. Levine, and H. H. Lu. 2006b. Development of controlled matrix heterogeneity on a triphasic scaffold for orthopedic interface tissue engineering. *Tissue Engineering* 12:3497–3508.

Spalazzi, J. P., A. L. Boskey, and H. H. Lu. 2007. Region-dependent variations in matrix collagen and mineral distribution across the femoral and tibial anterior cruciate ligament-to-bone insertion sites. *Transactions of the 53rd Annual Meeting of the Orthopeadic Research Society.*

Spalazzi, J. P., E. Dagher, S. B. Doty, X. E. Guo, S. A. Rodeo, and H. H. Lu. 2008a. *In vivo* evaluation of a multiphased scaffold designed for orthopaedic interface tissue engineering and soft tissue-to-bone integration. *Journal of Biomedical Material Research A* 86:1–12.

Spalazzi, J. P., M. C. Vyner, M. T. Jacobs, K. L. Moffat, and H. H. Lu. 2008b. Mechanoactive scaffold induces tendon remodeling and expression of fibrocartilage markers. *Clinical Orthopaedics and Related Research* 466:1938–1948.

Subramony, S. D., B. R. Dargis, M. Castillo, E. U. Azeloglu, M. S. Tracey, and H. H. Lu. 2010. Mechanical stimulation of hMSC differentiation on nanofiber scaffolds for ligament tissue engineering. *Transactions of the 56th Annual Meeting of the Orthopaedic Research Society.*

Thomopoulos, S., G. R. Williams, J. A. Gimbel, M. Favata, and L. J. Soslowsky. 2003. Variations of biomechanical, structural, and compositional properties along the tendon to bone insertion site. *Journal of Orthopedic Research* 21:413–419.

Ventura, A., C. Terzaghi, C. Legnani, E. Borgo, and W. Albisetti. 2010. Synthetic grafts for anterior cruciate ligament rupture: 19-year outcome study. *The Knee* 17(2): 108–113.

Venugopal, J. R., S. Low, A. T. Choon, A. B. Kumar, and S. Ramakrishna. 2008. Nanobioengineered electrospun composite nanofibers and osteoblasts for bone regeneration. *Artificial Organs* 32:388–397.

Vitale, M. A., M. G. Vitale, J. G. Zivin, J. P. Braman, L. U. Bigliani, and E. L. Flatow. 2007. Rotator cuff repair: An analysis of utility scores and cost-effectiveness. *Journal of Shoulder and Elbow Surgery* 16:181–187.

Wang, I. E., S. Mitroo, F. H. Chen, H. H. Lu, and S. B. Doty. 2006. Age-dependent changes in matrix composition and organization at the ligament-to-bone insertion. *Journal of Orthopedic Research* 24:1745–1755.

Wei, X. and K. Messner. 1996. The postnatal development of the insertions of the medial collateral ligament in the rat knee. *Anatomy and Embryology* 193:53–59.

Woo, S. L. and J. A. Buckwalter. 1988. AAOS/NIH/ORS workshop. Injury and repair of the musculos-keletal soft tissues. Savannah, GA, June 18–20, 1987. *Journal of Orthopedic Research* 6:907–931.

Woo, S. L., M. A. Gomez, Y. Seguchi, C. M. Endo, and W. H. Akeson. 1983. Measurement of mechanical properties of ligament substance from a bone-ligament-bone preparation. *Journal of Orthopedic Research* 1:22–29.

Woo, S. L., J. Maynard, D. L. Butler, R. M. Lyon, P. A. Torzilli, W. H. Akeson, R. R. Cooper, and B. Oakes. 1988. Ligament, tendon, and joint capsule insertions to bone. In Woo, S. L., and Bulkwater, J. A. (Eds.), *Injury and Repair of the Musculosketal Soft Tissues.* American Academy of Orthopaedic Surgeons, Savannah, GA, pp. 133–166.

Woo, S. L-Y., G. A. Johnson, and B. A. Smith. 1993. Mathematical modeling of tendons and ligaments. *Transactions of the ASME* 115:468–473.

Yang, F., J. G. C. Wolke, and J. A. Jansen. 2008. Biomimetic calcium phosphate coating on electrospun poly(e-caprolactone) scaffolds for bone tissue engineering. *Chemical Engineering Journal* 137:154–161.

Yoshimoto, H., Y. M. Shin, H. Terai, and J. P. Vacanti. 2003. A biodegradable nanofiber scaffold by electro-spinning and its potential for bone tissue engineering. *Biomaterials* 24:2077–2082.

3

Polycaprolactone Nanowires for Controlling Cell Behavior at the Biointerface

Sarah L. Tao
*The Charles Stark Draper
Laboratory*

3.1 Introduction

Surface topography plays a crucial role in cell–substrate interactions. In a physiological environment, cells respond to nanometric topologies such as fibrous and porous materials formed by components of the extracellular matrix. Response to nanotopographic features (such as grooves, pores, pits, and pillars), though variable from cell type to cell type, has been reported in almost all mammalian cells and expertly reviewed in the literature (Bettinger et al., 2009; Kriparamanan et al., 2006; Martinez et al., 2009; Yim and Leong, 2005). Nanostructure shape and dimension, symmetry, and surface area coverage as well as base material play a large part in dictating cell response and changing basic cell behavior—how the cell may adhere, spread, and align, to subsequent downstream responses in proliferation, morphology, and differentiation.

Nanostructuring of medical devices, although not yet truly realized, offers great potential for enhancing device performance. By developing structured nanoscale topographies in synthetic materials, the interface between tissue and device can be specifically designed to increase or reduce cell adhesion and response. For example, an artificial scaffold which recreates the natural nanotopographical environment of a specific cell type as seen in the body may be essential in directing cells toward the creation of functional engineered tissues. Similarly, nanosurfacing medical implants may play a critical role in directing host–tissue response and reactivity toward a particular implant.

Rapid expansion in the fabrication of inorganic nanomaterials, such as oriented carbon nanotubes and nanostructures of semiconductors and metals, has led to great progress in developing materials for miniaturized devices. This interest in ordered, nanostructured materials has translated to applications in biology and medicine with recent findings that cellular responses can be directed by nanotopography. Although inorganic materials are of choice for electronic and mechanical devices, these materials are not necessarily appropriate for applications in biology and medicine. Nanostructures fabricated from polymeric biodegradable materials on the other hand, have great potential for biomedical applications in areas such as tissue engineering and drug delivery. Established methods for generating nanotopography, such as electron beam lithography, are costly and time consuming, particularly when generating large area patterns. The ability to produce nanosurfaces easily and inexpensively will likely increase the number of practical applications where nanotopography can be utilized.

In this chapter, the technique of nanotemplating polymer melts will be discussed. Nanotemplating is a simple method which can be used to nanostructure biodegradable materials without the use of organic solvents, pressure assistance, or custom instrumentation (Tao and Desai, 2007). Specifically, the fabrication of perpendicularly aligned polycaprolactone (PCL) nanowires will be discussed, along with cell response toward these nanowire structures, and the potential for their use in tissue engineering, regenerative medicine, and other biomedical applications.

3.2 Nanotemplating of Polymer Melts

Templating entails synthesizing a desired material within the pores of a membrane (Martin, 1994). Using a template of aligned and ordered pores produces ordered nanowire arrays perpendicular to the attached substrate. Template synthesis has been previously used to prepare nanotubes and wires from metals and semiconductor materials (Banerjee et al., 2002; Fan et al., 2006; Kline et al., 2006; Lombardi et al., 2006; Ma et al., 2004). By exploiting methods of electrochemical oxidation, phase separation, extrusion, or wetting in combination with template synthesis, similar structures have also been fabricated in various nondegradable polymers (Feng et al., 2002, 2003; Li et al., 2006; Martin, 1994; Parthasarathy and Martin, 1994; Qiao et al., 2005; Rynes and Demoustier-Champagne, 2005; Steinhart et al., 2002, 2003, 2004). However, these materials are not ideal for biomedical applications such as tissue engineering and drug delivery. For these applications, it would instead be advantageous to create nano-engineered constructs which are able to degrade and be resorbed by the body naturally over a period of time. Nonetheless, template-synthesized nanowires from biodegradable polymers are scarcely reported. Although Chen et al. have described a method of fabricating PCL nanofibers by extrusion of a precursor solution through a template into a solidifying solvent under pressure utilizing custom instrumentation (Chen et al., 2006), Tao et al. demonstrated that template synthesis can be used as a fast and inexpensive method to form perpendicularly oriented high aspect ratio (greater than 1:10) nanowire and nanofiber arrays from biodegradable and biocompatible polymers, including poly(lactic-*co*-glycolic acid), PCL, and poly(lactic-*co*-caprolactone), without the use of organic solvents, pressure assistance, or custom instrumentation (Tao and Desai, 2007).

The nanotemplating method used to form PCL nanowires in an aluminum oxide template is depicted in Figure 3.1. In general, anodic aluminum oxide films are formed by the electrochemical oxidation of aluminum. Depending on the type of anodization process and growth regime used, aluminum oxide membranes can be fabricated to contain nanopores in a wide range of diameters, lengths, and interpore distances (Lee et al., 2006; Li et al., 1998; Masuda and Fukada, 1995), and can be selectively etched with sodium hydroxide in the presence of PCL.

In order to overcome the need for fabricating nanoporous aluminum oxide membranes of varying thickness to produce differing nanowire lengths, nanowire length is instead tuned as a function of melt time and temperature. PCL is a semicrystalline polymer which melts in the range of 59–65°C depending on crystallite size, with a glass transition of −60°C, resulting in the polymer being in a rubbery state at room temperature. At a melt temperature of 130°C, nanowire lengths 2.5–27.0 μm could be produced in less than 60 min by varying melt time (Figure 3.2a). At a melt temperature of 65°C similar structures were formed, however increase in nanowire length took place over longer intervals. Nanowires less than 10 μm in length were found to be freestanding, though the wires shift to pack in loose clusters (Figure 3.2c and d). When greater than 10 μm in length, the nanostructures instead folded over to form long strands of arrayed, flexible nanofibers layered over the substrate base. The diameter of the PCL

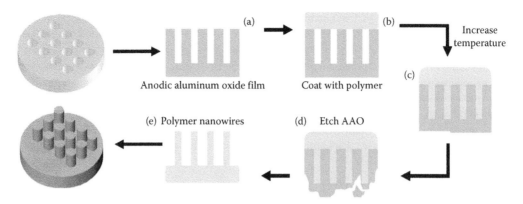

FIGURE 3.1 Nanotemplating method used to form perpendicularly aligned polymer nanowires from a polymer melt. (a) An aluminum oxide nanoporous membrane, (b) coated with a solid polymer. (c) When the temperature is increased above melt point, the polymer melt fills the pores of the membrane. (d) The aluminum oxide membrane is selectively etched, (e) until only the polymer nanowires remain.

nanowires was approximately 200 nm. The heat treatment and exposure to sodium hydroxide did not significantly change the wettability or the surface chemistry of PCL.

Previous studies have shown that melt encapsulation of proteins within PCL produces feasible systems for controlled delivery of stable proteins (Jameela et al., 1997; Lin and Yu, 2001). Combined with nanotemplating, this provides a method of encapsulating potential therapeutic substances such as

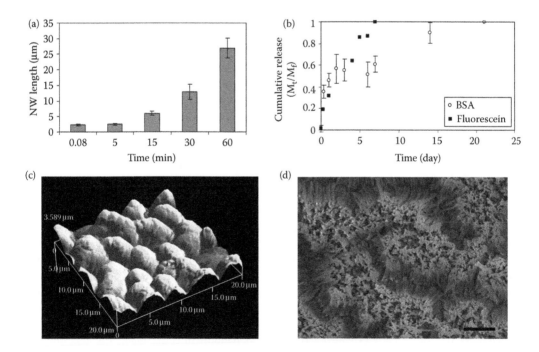

FIGURE 3.2 (a) Change in nanowire PCL length at a melting temperature of 130°C as a function of melt time. (b) Release of small molecule and proteins from nanowire PCL. (c) 20 μm intermittent contact atomic force microscope image (AFM) 3D image of PCL nanowires 2.5 μm in length. (d) Scanning electron microscope (SEM) image of free-standing PCL nanowires 2.5 μm in length. (Reprinted from Tao, S. L. and T. A. Desai. 2007. *Nano Lett* 7 (6):1463–1468. With permission. ©2007 American Chemical Society.)

proteins and peptides in the PCL nanowires for sustained release (Figure 3.2b) (Tao and Desai, 2007). Release of small molecules from the nanowire PCL was found to be controlled by Fickian diffusion, whereas sustained release of proteins due to a combination of diffusion through the matrix and partial diffusion through water-filled pores. An initial burst in protein release occurred due to drug desorption at the nanowire surface where the surrounding fluid begins to dissolve the exposed protein immediately, whereas the diffusion release phase is attributed to molecule diffusion from near the surface. As the protein at the surface dissolved, the porosity of the PCL nanowires increased, allowing fluid to dissolve protein molecules embedded in the nanowire. Protein molecules fully coated and embedded within the nanowire, are gradually released due to hindrance of diffusion from the inner core of the nanowire.

3.3 Cell Response to PCL Nanowires

3.3.1 Endothelial

Endothelial cell activation is essential for many processes including vascular remodeling and vessel growth. In response to certain stimuli, endothelial cells proliferate, migrate, and coalesce to form primitive vascular labyrinths that undergo maturation and remodeling. The ability to control endothelial response could greatly impact the treatment of diseases associated with pathological angiogenesis and tissue remodeling, or conversely to direct angiogenesis or vasculogenesis during the formation of *de novo* tissue for regenerative medicine applications. Alternatively, enhanced endothelialization could play an important role in vascular grafts, cardiovascular implants, and other blood-contacting devices where effective endothelial seeding could provide a reduction in platelet adhesion, fibrin formation, and thromboembolism, thus potentially increasing device performance.

Endothelial cells have been shown to respond to various nanotopographic cues (Bettinger et al., 2008; Dalby et al., 2002; Lee et al., 2008; Lu et al., 2008; Miller et al., 2004). These studies found endothelial cells to spread arcuately on low aspect ratio (1:1) nanostructures compared with flat surfaces, however cytoskeleton definition, stress fiber formation rate, and overall spreading decreased with an increase in nanostructure height (Dalby et al., 2002). For nanostructures of high aspect ratio (at least 1:10), a decrease in cell number and spreading was observed (Lee et al., 2008).

Human umbilical vein endothelial cells were found to be similarly adherent on glass, smooth PCL, and nanowire PCL. Furthermore, the majority of cells across all substrates were found to be spreading (defined as exhibiting a nonrounded morphology) after 24 h. Subconfluent cells cultured on glass and smooth PCL appear to be flat, widely spread, and highly motile. These cells exhibit both clear filopodia and lamellipodia that contain a thick cortical network of actin filaments, as well as discrete stress fibers. The endothelial cells were found to form direct interactions with neighboring cells and cell density increased over a period of time (Figure 3.3).

Cells cultured on the nanowire PCL, though spreading, appear to have a different morphology. Instead of forming lamellipodia, these cells were instead found to polarize with little alignment and extend long processes. Furthermore, these cells were found to sprout multiple processes which in turn, branched in varying direction and random orientation. Cell–cell contact was restricted to interaction between these branched processes. There appeared to be no arrangement of actin stress fibers, but actin condensation was found in the cell body, with a gradient of decreasing concentration from the sprout site toward the distal end of each branched process. In some cases, flecks of actin were found to be distributed along the process. These actin accumulations are commonly thought to represent the foci of a hypercontraction of formerly extended actin networks (Goodman et al., 1980). The long branched processes exhibited by these cells may enable them to sample their environment in the absence of a continuous surface. This form of endothelial pseudopodial branching is typically associated with local regulation of directional guidance during angiogenesis (Fischer et al., 2009); therefore, further studies must be performed in order to fully understand the implications of endothelial cell response to this particular nanowire PCL substrate.

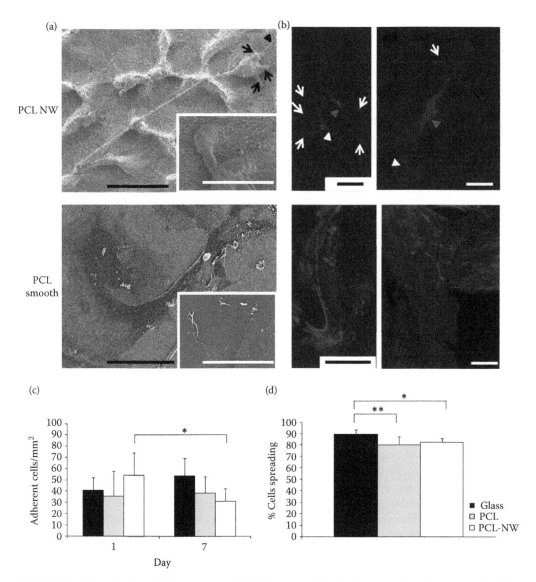

FIGURE 3.3 **(See color insert following page 10-24.)** Human umbilical vein endothelial cells cultured for 7 days. (a) SEM image of cells on smooth and nanowire PCL. Cells cultured on nanowire PCL sprout and extend multiple long, narrow processes with round tips, whereas cells cultured on smooth PCL are flat and well spread, forming lamellipodia for motility. Black arrows point to examples of sprouting. Black arrowhead points to filopodia associated with new sprouting process. (b) Cells cultured on nanowire and smooth PCL stained for actin by rhodamine phalloidin and nucleus by DAPI. White arrows point to examples of branched processes. Gray arrow heads point to concentrated actin at growth sprout, white arrowheads point to actin aggregates. (c) Number of adherent live cells after 1 and 7 days in culture. (d) Percent of spreading (nonrounded) cells after 24 h in culture. Black scale bars = 50 μm, white scale bars = 20 μm. $^{*}p < 0.05$, $^{**}p < 0.01$.

3.3.2 Neural

The most difficult cells and tissues to derive for use in tissue engineering strategies are the complex networks of the central nervous system (CNS). The capacity of stem cells to differentiate into a number of cell types, however, holds out the promise that eventually it may be possible to repair CNS damage from degenerative diseases, as well as traumatic injury. The retina is an ideal CNS structure for investigation as it is a highly organized and easily accessible for experimental manipulation. Photoreceptor degeneration initially leaves the inner retinal circuitry intact and new photoreceptors need only make single, short synaptic connections. Recent advances in stem cell transplantation have shown that limited photoreceptor replacement is possible in animal models using expandable cell populations (Klassen et al., 2004; Lamba et al., 2009; Osakada et al., 2008).

Multipotent tissue-specific progenitor cells, derived either from the brain (BPCs) or retina (RPCs), represent types of potential donor cell. These cells were the first to show evidence of integration into the neural retina (Klassen et al., 2004; Takahashi et al., 1998; Young et al., 2000). Integration of stem cells into the host retina, however, appears to be enhanced by the presence of developing or residual host neurons and glia that very likely provide guidance cues and may be functioning as a template with which the donor cells can engage. In clinical situations where the resident cell population has been severely depleted or when the local laminar cytoarchitecture has been disrupted, an alternative mechanism will be needed to confer organization to the grafted cells. One possible mechanism may be guidance cues provided by nanotopography.

Mouse RPCs cultured on nanowire PCL were found to remain robustly adherent to the substrate surface over an initial culture period of 72 h, whereas, cells cultured on glass and smooth PCL generally remained as suspended neurospheres in culture (Figure 3.4d), although adherent properties could be altered by coating the surface with adhesion proteins such as laminin. The RPCs seeded on smooth PCL were randomly adherent and remained relatively spheroid in shape. Processes were shown to extend between select cells by day 3, though they exhibited no direct alignment with specific surface regions. The densely packed, free-standing nanowires decreased the overall contact area of the PCL available for cell attachment. Consequently, RPCs were found to primarily attach as individual cells on the tips of nanowire clusters. After 3 days in culture, these cells were found to spread fan-like processes out to neighboring cells, creating apparent cell-to-cell contacts. After 7 days in culture, the cells were shown to form a dense monolayer across the nanowire surface, with rope-like extensions connecting the individual cells (Figure 3.4a–c). Analysis of RNA synthesis revealed marked downregulation of stem and neural stem cell markers Pax6, Hes1, nestin, and Sox2 in RPCs cultured on nanowire PCL, suggesting these cells were differentiating toward more mature states. Immunohistochemical analysis revealed that scaffold topology influenced protein expression levels. RPCs consistently labeled positively for nestin and neural filament marker nf-200, indicating the presence of undifferentiated cell populations. However, only RPCs cultured on nanowire PCL demonstrated evidence of differentiation by expression of the bipolar cell marker PKC, the photoreceptor marker recoverin, and the rod photoreceptor marker rhodopsin. RPCs cultured on nanowire PCL resulted in high levels of migration into the inner nuclear and ganglion cell layers of rhodposin knockout (Rho −/−) explants, whereas RPCs cultured on smooth PCL did not (Figure 3.4e and f). When transplanted subretinally in Rho −/−mice, RPCs cultured on nanowire PCL migrated into the retina outer nuclear layer (ONL) and inner nuclear layer (INL) and developed an apparent cell polarity with early photoreceptor-like morphology and expression of recoverin (Redenti et al., 2008).

3.3.3 Monocyte

Monocytes recruited and adherent to the surface of implanted biomedical devices can recognize the material as a foreign body. Their interaction at the biointerface can elicit a number of responses, including differentiation into macrophages and fusion into foreign body giant cells. Consequently, implants can become degraded, cause chronic inflammation, or become isolated by fibrous encapsulation, affecting the biocompatibility and overall performance of the implant. Considerable efforts have been made to produce material surfaces that control inflammation in a predictable way. By defining the relationships between physical cues and monocyte activation, established criteria for designing biomaterials can be utilized in future medical device and implant applications. Recent

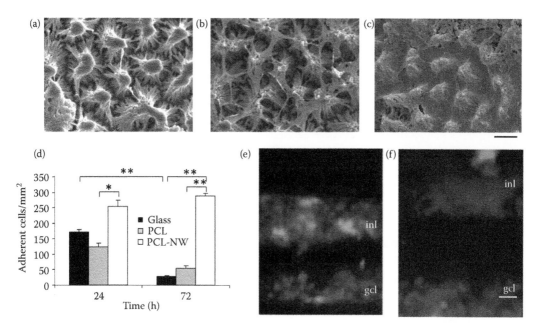

FIGURE 3.4 **(See color insert following page 10-24.)** SEM images of mouse retinal progenitor cells cultured on nanowire PCL at (a) day 1, (b) day 3, and (c) day 7. (d) Number of adherent cells after 24 and 72 h in culture on glass, smooth PCL, and nanowire PCL. (e) Integration of RPCs cultured on nanowire PCL into Rho –/– retinal explants, with high migration into the inner nuclear and ganglion cell layers. (f) RPCs cultured on smooth PCL with little integration of RPCs into Rho –/– retinal explants. Note that the ONL is absent from the 8- to 10-week Rho –/– retina due to degeneration. Black scale bar = 2 μm. White scale bar = 100 μm. (With kind permission from Springer Science+Business Media: Redenti, S. et al. 2008. *Journal of Ocular Biology, Dieases, and Informatics* 1(1):19–29. Copyright 2008.)

research has focused on understanding how nanostructuring of a biomaterial surface directs adherent monocyte activity and behavior as a means to direct subsequent biological responses (i.e., inflammation and wound healing) to implanted biomaterials (Ainslie et al., 2008a, 2008b; Hsu et al., 2004; Riedel et al., 2001). From these studies it was demonstrated that in almost all materials, including polymers, metals, and semiconductor materials, nanostructured counterparts gave rise to less inflammatory reactions.

Primary human blood-derived monocytes were isolated and seeded onto PCL surfaces. After 48 h in culture, cell response to nanowire topography was measured in terms of relative monocyte viability and morphology, in addition to production of inflammatory cytokines and reactive oxygen species. Activated cells generally display migratory ruffles or pseudopodia associated with cytoplasmic spreading. Adherent monocytes on control, smooth PCL, and nanowire PCL all displayed, to an extent, morphology associated with monocyte activation. However, cytoplasmic spreading and ruffling was more highly associated with smooth PCL, whereas the monocytes cultured on nanowire PCL were associated with pseudopodia projections extending into the nanowires of the substrate. Monocytes cultured on PCL surfaces were found to be generally smaller and more circular compared to tissue culture plastic (TCPS) and glass, a morphology associated with nonstimulated cells (Figure 3.5).

All cytokine levels were significantly lower on PCL surfaces in comparison to monocytes activated by lipopolysaccharide, a bacterial coat sugar. Cytokine production levels in monocytes cultured on PCL (both smooth and nanowire), with little exception, do not appear to be significantly different than monocytes cultured on TCPS. TNF-α production was downregulated in monocytes cultured on PCL surfaces in comparison to those cultured on TCPS. TNF-α is a cytokine with a role in the reduction of

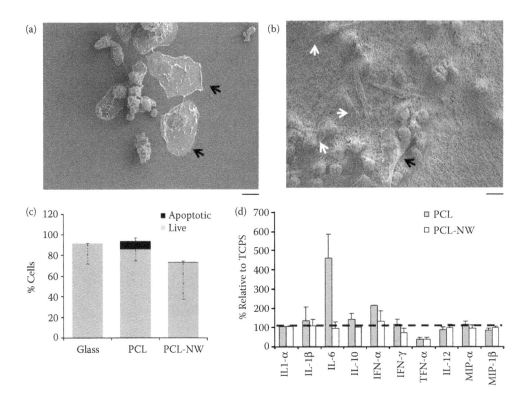

FIGURE 3.5   SEM images of human blood-derived monocytes on (a) smooth PCL, and (b) nanowire PCL. Black arrows point to examples of ruffled, spread cells. White arrows point to examples of pseudopodia extensions. (c) Percent monocytes which were apoptotic or alive. (d) Percent difference in cytokine production relative to control TCPS. Scale bar = 20 μm.

apoptosis. Monocytes become apoptotic when nonstimulated, which correlates with the higher degree of apoptotic cells seen on PCL and significantly lower levels of TNF-α. IL-6 production was upregulated in monocytes cultured on smooth PCL, but not nanowire PCL. As IL-6 is a monocyte proinflammatory cytokine, this suggests that the nanowire architecture may play a role in decreasing levels of inflammatory response (Ainslie et al., 2008a).

3.3.4 Fibroblast

Following inflammation, the end-stage healing response to the implantation of a material is the formation of a fibrotic capsule. This process may become pathological, however, if the fibroblasts proliferate too extensively and cause fibrotic hyperplasia, which in turn can directly impact implant failure. Because they play such an important role in implant integration and the healing process, fibroblasts are one of the most studied cells in terms of response to nanotopography (Berry et al., 2005; Correa-Duarte et al., 2004; Curtis et al., 2001, 2004; Dalby et al., 2004a, 2004b, 2008; Kaiser et al., 2006; Lee et al., 2008). Fibroblasts have shown different responses toward various nanotopographies, randomness, and symmetry. However, adhesion was commonly found to increase with decreasing feature size or height, causing subsequent changes in morphology and cytoskeleton arrangement (Yim and Leong, 2005).

Human lung fibroblasts seeded on nanowire PCL were found to be similarly adherent to fibroblasts grown on control surfaces (glass and smooth PCL). After 24 h, the numbers of spreading cells were quantified and it was found that while two thirds of the population was spread on glass, nearly no cells were found to spread on the nanowire PCL. After 72 h, the adherent live cell density was increased on all substrates. However, although the number of cells on each of the surfaces was comparable, it was apparent that the shape and morphology of the fibroblasts were different. Cells cultured on the glass substrates were characteristic in terms of cell type. They appeared elongated from the poles of the cells and with aligned actin fibers. The cell and nuclear morphology were coupled in terms of larger area and elongated shape (nuclear circularity ≈ 0.8). The morphology of these cells was flat and well-spread, with numerous cytoplasmic extensions forming and at times, connecting to other neighboring cells (Figure 3.6).

Fibroblasts cultured on smooth PCL, although spread, took on a triangular shape, with visible actin stress fibers, and a more circular nucleus (nuclear circularity ≈ 0.95). Upon examination of morphology, the lamellipodia and retraction fibers were clearly visible, suggesting directional motility. Fibroblast migration is known to be influenced by substrate compliance, and greater on surfaces of decreasing stiffness. It is possible that the higher degree of motility on the smooth PCL may be attributed to the relative decrease in stiffness, two orders of magnitude less than the glass.

While fibroblasts cultured on glass and smooth PCL appeared to spread and elongate, fibroblasts cultured on the PCL nanowires remained small and circular (nuclear circularity ≈ 0.92), with no visible actin stress fibers. Two distinct morphologies could be seen in the fibroblasts grown on the nanowire surface. The majority of cells were flat and conformed to the top of a cluster of nanowires. Few of the cells were stretched between clusters, with filopodia extending from around the circumference and the underside. In both cases, microvilli were more apparent than on those cells cultured on glass or smooth PCL. The decrease in cell area and lack of stress fibers in these cells, however, are not an indication of toxicity as cells remain live and adherent. However, cell spreading is a necessary mechanism for cell division. Although the nanowire topography increases the overall surface area of the PCL, the high aspect nanowires effectively reduces the contact area which the cell can effectively sense and adhere to. In fact, the ratio of the planar contact area presented to the cell in comparison to total surface area is approximately $1:3 \times 10^9$. Reduction of the cell contact area most likely limits the ability of the fibroblasts to spread and proliferate. Similar response was demonstrated in fibroblasts cultured on other high aspect ratio structures (Lee et al., 2008). The ability for high aspect ratio nanostructures to limit fibroblast spreading and proliferation may have some potential application then as surface coatings which can limit the fibrotic response toward implanted medical devices.

3.3.5 Bone

Since the initial introduction of PCL nanowires as a suitable biointerface, other groups have integrated its use into applications in orthopedic tissue engineering. Porter et al. have utilized this same nanowire PCL strategy as a building block for the development of three-dimensional bone scaffolds (Porter et al., 2009a, 2009b). Nanowire PCL surfaces were shown to enhance mesenchymal stem cell (MSC) response in terms of survivability, viability, cytoskeleton changes, and morphology as compared with control surfaces of smooth PCL and TCPS. Nanowire PCL also induced a rapid production of bone extracellular matrix by differentiated MSCs, indicated by accelerated calcium phosphate mineralization, and osteocalcin and osteopontin production.

3.4 Conclusion

Nanotemplanting provides a rapid and inexpensive method of producing nanostructures in biodegradeable and biocompatible polymers, such as PCL. The examples presented in this chapter clearly indicate that various cell types respond to nanowire PCL in different ways. The nanowire features were shown to alter cell behavior in terms of adhesion, proliferation, migration, as well as RNA synthesis, and protein production. This is entirely consistent with the large body of literature demonstrating the ability of

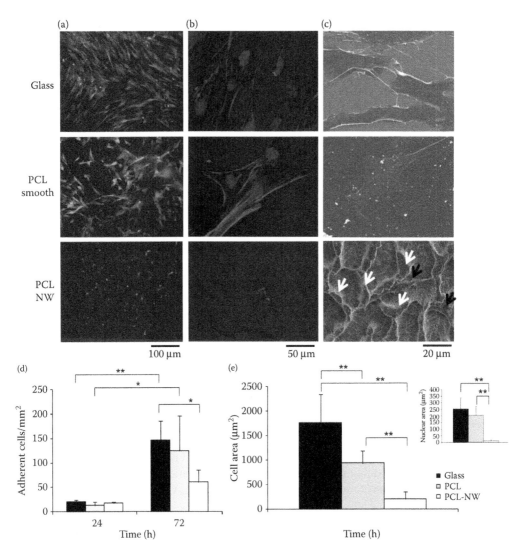

FIGURE 3.6   (See color insert following page 10-24.) Human lung fibroblasts cultured on glass, smooth PCL, and nanowire PCL substrates for 72 h. (a) Live cells stained by 5-chloromethylfluorescein diacetate. (b) Actin stained by rhodamine phalloidin and nucleus stained by DAPI. (c) SEM image of cell morphology. Cells cultured on glass elongated, while cells on smooth PCL appeared triangular and motile. Cells cultured on nanowire PCL were either conformed to the top of the nanowire cluster (white arrows) or were spread between clusters (black arrows). (d) Number of adherent live cells after 24 and 72 h in culture. (e) Cell area after 72 h in culture. Inset shows nuclear area. $*p < 0.05$, $**p < 0.01$. (Reprinted from Tao, S. L. and T. A. Desai. 2007. *Nano Lett* 7 (6):1463–1468. With permission. © 2007 American Chemical Society.)

nanoscale features to directly influence cell response. However, much investigation is still needed before the mechanisms behind nanotopographic influence on cell behavior can be well understood. Harnessing the full potential of nanotopographical guidance will most likely require additional attention to many detailed aspects of the complex and dynamic relationship between the cell and its microenvironment. But as the field advances, the ability to precisely control cell response using nanotopography will largely have a profound impact in the design and development of medical device implants and functional engineered tissues.

Acknowledgments

The author gratefully acknowledges funding from the Sandler Family Foundation Translational Research Fellowship, Knights Templar Eye Foundation, Lincy Foundation, Discover Eye Foundation, Foundation Fighting Blindness, and the Stanford CIS Grant Program.

References

Ainslie, K. M., S. L. Tao, K. C. Popat, H. Daniels, V. Hardev, C. A. Grimes, and T. A. Desai. 2008a. *In vitro* inflammatory response of nanostructured titania, silicon oxide, and polycaprolactone. *J. Biomed. Mater. Res. A*, 91(3):647–55.

Ainslie, K. M., S. L. Tao, K. C. Popat, and T. A. Desai. 2008b. *In vitro* immunogenicity of silicon-based micro- and nanostructured surfaces. *ACS Nano* 2 (5):1076–1084.

Banerjee, S., A. Dan, and D. Chakravorty. 2002. Synthesis of conducting nanowires. *J. Mater. Sci.* 37 (20):4261–4271.

Berry, C. C., M. J. Dalby, D. McCloy, and S. Affrossman. 2005. The fibroblast response to tubes exhibiting internal nanotopography. *Biomaterials* 26 (24):4985–4992.

Bettinger, C. J., R. Langer, and J. T. Borenstein. 2009. Engineering substrate topography at the micro- and nanoscale to control cell function. *Angew. Chem. Int. Ed. Engl.* 48 (30):5406–5415.

Bettinger, C. J., Z. Zhang, S. Gerecht, J. T. Borenstein, and R. Langer. 2008. Enhancement of *in vitro* capillary tube formation by substrate nanotopography. *Adv. Mater. Deerfield* 20 (1):99–103.

Chen, Y., L. N. Zhang, X. Y. Lu, N. Zhao, and J. Xu. 2006. Morphology and crystalline structure of poly(epsilon-caprolactone) nanofiber via porous aluminium oxide template. *Macromol. Mater. Eng.* 291 (9):1098–1103.

Correa-Duarte, M. A., N. Wagner, J. Rojas-Chapana, C. Morsczeck, M. Thie, and M. Giersig. 2004. Fabrication and biocompatibility of carbon nanotube-based 3D networks as scaffolds for cell seeding and growth. *Nano Lett* 4 (11):2233–2236.

Curtis, A. S., B. Casey, J. O. Gallagher, D. Pasqui, M. A. Wood, and C. D. Wilkinson. 2001. Substratum nanotopography and the adhesion of biological cells. Are symmetry or regularity of nanotopography important? *Biophys. Chem.* 94 (3):275–283.

Curtis, A. S., N. Gadegaard, M. J. Dalby, M. O. Riehle, C. D. Wilkinson, and G. Aitchison. 2004. Cells react to nanoscale order and symmetry in their surroundings. *IEEE Trans. Nanobiosci.* 3 (1):61–65.

Dalby, M. J., N. Gadegaard, M. O. Riehle, C. D. Wilkinson, and A. S. Curtis. 2004a. Investigating filopodia sensing using arrays of defined nano-pits down to 35 nm diameter in size. *Int. J. Biochem. Cell Biol.* 36 (10):2005–2015.

Dalby, M. J., N. Gadegaard, and C. D. Wilkinson. 2008. The response of fibroblasts to hexagonal nanotopography fabricated by electron beam lithography. *J. Biomed. Mater. Res. A* 84 (4):973–979.

Dalby, M. J., D. Giannaras, M. O. Riehle, N. Gadegaard, S. Affrossman, and A. S. Curtis. 2004b. Rapid fibroblast adhesion to 27 nm high polymer demixed nano-topography. *Biomaterials* 25 (1):77–83.

Dalby, M. J., M. O. Riehle, H. Johnstone, S. Affrossman, and A. S. Curtis. 2002. *In vitro* reaction of endothelial cells to polymer demixed nanotopography. *Biomaterials* 23 (14):2945–2954.

Fan, H. J., W. Lee, R. Hauschild, M. Alexe, G. Le Rhun, R. Scholz, A. Dadgar et al. 2006. Template-assisted large-scale ordered arrays of ZnO pillars for optical and piezoelectric applications. *Small* 2 (4):561–568.

Feng, L., S. Li, H. Li, J. Zhai, Y. Song, L. Jiang, and D. Zhou. 2002. Super-hydrophobic surface aligned polyarylonitrile nanofibers. *Angew. Chem. Int. Ed.* 41 (7):1221–1223.

Feng, L., Y. Song, J. Zhai, B. Liu, J. Xu, L. Jiang, and D. Zhu. 2003. Creation of superhydrophobic surface from an amphiphilic polymer. *Angew. Chem. Int. Ed.* 42 (7):800–802.

Fischer, R. S., M. Gardel, X. Ma, R. S. Adelstein, and C. M. Waterman. 2009. Local cortical tension by myosin II guides 3D endothelial cell branching. *Curr. Biol.* 19 (3):260–265.

Goodman, G., B. Woda, and R. Klolberg. 1980. Redistribution of contractile and cytoskeletal components induced by cytochalasin. *Eur. J. Cell Biol.* 22:733–744.

Hsu, S. H., C. M. Tang, and C. C. Lin. 2004. Biocompatibility of poly(epsilon-caprolactone)/poly(ethylene glycol) diblock copolymers with nanophase separation. *Biomaterials* 25 (25):5593–5601.

Jameela, S. R., N. Suma, and A. Jayakrishnan. 1997. Protein release from poly(e-caprolactone) microspheres prepared by melt encapsulation and solvent evaporation techniques: A comparative study. *J. Biomater. Sci. Polymer Edn.* 8 (6):457–466.

Kaiser, J. P., A. Reinmann, and A. Bruinink. 2006. The effect of topographic characteristics on cell migration velocity. *Biomaterials* 27 (30):5230–5241.

Klassen, H. J., T. F. Ng, Y. Kurimoto, I. Kirov, M. Shatos, P. Coffey, and M. J. Young. 2004. Multipotent retinal progenitors express developmental markers, differentiate into retinal neurons, and preserve light-mediated behavior. *Invest. Ophthalmol. Vis. Sci.* 45 (11):4167–4173.

Kline, T. R., M. L. Tian, J. G. Wang, A. Sen, M. W. H. Chan, and T. E. Mallouk. 2006. Template-grown metal nanowires. *Inorg. Chem.* 45 (19):7555–7565.

Kriparamanan, R., P. Aswath, A. Zhou, L. Tang, and K. T. Nguyen. 2006. Nanotopography: Cellular responses to nanostructured materials. *J. Nanosci. Nanotechnol.* 6 (7):1905–1919.

Lamba, D. A., J. Gust, and T. A. Reh. 2009. Transplantation of human embryonic stem cell-derived photoreceptors restores some visual function in Crx-deficient mice. *Cell Stem Cell* 4 (1):73–79.

Lee, J., B. S. Kang, B. Hicks, T. F. Chancellor, Jr., B. H. Chu, H. T. Wang, B. G. Keselowsky, F. Ren, and T. P. Lele. 2008. The control of cell adhesion and viability by zinc oxide nanorods. *Biomaterials* 29 (27):3743–3749.

Lee, W., R. Ji, U. Gosele, and K. Nielsch. 2006. Fast fabrication of long range ordered porous alumina membranes by hard anodization. *Nat. Mater.* 5:741–747.

Li, A. P., F. Muller, A. Birner, K. Nielsch, and U. Gosele. 1998. Hexagonal pore arrays with a 50–420 nm interpore distance formed by self-organization in anodic alumina. *J. Appl. Phys.* 84:6023–6026.

Li, H. Y., Y. C. Ke, and Y. L. Hu. 2006. Polymer nanofibers prepared by template melt extrusion. *Journal of Applied Polymer Science* 99:1018.

Lin, W. J. and C. C. Yu. 2001. Comparison of protein loaded poly(e-caprolactone) microparticles prepared by the hot-melt technique. *J. Microencapsulation* 18 (5):585–592.

Lombardi, I., A. I. Hochbaum, P. D. Yang, C. Carraro, and R. Maboudian. 2006. Synthesis of high density, size-controlled Si nanowire arrays via porous anodic alumina mask. *Chem. Mater.* 18 (4):988–991.

Lu, J., M. P. Rao, N. C. MacDonald, D. Khang, and T. J. Webster. 2008. Improved endothelial cell adhesion and proliferation on patterned titanium surfaces with rationally designed, micrometer to nanometer features. *Acta Biomater.* 4 (1):192–201.

Ma, H., Z. L. Tao, F. Gao, and J. Chen. 2004. Template synthesis of transition-metal Ru and Pd nanotubes. *Chinese J. Inorg. Chem.* 20 (10):1187–1190.

Martin, C. R. 1994. Nanomaterials: A membrane-based synthetic approach. *Science* 266 (5193):1961–1966.

Martinez, E., E. Engel, J. A. Planell, and J. Samitier. 2009. Effects of artificial micro- and nano-structured surfaces on cell behaviour. *Ann. Anat.* 191 (1):126–135.

Masuda, H. and K. Fukada. 1995. Ordered metal nanohole arrays made by a two-step replication of honeycomb structures of anodic alumina. *Science* 268:1466–1468.

Miller, D. C., A. Thapa, K. M. Haberstroh, and T. J. Webster. 2004. Endothelial and vascular smooth muscle cell function on poly(lactic-*co*-glycolic acid) with nano-structured surface features. *Biomaterials* 25 (1):53–61.

Osakada, F., H. Ikeda, M. Mandai, T. Wataya, K. Watanabe, N. Yoshimura, A. Akaike, Y. Sasai, and M. Takahashi. 2008. Toward the generation of rod and cone photoreceptors from mouse, monkey and human embryonic stem cells. *Nat. Biotechnol.* 26 (2):215–224.

Parthasarathy, R. V. and C. R. Martin. 1994. Template-synthesized polyaniline microtubules. *Chem Mater.* 6 (10):1627–1632.

Porter, J. R., A. Henson, and K. C. Popat. 2009a. Biodegradable poly(epsilon-caprolactone) nanowires for bone tissue engineering applications. *Biomaterials* 30 (5):780–788.

Porter, J. R., A. Henson, S. Ryan, and K. C. Popat. 2009b. Biocompatibility and mesenchymal stem cell response to poly(epsilon-caprolactone) nanowire surfaces for orthopedic tissue engineering. *Tissue Eng. Part A* 15 (9):2547–2559.

Qiao, J., Z. Zhang, X. Meng, S. Zhou, S. Wu, and S. Lee. 2005. Morphology-controllable preparation of 1D poly(vinyl pyrrolidone) nanostructured arrays. *Nanotechnology* 16:433–436.

Redenti, S., S. Tao, J. Yang, P. Gu, H. Klassen, S. Saigal, T. Desai, and M. J. Young. 2008. Retinal tissue engineering using mouse retinal progenitor cells and a novel biodegradable, thin-film poly(e-caprolactone) nanowire scaffolds. *J. Ocular Biol., Diseases, Inform.* 1 (1):19–29.

Riedel, M., B. Muller, and E. Wintermantel. 2001. Protein adsorption and monocyte activation on germanium nanopyramids. *Biomaterials* 22 (16):2307–2316.

Rynes, O. and S. Demoustier-Champagne. 2005. Template electrochemical growth of polypyrrole and gold-polypyrrole-gold nanowire arrays. *Journal of the Electrochemical Society* 152: D130–D135.

Steinhart, M., J. H. Wendorff, A. Grenier, R. B. Wehrspohn, K. Nielsch, J. Schilling, J. Choi, and U. Gosele. 2002. Polymer nanotubes by wetting of ordered porous templates. *Science* 296:1997.

Steinhart, M., J. H. Wendorff, and R. B. Wehrspohn. 2003. Nanotubes a la carte: Wetting of porous templates. *ChemPhysChem* 4:1171–1176.

Steinhart, M., R. B. Wehrspohn, U. Gosele, and J. H. Wendorff. 2004. Nanotubes by template wetting: A modular assembly system. *Angew. Chem. Int. Ed.* 43:1334–1344.

Takahashi, M., T. D. Palmer, J. Takahashi, and F. H. Gage. 1998. Widespread integration and survival of adult-derived neural progenitor cells in the developing optic retina. *Mol. Cell Neurosci.* 12:340–348.

Tao, S. L. and T. A. Desai. 2007. Aligned arrays of biodegradable poly(epsilon-caprolactone) nanowires and nanofibers by template synthesis. *Nano Lett* 7 (6):1463–1468.

Yim, E. K. and K. W. Leong. 2005. Significance of synthetic nanostructures in dictating cellular response. *Nanomedicine* 1 (1):10–21.

Young, M. J., J. Ray, S. J. Whiteley, H. Klassen, and F. H. Gage. 2000. Neuronal differentiation and morphological integration of hippocampal progenitor cells transplanted to the retina of immature and mature dystrophic rats. *Mol. Cell Neurosci.* 16:197–205.

4

Electrospun Nanofibers for Neural Applications

Yee-Shuan Lee
New Jersey Institute of Technology

Treena Livingston Arinzeh
New Jersey Institute of Technology

This chapter includes recent progress in the use of electrospinning processing techniques for fabricating nanofiber scaffolds for neural applications. Electrospinning is a process developed in the textile industry and has recently been used in the medical field for fabricating sheets of fibers at the nanoscale. Central and peripheral nervous system injuries may benefit from the use of scaffolds to facilitate the regrowth of nerves. This chapter reviews the challenges in neural tissue engineering and studies using electrospun scaffolds as an approach in nerve repair.

4.1 Neural Repair

The complex physiology of the nervous system presents unique challenges and increases the difficulty in finding effective treatments for the functional recovery of nerve related diseases and injuries. The human nervous system is organized into two components, the central nervous system (CNS) and the peripheral nervous system (PNS) (Tortora and Derrickson, 2009). The following section describes neural repair with respect to brain, spinal cord, and PNS injuries.

4.1.1 Brain Tissue Repair

Neurodegenerative disease and traumatic brain injury are the leading causes of brain tissue damage. Alzheimer's and Parkinson's diseases occur in at least 2.4 and 1 million people in the United States, respectively, and are the most common neurodegenerative diseases that target a specific group of neurons (Parkinson's Disease Foundation, 2008; Alzheimer's Foundation of America, 2009). Common pathological onset for neurodegenerative disease is the accumulation of insoluble filamentous aggregates which underlie early axonal dysfunction and pathology, leading to potentially irreversible neuron degeneration (Skovronsky et al., 2006; Vickers et al., 2009; Brandt, 2001). Unlike the PNS, the CNS provides very limited self-repair capability. Current therapeutic strategies focus on stabilizing symptoms and slowing the progression of the disease. Treatment intervention researches are mainly pharmacological or cellular based (Park et al., 2009). Brain damage caused by traumatic brain injury results in immediate and delayed cell death leading to a cavity formation and glial scaring (Fitch et al., 1999). Therapeutic strategy for brain repair can be described in three steps: (1) provide neuroprotection to reduce inflammation and prevent secondary cell death, (2) replace damaged neurons and provide appropriate factors, and (3) promote neurite regeneration and growth to restore original neural structure (Orive et al., 2009).

Neuroprotective and other drugs are usually delivered systemically but are limited by the blood–brain barrier (BBB) and the prolonged traveling time reduces its stability (Pardridge, 2005a, 2005b, 2007). Liposomes and polymeric nanoparticles (NPs) are the most investigated delivery vehicle for brain drug delivery (Garcia-Garcia et al., 2005). Liposomes with site-specific ligands allow better penetration through the BBB and increase the stability of the drug before reaching the target (Garcia-Garcia et al., 2005; Béduneau et al., 2007; Weinstein et al., 1978). NPs have been shown to be more stable than liposomes in the body and are easier to manipulate the drug delivery profile (Zhong and Bellamkonda, 2008). It is hypothesized that the NPs pass through the BBB by site-specific phagocytosis or passive diffusion (Lockman et al., 2002; Misra et al., 2003). Micro and nanoparticles prepared with poly (ethylene-*co*-vinylacetate) (EVAC) (During et al., 1989; Freese et al., 1989; Hoffman et al., 1990; Krewson et al., 1995; Krewson and Saltzman, 1996; Mahoney and Saltzman, 1999; Powell et al., 1990) and poly(lactic-*co*-glycolic acid) (PLGA) (Aubert-Pouessel et al., 2004; Bible et al., 2009; Kim and Martin, 2006; McRae and Dahlström, 1994; Menei et al., 2000; Schubert et al., 2006) have been previously investigated. Local administration of PLGA microspheres have been used to deliver nerve growth factor and neurotransmitters (dopamine or noradrenaline) for potential treatment for Huntington's and Parkinson's diseases, respectively (Benoit et al., 2000; McRae and Dahlström, 1994). The advantages of local delivery are reduced systemic side-effects, limiting passage through the BBB, and increasing therapeutic effects. However, local delivery is an invasive administration and the dose cannot be adjusted. NPs can be used as a cell delivery vehicle for tissue repair to enhance survival (Orive et al., 2009). PLGA particles seeded with neural stem cells (NSCs) were injected into rats with a stroke induced lesion and demonstrated good host interaction (Bible et al., 2009). Encapsulated genetically engineered cells releasing trophic factors demonstrated neuroprotection and behavioral and morphological improvement in diseases such as Parkinson's (Sajadi et al., 2006; Yasuhara et al., 2005), Huntington's (Emerich et al., 1997), Alzheimer's (Winn et al., 1994), and amyotrophic lateral sclerosis (Tan et al., 1996). Clinical trials of encapsulated genetically modified fibroblast delivering ciliary neurotrophic factors (CNTF) for Huntington's disease and amyotrophic lateral sclerosis showed sustained release of CNTF, but the survival of implanted cells and the administration method still needs improvement (Aebischer et al., 1996; Bloch et al., 2004; Orive et al., 2009; Zurn et al., 2000). In summary, encapsulated genetically engineered cells releasing protective or stimulating factors is a promising method in providing neuroprotection, morphological, and behavioral improvement in neurodegenerative diseases.

4.1.2 Spinal Cord Repair

Similar to traumatic brain injury, in spinal cord injury, the initial neurological damage provokes a series of cellular and biochemical responses leading to further damage, commonly known as the secondary injury. The secondary response will further prohibit nerve regeneration and cause further cell death. The initial cell death will create a cavity lesion at the injury site and glial scar around the lesion. Shortly after the injury, spontaneous axonal sprouting occurs. However, the unpleasant microenvironment, especially the glial scar at the site of injury, inhibits further regeneration. Current therapeutic interventions for spinal cord injury include pharmacological interventions, neutralizing inhibitory signals, and gene therapy, which all emphasize secondary injury prevention and neuroprotection (Samadikuchaksaraei, 2007). Functional reconstruction has been approached by the blockage of molecules that inhibit axon regeneration (Buchli and Schwab, 2005; Cai et al., 2001; Chen et al., 2000a; Decherchi et al., 1997; Dergham et al., 2002; Fournier et al., 2003; Gautier et al., 1998; Hadlock et al., 1999; Mukhopadhyay et al., 1994; Schwab, 2004; Yamashita and Tohyama, 2003; Yoshii et al., 2004; Zhang et al., 2005), prevention of scar formation (48), and injection of activated macrophages (Schwartz et al., 1999a, 1999b) and human stem cells (Hofstetter, 2005; Karimi-Abdolrezaee et al., 2006; McDonald and Howard, 2002; McDonald et al., 1999). Lesion site bridging with olfactory ensheathing cells (Li et al., 1997) or Schwann cells (Bunge, 2002; Bunge and Pearse, 2003; Pearse et al., 2004) in combination with neurotrophic factors (Bradbury et al., 1999) also enhances neurite regeneration.

4.1.3 Peripheral Nerve Repair

The most severe PNS injury is complete transection of the nerve fiber. After the injury, protease activity increases at the site of injury initiating a series of degradation events at the distal ends of the injury. The cytoskeleton begins to break down leading to membrane rupture. Schwann cells in the distal end will trigger demyelination of the injured axons. The Schwann cells and macrophages will clean up the axonal and myelin debris (Stoll et al., 1989) and also release cytokines that promote axonal growth (Chaudhry et al., 1992). New axonal formation is usually initiated from the unmyelinated region, the nodes of Ranvier and in humans, axon regeneration rate is about 2–5 mm per day (Jacobson and Guth, 1965). For large nerve defects, the recovery rate is prolonged.

For PNS repair of short distances, the standard method is to suture the two ends together. This method is not suitable for large defects because it would introduce undesirable tension causing cell death to the remaining nerve fiber (Millesi et al., 1966). An autologous nerve graft is commonly used to repair large nerve gaps (Lundborg, 1988; Mackinnon and Dellon, 1988), but its disadvantage is the loss of function at donor site. Alternative bridging devices approved by the FDA are Neurotube (polyglycolic acid, Synovis Micro Companies Alliance, Birmingham, AL) (Schlosshauer et al., 2006), NeuroMatrix-Neuroflex (Type-1 collagen, Coolagne Matrix Inc., Franklin Lakes, NJ) (Schlosshauer et al., 2006), Neurolac (poly-D,L-lactide-caprolactone, Polyganics BV, The Netherlands) (Schlosshauer et al., 2006), NeuraGen Nerve Guide (Type-1 collagen, Integra Neuroscience, Plainsboro, NJ) (Archibald et al., 1995; Schlosshauer et al., 2006), and SaluBridge nerve cuff (polyvinyl alcohol hydrogel, SaluMedica LLC, Atlanta, GA) (Lundborg et al., 1997; Schlosshauer et al., 2006), but the last two are only suitable for nerve defects up to several millimeters long while others are still under investigation.

Poly-glycolide (PGA) nerve guide implants for defect lengths between 2 and 65 mm in humans have better or similar outcomes as nerve coaptation or autologous transplantation (Battiston et al., 2005; Crawley and Dellon, 1992; Hagiwara et al., 2002; Inada et al., 2004, 2005; Kim and Lee Dellon, 2001; Mackinnon and Dellon, 1990; Navissano et al., 2005; Schlosshauer et al., 2006; Weber et al., 2000). Silicone and polytetrafluoroethylene (PTFE) are both bio-inert material and have been considered for nerve conduits in humans. Silicone was not as successful as PGA in patient response (Braga-Silva, 1999; Dahlin et al., 2001; Lundborg et al., 1991, 1994, 1997, 2004; Luo et al., 1997; Merle et al., 1989; Schlosshauer et al., 2006). It was suggested that the delayed complication may be due to compression of the newly myelinated axon, increasing the cross sectional area in the conduit. GoreTex (PTFE) implantation in humans support neuronal regeneration but may cause compression on pressure-sensitive axons long after implantation (Schlosshauer et al., 2006). GoreTex in large defects showed poor results (Stanec and Stanec, 1998a) and no significant recovery in smaller defects (Pitta et al., 2001; Pogrel et al., 1998; Stanec and Stanec, 1998b).

4.1.4 Tissue Engineering Approach

A tissue engineering approach is to use a scaffold, either in combination with cells and other extrinsic factors to simulate the environment at the site of the injury. This tissue-engineered construct will help repair and restore the function of the damage tissue. The scaffold, which can be fabricated with either a natural or synthetic polymer, should have properties similar to the native extracellular matrix (ECM) to promote cell proliferation and differentiation.

After spinal cord injury, unidirectional aligned structure of the axons in the spinal cord is disrupted and this structural change affects the spared neurons surviving after the injury (Zhang et al., 2005). Unlike the CNS, the PNS has some capability of self-repair postinjury but is restricted to minimal damage. Hence the bioengineering strategy for CNS repair is to create a suitable environment providing mechanical, physical, or chemical cues to promote axonal regeneration.

Biomaterial bridges shaped into a tubular structure with guidance channels of nondegradable polymers including polyethylene (Decherchi et al., 1997), polyvinylidene fluoride (PVDF) (Aebischer et al., 1987), polyvinylidene fluoride-trifluoroethylene (PVDF-TrFE) (Fine et al., 1991), and biodegradable polymers such as PLLA (Patist et al., 2004), PGA (Gautier et al., 1998), and collagen (Yoshii et al., 2004) have supported regeneration after CNS injury. In a bridging device, the cell favors the implantation site more than the surrounding environment, thus, depicting low host–implant interaction (Zhang et al., 2005). Crosslinked collagen and collagen filament conduits improved axonal regeneration and function (Yoshii et al., 2003, 2004). However, the axons were entangled at the distal host–implant interface. Acellular collagen conduit directed axon regrowth into the ventral root in rat (Liu et al., 2001) and had axon regeneration and function recovery in a transected cat (Goldsmith et al., 2005). A collagen conduit with neurotrophin-3 (NT-3) increased axonal growth in local axon growth only but inhibited brainstem motor neurons (Tsai et al., 2006) and the corticospinal tract (Houweling et al., 1998). When applied with fibroblast growth factor 1 (FGF-1), it promoted reticular and vestibular brainstem motor neuron axon regrowth (Tsai et al., 2006).

Alginate is a linear homopolymer and abundant in brown algae. It is biocompatible, has a high water absorbance and, hence widely used for cell immobilization and encapsulation. Alginate sponge promoted axonal elongation penetrating both rostral and caudal ends forming synapses with local neurons (Kataoka et al., 2001; Suzuki et al., 1999; Tian et al., 2005). The advantage of alginate is the reduction of glial scarring at conduit–host interface. Axonal growth into the sponge significantly increased in comparison to collagen (Kataoka et al., 2004). Anisotropic capillary hydrogel (ACH) made with alginate increased robust growth longitudinally.

Bioengineering strategies for PNS repair are to find alternatives to the autologous nerve graft especially for large nerve defects which will lead to functional recovery and will accelerate the recovery rate. Present research focus on creating a scaffold that provides chemical and physical guidance across the site of injury. The initial approach was to use various autologous tissue grafts for repair but it was limited by poor feasibility and isolation (Schmidt and Leach, 2003). Certain natural materials found in the ECM can influence axonal development and repair (Grimpe and Silver, 2002; Rutishauser, 1993). These materials such as collagen (Archibald et al., 1991; Ceballos et al., 1999; Dubey et al., 1999; Yoshii et al., 2002), laminin (Ahmed and Brown, 1999; Chen et al., 2000b; Kauppila et al., 1993; Toba et al., 2002; Tong et al., 1994; Whitworth et al., 1995; Yoshii and Oka, 2001), and fibronectin (Ahmed and Brown, 1999; Whitworth et al., 1995) have been fabricated into nerve conduits and grafts providing a suitable matrix for promoting neural regeneration. Synthetic biodegradable polymers like polyethylene glycol (PEG) (Borgens et al., 2002; Krause and Bittner, 1990; Lore et al., 1999), EVAC (Bloch et al., 2001; Fine et al., 2002), PLGA (Bryan et al., 2004; Hadlock et al., 1998; Molander et al., 1982), PLLA (poly-lactic acid) (Evans et al., 2000; Evans et al., 1999; Hadlock et al., 1998), poly(glycerol sabacate) (Sundback et al., 2005), and hyaluronic acid (Seckel et al., 1995) have been investigated for their potential as PNS nerve conduits. The advantage of using synthetic polymers is to be able to process them to create unique three-dimensional structures that will promote Schwann cell migration and neurite extension. Piezoelectric PVDF and PVDF-TrFE (Valentini et al., 1993) and electrically conductive pyrrole (Schmidt et al., 1997) are investigated to enhance neurite extension by electrical stimulation.

Fabricating a well-designed three-dimensional scaffold mimicking the architecture of the natural ECM is essential for tissue engineering applications. Biological and topological cues provided by various ECM components influence the regulation of cellular behavior. The spinal cord is a well-organized aligned fibrous structure. A tube with an aligned-lumen structure is desired to create a similar micro-environment for neural regeneration. This can be fabricated using various methods such as freeze-drying, selfassembly, and electrospinning. Electrospinning is a material fabrication method that has gained considerable interest for various tissue engineering applications. It is a unique processing technique allowing for greater flexibility in scaffold design.

4.2 Electrospinning

4.2.1 Introduction to Electrospinning

In the 1500s, William Gilbert observed that whenever an electrostatic force was presented above a spherical water droplet within a certain distance on a dry surface, the water droplet will become conical (Taylor, 1966). The concept was further developed by Lord Rayleigh in 1882 (Taylor, 1966) when he showed instability of liquid droplets due to in the presence of an electric field. When the electric field overcomes the surface tension, the unstable, charged liquid droplets would form a series of droplets and eject as a fine jet. Later in 1902, John Colley patented the electrospraying process and apparatus (Cooley, 1902). In his apparatus, a fluid charged with a high voltage was dispensed into a chamber filled with fluid. The charged fluid would become fibers and were collected in the secondary fluid chamber. In 1914, John Zelany published his attempt on a mathematical model describing the electrical discharge of fluid in the electrospraying process (Zeleny, 1914). The electrospinning apparatus and process was first patented by Anton Formhals in 1934 and he was able to spin cellulose acetate fibers (Formhals, 1934). He later patented other apparatuses to improve the fiber collection and quality in 1939 and 1940 (Formhals, 1939, 1940). Sir Geoffrey Taylor in 1969 observed that when a polymer solution was subjected to a high voltage, the injected charge will introduce an opposite force to the surface tension of the liquid. When the applied electric field increased, the polymer at the surface would elongate and form a conical shape known as the Taylor cone (Taylor, 1966). In 1993, Doshi and Reneker attempted to describe the influence of various electrospinning parameters in PEO fiber morphology (Doshi and Reneker, 1995). His parameters are the guidelines for optimizing the electrospinning conditions for a polymer of interest that are still used today.

A typical setup for electrospinning is shown in Figure 4.1. The setup consists of a high voltage power source, syringe pump, syringe, needle, and grounded collection device. A general procedure can be described for fabricating electrospun scaffolds. The polymer solution is loaded into the syringe attached with a needle. A high voltage is applied to the polymer solution and is eluted at the desired rate (controlled by the syringe pump). When a high voltage is injected into the polymer solution, the electrostatic force overcomes the surface tension of the polymer solution at the tip of the needle, and eventually a Taylor cone is formed and then further elongated into the fluid jet. The charged fluid jet is collected on the grounded device due to the electric potential difference between the polymer solution at the tip of the syringe and the grounded collecting device. The whipping motion of the polymer jet that takes place between the needle and the plate allows for the solvent to evaporate hence collecting dried polymer fiber meshes on the collection plate.

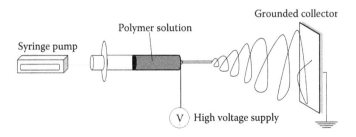

FIGURE 4.1 A typical electrospinning setup.

Fiber morphology and size can be altered by controlling the various electrospinning parameters such as, polymer solution concentration, the distance between the collection plate and needle, the needle size and tip, voltage field applied, and the flow rate of the polymer solution. Each variable is not entirely independent of one another hence, optimizing the parameter settings is essential in achieving the desired fiber size and morphology. The polymer solution concentration influences the fiber size significantly. The change in concentration will influence the viscosity of the solution therefore ultimately affecting the surface tension of the solution in the needle. A lower polymer concentration usually results in beading in the fibers. In some cases, fiber jets fail to form resulting in spraying. A concentration of polymer solution that is too high will be unable to electrospin because of high surface tension inhibiting polymer jet formation resulting in dripping of the polymer solution at the tip of the needle. The correct combination of polymer–solvent system is also important. An organic solvent is often used due to its dielectric constant allowing charging of the solution. External factors such as temperature and humidity can also affect fiber morphology significantly. Solvent evaporation during the whipping process is essential for good fiber morphology. Both the temperature and humidity can influence the rate of evaporation.

Two pairs of parameters highly influence the electrospinning procedure. First pair is the needle size and the polymer solution concentration. Their choice is dependent upon the desired fiber size. For smaller fibers, smaller needles are often used with lower concentrations of polymer solution. For larger fibers, larger needles are used with higher concentrations of polymer solution. The second pair is the voltage field applied and the distance between the needle and the collector. They influence the whipping process that is directly associated with the solvent evaporation. Poor solvent evaporation leads to wet fiber collection and fibers may fuse together after solvent evaporation, postspinning. A higher voltage applied results in an increased potential difference leading to faster whipping process. Usually, a higher potential difference requires a larger distance between the needle and the collector and vice versa to increase the whipping distance. Adjustment of whipping distance related to voltage applied results in optimal fibers. This pair of parameters is often dependent upon the polymer–solvent system used for the electrospinning process and can be manipulated for fiber size optimization. Optimized parameters allow for a quick method to fabricate nano- to micron-sized fibrous meshes.

Scanning electron microscopy (SEM) images of random and aligned electrospun fibrous meshes are shown in Figures 4.2a and b, respectively. Random nonwoven fibrous meshes are the most common product of electrospinning. It is achieved by collecting the fibers on a grounded metal plate. Aligned fibrous mesh can be achieved by varying the collection method. The most common method is collecting on a high-speed rotating drum or disk (Teo and Ramakrishna, 2006) (Figure 4.3). This allows the fiber collection along the direction of rotation. Small diameter tubes can also be fabricated by this method and is useful in vascular studies (Wen and Tresco, 2006). A high rotation speed has better fiber

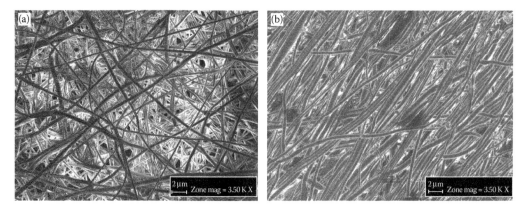

FIGURE 4.2 Scanning electron microscopy images of electrospun (a) random and (b) aligned fibrous meshes.

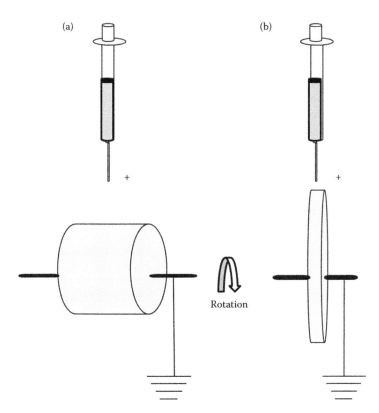

FIGURE 4.3   Popular collection methods for aligned fibrous scaffolds: (a) rotating drum and (b) rotating disk.

alignment compared to lower rotation speed but may cause fiber discontinuity (Teo and Ramakrishna, 2006; Wang et al., 2009). Other collection methods are, between two blades, rings, or needles, using auxiliary electrode for guiding the fibers (Teo and Ramakrishna, 2006). Continuous improvement of aligned fibrous scaffold fabrication is essential in achieving a high degree of alignment and thickness of the fibrous mats.

The electrospun nanofiber scaffold architecture is similar to the naturally occurring protein fibrils in the ECM (Li et al., 2002; Ma et al., 2005). Each individual nanoscale fiber has high surface to volume and aspect ratio allowing more surface contact between the cell and each fiber. Increase in porosity also allows greater cellular and media penetration. Electrospun scaffolds should resemble the ECM environment biologically and physically to achieve a successful tissue engineering application. The physical and biological properties of the scaffold are dependent on the material used for electrospinning and material properties such as hydrophilicity, mechanical properties, biodegradability, and level of cellular interaction are important. The properties of the scaffolds can be manipulated by copolymerization or polymer blending of various biodegradable or nonbiodegradable and synthetic or natural materials. The advantage of using a synthetic polymer is its low batch-to-batch variation with better manipulation, prediction, and reproducible mechanical and physical properties. Electrospinning allows the fabrication of a variety of polymers. It also allows easy manipulation of scaffold architectural features such as fiber diameter, morphology, and porosity which is important in neural applications where submicron filament size has been shown to have the highest dorsal root ganglion (DRG) neuronal outgrowth when compared to larger size filaments (Wen and Tresco, 2006). Postspinning modification can also enhance biological or physical properties. For example, hot-stretched electrospun polyacrylonitrile (PAN) nanofibers enhance the crystallinity and fiber alignment improving the mechanical modulus and tensile strength (Hou et al., 2008). Electrospun synthetic fibrous scaffolds are often treated with ECM components to further promote cell adhesion, proliferation, differentiation, and axonal regeneration (Koh et al., 2008).

4.2.2 Electrospun Scaffolds for Neural Applications

Nerve regeneration across the glial scar and lesion site has been achieved by using various bridging device in both CNS and PNS. Increasingly, unidirectional aligned topography has been incorporated into the bridging device to provide contact guidance enhancing axonal regeneration across the lesion area. A successful tissue engineering strategy for neural repair is to create aligned fibrous scaffolds to provide a cellular level of guidance for cell migration and directional axonal regeneration across the lesion site. Common aligned fibrous scaffold fabrication methods are listed in Table 4.1. Two main factors influence neural contact guidance: degree of alignment and aligned fiber density. The increase in aligned fiber density has been shown to correlate to higher neurite density where the average neurite length was not affected (Wang et al., 2009). However, crossed fiber orientation diverted the DRG neurite

TABLE 4.1 Summary of Collection Devices and Parameters Used to Fabricate Electrospun, Aligned Scaffolds

Collecting device	Rotation Speed	Distance	Voltage	Polymer	Ref.
1. Disk:					
with coverslip	1000 rpm	—	—	PCL and PCL/gelatin	(Ghasemi-Mobarakeh et al., 2008)
with coverslip	1000 rpm	10 cm	12 kV	PLLA	(Yang et al., 2005)
2. Wheel:					
	30, 110, 250 rpm	7 cm	6–9 kV	PLLA	(Corey et al., 2007)
with PLGA coated coverslip	285 rpm	5 cm	10 kV	PLLA	(Corey et al., 2008)
3. Drum:					
	1000 rpm	20 cm	12 kV	PHB and PHBV	(Suwantong et al., 2007)
	2200 rpm	5–6 cm	8 kV	PCLEEP with GDNF	(Chew et al., 2007)
	6.4 m/s	15 cm	15 kV	PLGA	(Lee et al., 2009)
	—	—	15 kV	PAN-MA	(Kim et al., 2008)
with PLGA-coated coverslip	4.9 and 10.0 m/s	15 cm	15 kV	PLGA	(Lee, Bashur, Gomez et al., 2009)
4. Undefined target:					
with laminin-coated coverslip	4.2 m/s	6.5 cm	10 kV	PLGA	(Kim et al., 2006)
with PCL film	200 rpm	5 cm	7 kV	PCL	(Chew et al., 2008)
5. Bar:	120 rpm	10–20 cm	20–30 kV	chitosan	(Ahmed et al., 2006)
6. Dual collector:					
	4 cm apart	20 cm	20 kV	PCL, PCL/collagen	(Schnell et al., 2007)
with PEG coverslip	4 cm apart	20 cm	20 kV	PCL, PCL/collagen	(Gerardo-Nava et al., 2009)
7. Rectangular drum	~10 rpm for random, 5000 rpm for aligned	20 cm		polydioxanone	(Chow et al., 2007)
8. Mandrel with four perpendicular symmetrically arranged rods	100 and 1000 rpm	—	15 kV	PCL	(Yao et al., 2009)
9. Stainless-steel frame (open void of 2 cm × 5 cm)	—	—	12 kV	PCL	(Xie et al., 2009b, 2009c)

extension away from the axis of alignment and in some case restricted extension. Selecting a suitable material for electrospinning with the appropriate physical and biological properties can reduce inflammatory response and provide support and guidance for neural regeneration (Cao et al., 2009). Various synthetic and natural polymers have been investigated for fabricating scaffolds for neural applications. The following is a summary of *in vitro* and *in vivo* studies of electrospun scaffolds for neural application (Table 4.1).

4.3 *In Vitro* Applications

4.3.1 Synthetic Polymer and Blends

PLLA, PGA, and poly (ε-caprolactone) (PCL) are the most commonly used synthetic, biodegradable, and biocompatible polymers in neural applications (see Table 4.2). Yang et al. first published electrospun aligned PLLA scaffolds for neural application in 2005. Since then, there has been a gradual increase in research interest in developing an electrospun-based conduit for neural repair. The majority of these studies have focused on evaluating neural proliferation, differentiation, and neurite extension of various cell types on aligned fibrous scaffolds fabricated with different materials and fiber sizes.

Mouse embryonic stem cell preferred differentiation into oligodendrocytes on 3D electrospun PCL scaffolds compared to 2D laminin-coated surface suggesting the importance of scaffold matrix (Xie et al., 2009c). No neuron was observed and the astrocytes had longer processes on the PCL scaffold. Aligned and random PCL fiber also induced mice embryonic stem cells to differentiate into neurons, astrocytes, and oligodendrocytes (Xie et al., 2009c). In other studies, aligned PLLA nanofibrous scaffold also supported the growth and extension of DRGs (Corey et al., 2007, 2008) and primary motor neurons (Corey et al., 2008). Varying degrees of PLLA fiber alignment influenced DRG neurite extension and Schwann cell morphology (Corey et al., 2007). Growth cones in axons are directed by surface molecules and influence axon growth significantly. Aligned polydioxanone mesh promoted directional and growth dynamics of rat DRGs cocultured with glial cells (Chow et al., 2007). Random and aligned electrospun PCL scaffold induced upregulation of myelin-associated glycoprotein (MAG), an early myelination marker and downregulation of NCAM-1 (immature Schwann cell marker) as predicted (Chew et al., 2008). However, upregulation of P0, myelin-specific gene was only observed on the aligned PCL scaffolds suggesting promotion of Schwann cell maturation (Chew et al., 2008). PC12 cells showed maximum alignment to the microaligned PLGA mesh and largest neurite outgrowth was observed when a pressure of 0.50 and 0.25 Pa, respectively, were applied (Kim et al., 2006). This finding suggested combined fiber morphology with low fluid stress is a promising method for neurite outgrowth stimulation.

It is believed that fiber diameter influences cell adhesion, proliferation, migration, and differentiation. Yang et al. demonstrated electrospun nano-sized fibers (300 nm) of PLLA enhanced neural differentiation of neonatal mouse cerebellum C17.2 stem cells (C17.2 cells) as compared to the microsized (1.25 μm) fibers. Both cell types elongated and oriented neurites along the direction of the aligned fibers. Cells on nano-aligned fibers had the longest neurite extension (Yang et al., 2005). Rat NSCs were shown to differentiate into oligodendrocytes and neurons on 283 and 749 nm electrospun polyethersulfone fibrous scaffolds, respectively (Christopherson et al., 2009). Small-sized fibers promoted cell adhesion and migration whereas larger fibers had lower cell attachment and migration. PC12 neurite extension on aligned PCL fibers with diameters of 3.7 ± 0.5 and 5.9 ± 0.9 μm were significantly longer than on nonaligned fibers with diameter of $4.4 + 0.5$ μm and neurites extended along the fibers only when the fiber diameter was 0.8–0.9 μm (Yao et al., 2009). In the same study, a novel spinning technique was used to fabricate an 8 cm-conduit with 1.4 mm inner diameter, with an outer layer of random and an inner layer of aligned PCL fiber for mouse sciatic nerve model. Total neurite elongation length of rat embryonic hippocampal neuron was similar on smaller and larger poly-D-lysine coated PLGA fibers (Lee et al., 2009). However, neurite polarization was greater on smaller fibers and aligned fibers suggesting the degree of fiber alignment to be the key factor in axon formation and elongation (Lee et al., 2009).

TABLE 4.2 Summary of Recent *In Vitro* Studies of Electrospun Scaffolds for Neural Applications

Material	Solvent	Fiber		Cell Type	App.	Ref.
		Alignment	Diameter			
Poly (L-lactic acid) (PLLA)						
	70:30 DCM/DMF	R + A	300 nm(R/A) 1.5 μm(R/A)	C17.2	—	(Yang et al., 2005)
	1:1 THF/DCM	R[a]	0.51 μm	Mouse embryonic cortical neuron	—	(Nisbet et al., 2007)
	Chloroform	A[b]	524 ± 305 nm	rat DRG, SC	PNS	(Corey et al., 2007)
	Chloroform	A[c]	—	rat DRG, primary motor neuron	—	(Corey et al., 2008)
	Chloroform	A	1.2–1.6 μm	chick DRG	—	(Wang et al., 2009)
Laminin coated	HFIP	R	100–500 nm	PC12	PNS	(Koh et al., 2008)
PPy coated	DCM + 2 × 10[-3] M CTAB	R + A	200 ± 34 nm	chick DRG	—	(Xie et al., 2009b)
Poly(ε-caprolactone) (PCL)						
	HFIP	R + A	431 ± 118 nm	C17.2	—	(Ghasemi-Mobarakeh et al., 2008)
	75/25 chloroform/methanol	A	559 ± 300 nm	chick DRG, SC, OEC, fibroblast	PNS	(Schnell et al., 2007)
	75:25 chloroform/methanol	R	630 ± 40 nm	RT4-D6P2T	PNS	(Prabhakaran et al., 2008)
	75:25 chloroform/methanol	R + A	564 + 208.8 nm	hNP-Acs, U373, SH-SY5Y	CNS	(Gerardo-Nava et al., 2009)
	8:2 DCM:methanol	R + A	1.03 + 0.03 μm (A) 2.26 + 0.08 μm (R)	SC	PNS	(Chew et al., 2008)
	8:2 DCM:DMF	R + A[d]	~250 nm	chick DRG	—	(Xie et al., 2009a)
	8:2 DCM:DMF	R + A	~250 nm	Mouse embryonic stem cells	—	(Xie et al., 2009c)
Aminolysed by ethylenediamine	1:1 Chloroform/methanol	R	750 ± 100 nm	rat brain derived NSCs	CNS	(Nisbet et al., 2008)
Collagen coated	Chloroform	R + A	4.4 + 0.5 μm (R) 0.8 + 0.7 μm (A) 3.7 + 0.5 μm (A) 5.9 + 0.9 μm (A) 8.8 + 0.9 μm (A)	PC12	PNS	(Yao et al., 2009)
PCL + PPy coat	DCM + 2 × 10[-3] M CTAB (R), DCM:DMF (A)	R + A	220 + 36 nm	chick DRG	—	(Xie et al., 2009a)
75:25 PCL/chitosan	HFIP/75:25 TFA/DCM	R	190 ± 26 nm	RT4-D6P2T	PNS	(Prabhakaran et al., 2008)
75:25 PCL/collagen	HFIP	A	541 ± 164 nm	chick DRG, SC, OEC, fibroblast	PNS	(Schnell et al., 2007)

Material	Solvent	Alignment	Fiber diameter	Cell type	Application	Reference
75:25 PCL/collagen	HFIP	R + A	601.4 + 151.2 nm	hNP-Acs, U373, SH-SY5Y	CNS	(Gerardo-Nava et al., 2009)
70:30 PCL/gelatin	HFIP	R + A	189 ± 56 nm	C17.2	—	(Ghasemi-Mobarakeh et al., 2008)
Poly(lactic-*co*-glycolic acid) (PLGA)						
—	1:1 THF/DCM	R[a]	0.76 μm	Mouse embryonic cortical neuron	—	(Nisbet et al., 2007)
50:50	1:1 DMF/THF	A	3–5 μm (A)	PC12	—	(Kim et al., 2006)
75:25, PPy coated	HFIP	R + A	0.36 + 0.13 μm (R) 0.25 + 0.11 μm (A)	PC12 and hippocampal neurons	—	(Lee et al., 2009)
75:25, PLL coated	HFIP	A[b]	2.22 + 0.55 μm 1.51 + 0.56 μm 0.44 + 0.18 μm	Embryonic hippocampal neurons	—	(Lee et al., 2009)
Other materials						
PAN-MAs	DMF at 60°C	R + A	400–600 nm	rat DRG	PNS	(Kim et al., 2008)
Polydioxanone	HFIP	R + A	2–3 μm	DRG, Astrocyte-DRG	CNS	(Chow et al., 2007)
Polyamide ($C_{28}O_4N_4H_{47}$)$_n$ and ($C_{27}O_{4,4}N_4H_{50}$)$_n$	—	R	Average 180 nm	E15 cerebellar granule neurons, cortical, hippocampal, ventral spinal cord, and DRG	—	(Ahmed et al., 2006)
PHB and PHBV	Chloroform	A	3.7 μm, 2.3 μm	L929 and RT-D6P2T	—	(Suwantong et al., 2007)
PMMAAA, immobilized with collagen	Acetone	R	450 ± 88 nm	rat embryonic cortical neuron	—	(Li et al., 2008)
PES coat with laminin	DMSO	R	283 ± 45 nm 749 ± 153 nm 1452 ± 312 nm	Rat hippocampus-derived adult NSCs	—	(Christopherson et al., 2009)
15:85 Doped PANI: 70:30 PCL:gelatin	HFIP	R	112 ± 8 nm	Nerve stem cells	—	(Ghasemi-Mobarakeh et al., 2009)

[a] Hydrolyzed with KOH.
[b] Varying degree of alignment.
[c] Aligned or with PLGA glue.
[d] Varying degree of alignment + stacking, with or without laminin coating.

R—random; A—aligned; R + A—both; DCM—dichloromethane; DMF—dimethylformamide; C17.2—neural stem cell line; THF—tetrahydrofuran; SC—Schwann cells; DRG—dorsal root ganglia cells; HFIP–1,1,1,3,3,3-hexafluoro-2-propanol; PC12–rat adrenal pheochromocytoma cells; CTAB–ionic surfactant cetyltrimethyl-ammonium bromide; OEC–olfactory ensheathing cells; RT4-D6P2T–rat Schwann cells; PAN-MA–poly(acrylonitrile-*co*-methylacrylate); PHB–Poly(3-hydroxybutyrate); PHBV–Poly(3-hydroxybutyrate-*co*-3-hydroxyvalerate); PMMAAA–methyl methacrylate and acrylic acid; L929–mouse connective tissue, fibroblast-like cells; RT4-D6P2T–mouse Schwann cell; PANI–polyaniline.

Many synthetic polymers are hydrophobic which results in poor cell adhesion and proliferation. The scaffolds are often treated by chemical processes or ECM components are incorporated to improve hydrophilicity to improve cell attachment and neurite extension. Nisbet et al. hydrolyzed electrospun PLLA and PLGA creating scaffolds with varying surface tension. Scaffolds with lower surface tension induced cortical neuron–neurite extension and the scaffolds had a large interfiber distance allowing guidance for neurite extension (Nisbet et al., 2007). Collagen type-I was immobilized on electrospun poly-methyl methacrylate (PMMA) and acrylic acid (AA) (PMMAAA) nano-fibrous scaffolds. The amount of carboxyl contents of the materials influenced the collagen immobilization directly (Li et al., 2008). Cell viability and neurite extension of the cortical neurons were found to be dependent on the amount of carboxyl content (Li et al., 2008). Electrospun PCL treated with ethylenediamine (ED) increased the hydrophilicity, thus, affecting cell attachment but did not affect the differentiation of rat brain-derived NSCs (Nisbet et al., 2008). Laminin is a cell adhesion molecule that promotes neurite outgrowth through multiple adhesion sites (Powell and Kleinman, 1997). Incorporating laminin by physical absorption, covalent coupling, or blending with polymer solution into PLLA nanofibers showed similar PC12 neurite extension (Koh et al., 2008). Hence, all three are efficient functionalization techniques to incorporate ECM or other component to enhance the properties of the scaffolds.

It has been demonstrated that electrical stimulation through a polypyrrole (PPy) film improved PC12 neurite extension significantly (Schmidt et al., 1997). Electrospun aligned and random PLGA meshes were coated with PPy to provide electric stimulation to promote and guide neurite extension. Electrically stimulated PC12 cells had significantly longer neurites than cells on unstimulated scaffolds (Lee et al., 2009). Similarly, stimulated PC12 cells also had longer neurites on the stimulated aligned versus random PPy-PLGA scaffolds. Neither electric stimulation nor the fiber alignment influenced the neurite elongation and the number of neurite-bearing cells of hippocampal neurons. Electrospun PCL and PLLA nanofibers were coated with PPy by *in situ* polymerization to create a core-sheath fiber morphology (Xie et al., 2009b). The electrically stimulated random and aligned scaffold further enhanced the maximum neurite length by 83% and 47%, respectively. Another electrically conductive polymer, polyaniline (PANI), has been gaining recent interest in tissue engineering applications (Bidez et al., 2006; Guimard et al., 2007; Li et al., 2006). Electrospinning a polymer blend of PANI with PCL/gelatin enhanced nerve stem cell proliferation and neurite outgrowth, when electrically stimulated (Ghasemi-Mobarakeh et al., 2009). Overall, the studies suggest that electrical stimuli in electrospun fiber may enhance neurite extension.

4.3.2 Blend of Synthetic and Natural Materials

The use of synthetic polymers blended with natural materials in order to enhance cellular attachment and neurite extension has gained interest. PCL/chitosan blended electrospun scaffold have been shown to promote Schwann cell attachment and proliferation. Blending also improved the mechanical properties as compared to chitosan electrospun scaffolds (Prabhakaran et al., 2008). Aligned nanofibrous PCL/gelatin and PCL/collagen scaffolds promoted C17.2 (Ghasemi-Mobarakeh et al., 2008) and U373 (Gerardo-Nava et al., 2009) cell proliferation and differentiation, respectively. U373 cells and human neural progenitor-astrocyte committed cells had similar astrocyte processes alignment and extension on PCL and PCL/collagen aligned nanofibers but the former demonstrated stronger proliferation and collagen improved adhesion and migration significantly over the latter (Gerardo-Nava et al., 2009). Human neuroblastoma cell line (SH-SY5Y) had poor cellular attachment to both PCL and PCL/collagen fibers but had long axonal growth up to 600 µm (Gerardo-Nava et al., 2009). Schwann cell migration and process formation was also enhanced on collagen/PCL aligned scaffolds (Schnell et al., 2007). Incorporating ECM components such as collagen with electrospun PCL scaffolds improved process length of fibroblast and OECs (Schnell et al., 2007). DRGs however favored pure PCL scaffolds over collagen/PCL blends.

4.4 *In Vivo* Studies

The *in vivo* studies examining the use of electrospun scaffolds have been investigated for brain and PNS applications. Bilayered chitosan tube with an outer layer of chitosan film and inner layer aligned chitosan fibers promoted nerve regeneration in rat sciatic nerve (Ahmed et al., 2006). Aligned electrospun PCL and ethyl-ethylene phosphate (PCLEEP) with human glial cell-derived neurotrophic factor (GDNF) showed maximal electrophysiological recovery in rat sciatic nerve as compared with longitudinally or circumferentially oriented aligned PCLEEP (Chew et al., 2007). Polysulfone nerve conduit (Koch Membrane Systems) with either (1) saline filled conduit, (2) aligned, or (3) random PAN-MA fibrous mats were used as a rat tibial nerve bridge (Kim et al., 2008). The aligned construct improved functional outcome significantly in a 17 mm nerve defect as compared to the random construct implicating the important role of topography in neural regeneration. Aligned and random electrospun PCL scaffolds were implanted into the caudate putamen of the adult rat brain (Nisbet et al., 2009). The fiber alignment influenced the neurite infiltration by a minimal inflammatory response.

4.5 Summary

Nerve regeneration and repair is a complex and challenging problem. A better understanding of the molecular biology of neural development, pathology, and repair will aid in finding new potential targets for novel therapeutic intervention. This review of *in vitro* and *in vivo* studies of electrospun fibrous scaffolds has demonstrated its feasibility to promote neural cell differentiation and neurite extension. Electrospinning is an economical method for mass production of fibrous scaffolds that mimic the ECM architecture and provide physical cues for cell behavior manipulation. Incorporating the scaffolds with ECM components, growth factors, and cells will further enhance its potential to promote neurite extension and outgrowth. The tailored nanofibrous scaffolds hold great promise for neural tissue engineering.

References

Aebischer, P., M. Schluep, N. Déglon, J. M. Joseph, L. Hirt, B. Heyd, M. Goddard, et al. 1996. Intrathecal delivery of CNTF using encapsulated genetically modified xenogeneic cells in amyotrophic lateral sclerosis patients. *Nature Medicine* 2 (6):696–699.

Aebischer, P., R. F. Valentini, P. Dario, C. Domenici, and P. M. Galletti. 1987. Piezoelectric guidance channels enhance regeneration in the mouse sciatic nerve after axotomy. *Brain Research* 436 (1):165–168.

Ahmed, I., H. Y. Liu, P. C. Mamiya, A. S. Ponery, A. N. Babu, T. Weik, M. Schindler, and S. Meiners. 2006. Three-dimensional nanofibrillar surfaces covalently modified with tenascin-C-derived peptides enhance neuronal growth *in vitro*. *Journal of Biomedical Materials Research–Part A* 76 (4):851–860.

Ahmed, Z. and R. A. Brown. 1999. Adhesion, alignment, and migration of cultured Schwann cells on ultrathin fibronectin fibres. *Cell Motility and the Cytoskeleton* 42 (4):331–343.

Alzheimer's Foundation of America. 2009. Statistics about Alzheimer's Disease. Retrieved from http://www.alzfdn.org/AboutAlzheimers/statistics.html, June 2009.

Archibald, S. J., C. Krarup, J. Shefner, S. T. Li, and R. D. Madison. 1991. A collagen-based nerve guide conduit for peripheral nerve repair: An electrophysiological study of nerve regeneration in rodents and nonhuman primates. *Journal of Comparative Neurology* 306 (4):685–696.

Archibald, S. J., J. Shefner, C. Krarup, and R. D. Madison. 1995. Monkey median nerve repaired by nerve graft or collagen nerve guide tube. *Journal of Neuroscience* 15 (5 II):4109–4123.

Aubert-Pouessel, A., M. C. Venier-Julienne, A. Clavreul, M. Sergent, C. Jollivet, C. N. Montero-Menei, E. Garcion, D. C. Bibby, P. Menei, and J. P. Benoit. 2004. *In vitro* study of GDNF release from biodegradable PLGA microspheres. *Journal of Controlled Release* 95 (3):463–475.

Battiston, B., S. Geuna, M. Ferrero, and P. Tos. 2005. Nerve repair by means of tubulization: Literature review and personal clinical experience comparing biological and synthetic conduits for sensory nerve repair. *Microsurgery* 25 (4):258–267.

Béduneau, A., P. Saulnier, and J. P. Benoit. 2007. Active targeting of brain tumors using nanocarriers. *Biomaterials* 28 (33):4947–4967.

Benoit, J. P., N. Faisant, M. C. Venier-Julienne, and P. Menei. 2000. Development of microspheres for neurological disorders: from basics to clinical applications. *Journal of Controlled Release* 65 (1–2):285–296.

Bible, E., D. Y. Chau, M. R. Alexander, J. Price, K. M. Shakesheff, and M. Modo. 2009. The support of neural stem cells transplanted into stroke-induced brain cavities by PLGA particles. *Biomaterials* 30 (16):2985–2994.

Bidez, P. R., S. Li, A. G. Macdiarmid, E. C. Venancio, Y. Wei, and P. I. Lelkes. 2006. Polyaniline, an electroactive polymer, supports adhesion and proliferation of cardiac myoblasts. *Journal of Biomaterials Science, Polymer Edition* 17 (1):199–212.

Bloch, J., A. C. Bachoud-Lévi, N. Déglon, J. P. Lefaucheur, L. Winkel, S. Palfi, J. P. Nguyen, et al. 2004. Neuroprotective gene therapy for Huntington's disease, using polymer-encapsulated cells engineered to secrete human ciliary neurotrophic factor: Results of a phase I study. *Human Gene Therapy* 15 (10):968–975.

Bloch, J., E. G. Fine, N. Bouche, A. D. Zurn, and P. Aebischer. 2001. Nerve growth factor- and neurotrophin-3-releasing guidance channels promote regeneration of the transected rat dorsal root. *Experimental Neurology* 172 (2):425–432.

Borgens, R. B., R. Shi, and D. Bohnert. 2002. Behavioral recovery from spinal cord injury following delayed application of polyethylene glycol. *Journal of Experimental Biology* 205 (1):1–12.

Bradbury, E. J., S. Khemani, V. R. King, J. V. Priestley, and S. B. McMahon. 1999. NT-3 promotes growth of lesioned adult rat sensory axons ascending in the dorsal columns of the spinal cord. *European Journal of Neuroscience* 11 (11):3873–3883.

Braga-Silva, J. 1999. The use of silicone tubing in the late repair of the median and ulnar nerves in the forearm. *Journal of Hand Surgery* 24 B (6):703–706.

Brandt, R. 2001. Cytoskeletal mechanisms of neuronal degeneration. *Cell Tissue Research* 305 (2):255–265.

Bryan, D. J., J. B. Tang, S. A. Doherty, D. D. Hile, D. J. Trantolo, D. L. Wise, and I. C. Summerhayes. 2004. Enhanced peripheral nerve regeneration through a poled bioresorbable poly(lactic-*co*-glycolic acid) guidance channel. *Journal of Neural Engineering* 1 (2):91–98.

Buchli, A. D. and M. E. Schwab. 2005. Inhibition of Nogo: A key strategy to increase regeneration, plasticity and functional recovery of the lesioned central nervous system. *Annals of Medicine* 37 (8):556–567.

Bunge, M. B. 2002. Bridging the transected or contused adult rat spinal cord with Schwann cell and olfactory ensheathing glia transplants. *Progress in Brain Research* 137:275–282.

Bunge, M. B. and D. D. Pearse. 2003. Transplantation strategies to promote repair of the injured spinal cord. *Journal of Rehabilitation Research and Development* 40 (4 Suppl 1):55–62.

Cai, D., J. Qiu, Z. Cao, M. McAtee, B. S. Bregman, and M. T. Filbin. 2001. Neuronal cyclic AMP controls the developmental loss in ability of axons to regenerate. *Journal of Neuroscience* 21 (13):4731–4739.

Cao, H., T. Liu, and S. Y. Chew. 2009. The application of nanofibrous scaffolds in neural tissue engineering. *Advanced Drug Delivery Reviews* 61:1155–1164.

Ceballos, D., X. Navarro, N. Dubey, G. Wendelschafer-Crabb, W. R. Kennedy, and R. T. Tranquillo. 1999. Magnetically aligned collagen gel filling a collagen nerve guide improves peripheral nerve regeneration. *Experimental Neurology* 158 (2):290–300.

Chaudhry, V., J. D. Glass, and J. W. Griffin. 1992. Wallerian degeneration in peripheral nerve disease. *Neurologic Clinics* 10 (3):613–627.

Chen, M. S., A. B. Huber, M. E. D. Van Der Haar, M. Frank, L. Schnell, A. A. Spillmann, F. Christ, and M. E. Schwab. 2000a. Nogo-A is a myelin-associated neurite outgrowth inhibitor and an antigen for monoclonal antibody IN-1. *Nature* 403 (6768):434–439.

Chen, Y. S., C. L. Hsieh, C. C. Tsai, T. H. Chen, W. C. Cheng, C. L. Hu, and C. H. Yao. 2000b. Peripheral nerve regeneration using silicone rubber chambers filled with collagen, laminin and fibronectin. *Biomaterials* 21 (15):1541–1547.

Chew, S. Y., R. Mi, A. Hoke, and K. W. Leong. 2007. Aligned protein–polymer composite fibers enhance nerve regeneration: A potential tissue-engineering platform. *Advanced Functional Materials* 17 (8):1288–1296.

Chew, S. Y., R. Mi, A. Hoke, and K. W. Leong. 2008. The effect of the alignment of electrospun fibrous scaffolds on Schwann cell maturation. *Biomaterials* 29 (6):653–661.

Chow, W. N., D. G. Simpson, J. W. Bigbee, and R. J. Colello. 2007. Evaluating neuronal and glial growth on electrospun polarized matrices: Bridging the gap in percussive spinal cord injuries. *Neuron Glia Biol* 3 (2):119–126.

Christopherson, G. T., H. Song, and H. Q. Mao. 2009. The influence of fiber diameter of electrospun substrates on neural stem cell differentiation and proliferation. *Biomaterials* 30 (4):556–564.

Cooley, J. F. 1902. Apparatus for electrically dispersing fluids, US Patent No. 692, 631.

Corey, J. M., C. C. Gertz, B. S. Wang, L. K. Birrell, S. L. Johnson, D. C. Martin, and E. L. Feldman. 2008. The design of electrospun PLLA nanofiber scaffolds compatible with serum-free growth of primary motor and sensory neurons. *Acta Biomater* 4 (4):863–875.

Corey, J. M., D. Y. Lin, K. B. Mycek, Q. Chen, S. Samuel, E. L. Feldman, and D. C. Martin. 2007. Aligned electrospun nanofibers specify the direction of dorsal root ganglia neurite growth. *Journal of Biomedical Materials Research–Part A* 83 (3):636–645.

Crawley, W. A. and A. L. Dellon. 1992. Inferior alveolar nerve reconstruction with a polyglycolic acid bioabsorbable nerve conduit. *Plastic and Reconstructive Surgery* 90 (2):300–302.

Dahlin, L. B., L. Anagnostaki, and G. Lundborg. 2001. Tissue response to silicone tubes used to repair human median and ulnar nerves. *Scandinavian Journal of Plastic and Reconstructive Surgery and Hand Surgery* 35 (1):29–34.

Decherchi, P., N. Lammari-Barreault, P. Cochard, M. Carin, P. Réga, J. Pio, J. F. Péllissier, P. Ladaique, G. Novakovitch, and P. Gauthier. 1997. CNS axonal regeneration within peripheral nerve grafts cryopreserved by vitrification: Cytological and functional aspects. *Cryobiology* 34 (3):214–239.

Dergham, P., B. Ellezam, C. Essagian, H. Avedissian, W. D. Lubell, and L. McKerracher. 2002. Rho signaling pathway targeted to promote spinal cord repair. *Journal of Neuroscience* 22 (15):6570–6577.

Doshi, J. and D. H. Reneker. 1995. Electrospinning process and applications of electrospun fibers. *Journal of Electrostatics* 35 (2–3):151–160.

Dubey, N., P. C. Letourneau, and R. T. Tranquillo. 1999. Guided neurite elongation and Schwann cell invasion into magnetically aligned collagen in simulated peripheral nerve regeneration. *Experimental Neurology* 158 (2):338–350.

During, M. J., A. Freese, B. A. Sabel, W. M. Saltzman, A. Deutch, R. H. Roth, and R. Langer. 1989. Controlled release of dopamine from a polymeric brain implant: *In vivo* characterization. *Annals of Neurology* 25 (4):351–356.

Emerich, D. F., S. R. Winn, P. M. Hantraye, M. Peschanski, E. Y. Chen, Y. Chu, P. McDermott, E. E. Baetge, and J. H. Kordower. 1997. Protective effect of encapsulated cells producing neurotrophic factor CNTF in a monkey model of Huntington's disease. *Nature* 386 (6623):395–399.

Evans, G. R. D., K. Brandt, A. D. Niederbichler, P. Chauvin, S. Hermann, M. Bogle, L. Otta, B. Wang, and C. W. Patrick Jr. 2000. Clinical long-term *in vivo* evaluation of poly(L-lactic acid) porous conduits for peripheral nerve regeneration. *Journal of Biomaterials Science, Polymer Edition* 11 (8):869–878.

Evans, G. R. D., K. Brandt, M. S. Widmer, L. Lu, R. K. Meszlenyi, P. K. Gupta, A. G. Mikos, et al. 1999. *In vivo* evaluation of poly(L-lactic acid) porous conduits for peripheral nerve regeneration. *Biomaterials* 20 (12):1109–1115.

Fine, E. G., I. Decosterd, M. Papaloïzos, A. D. Zurn, and P. Aebischer. 2002. GDNF and NGF released by synthetic guidance channels support sciatic nerve regeneration across a long gap. *European Journal of Neuroscience* 15 (4):589–601.

Fine, E. G., R. F. Valentini, R. Bellamkonda, and P. Aebischer. 1991. Improved nerve regeneration through piezoelectric vinylidenefluoride-trifluoroethylene copolymer guidance channels. *Biomaterials* 12 (8):775–780.

Fitch, M. T., C. Doller, C. K. Combs, G. E. Landreth, and J. Silver. 1999. Cellular and molecular mechanisms of glial scarring and progressive cavitation: *In vivo* and *in vitro* analysis of inflammation-induced secondary injury after CNS trauma. *Journal of Neuroscience* 19 (19):8182–8198.

Formhals, A. 1934. Process and apparatus for preparing artificial threads, US Patent No. 1,975,504.

Formhals, A. 1939. Method and apparatus for spinning, US Patent No. 2,160,962.

Formhals, A. 1940. Artificial thread and method of producing same, US Patent No. 2,187,306.

Fournier, A. E., B. T. Takizawa, and S. M. Strittmatter. 2003. Rho kinase inhibition enhances axonal regeneration in the injured CNS. *Journal of Neuroscience* 23 (4):1416–1423.

Freese, A., B. A. Sabel, W. M. Saltzman, M. J. During, and R. Langer. 1989. Controlled release of dopamine from a polymeric brain implant: *In vitro* characterization. *Experimental Neurology* 103 (3):234–238.

Garcia-Garcia, E., K. Andrieux, S. Gil, and P. Couvreur. 2005. Colloidal carriers and blood–brain barrier (BBB) translocation: A way to deliver drugs to the brain? *International Journal of Pharmacology* 298 (2):274–292.

Gautier, S. E., M. Oudega, M. Fragoso, P. Chapon, G. W. Plant, M. B. Bunge, and J. M. Parel. 1998. Poly(alpha-hydroxyacids) for application in the spinal cord: Resorbability and biocompatibility with adult rat Schwann cells and spinal cord. *Journal of Biomedical Materials Research* 42 (4):642–654.

Gerardo-Nava, J., T. Führmann, K. Klinkhammer, N. Seiler, J. Mey, D. Klee, M. Möller, P. D. Dalton, and G. A. Brook. 2009. Human neural cell interactions with orientated electrospun nanofibers *in vitro*. *Nanomedicine (London, England)* 4 (1):11–30.

Ghasemi-Mobarakeh, L., M. P. Prabhakaran, M. Morshed, M. H. Nasr-Esfahani, and S. Ramakrishna. 2008. Electrospun poly(epsilon-caprolactone)/gelatin nanofibrous scaffolds for nerve tissue engineering. *Biomaterials* 29 (34):4532–4539.

Ghasemi-Mobarakeh, L., M. P. Prabhakaran, M. Morshed, M. H. Nasr-Esfahani, and S. Ramakrishna. 2009. Electrical stimulation of nerve cells using conductive nanofibrous scaffolds for nerve tissue engineering. *Tissue Engineering Part A* 15 (11):3605–3619.

Goldsmith, H. S., A. Fonseca Jr, and J. Porter. 2005. Spinal cord separation: MRI evidence of healing after omentum-collagen reconstruction. *Neurological Research* 27 (2):115–123.

Grimpe, B. and J. Silver. 2002. The extracellular matrix in axon regeneration. *Progress in Brain Research* 137:333–349.

Guimard, N. K., N. Gomez, and C. E. Schmidt. 2007. Conducting polymers in biomedical engineering. *Progress in Polymer Science (Oxford)* 32 (8–9):876–921.

Hadlock, T., J. Elisseeff, R. Langer, J. Vacanti, and M. Cheney. 1998. A tissue-engineered conduit for peripheral nerve repair. *Archives of Otolaryngology–Head and Neck Surgery* 124 (10):1081–1086.

Hadlock, T., C. Sundback, R. Koka, D. Hunter, M. Cheney, and J. Vacanti. 1999. A novel, biodegradable polymer conduit delivers neurotrophins and promotes nerve regeneration. *Laryngoscope* 109 (9):1412–1416.

Hagiwara, A., S. Nakashima, T. Itoh, C. Sakakura, E. Otsuji, H. Yamagishi, S. Okajima, et al. 2002. Clinical application of PGA-tube for regeneration of intrapelvic nerves during extended surgery for intrapelvic recurrent rectal cancer. *Japanese Journal of Cancer and Chemotherapy* 29 (12):2202–2204.

Hoffman, D., L. Wahlberg, and P. Aebischer. 1990. NGF released from a polymer matrix prevents loss of ChAT expression in basal forebrain neurons following a fimbria-fornix lesion. *Experimental Neurology* 110 (1):39–44.

Hofstetter Cp, H. N. 2005. Allodynia limits the usefulness of intraspinal neural stem cell grafts; directed differentiation improves outcome. *Nature Neuroscience* 8 (3):346–353.

Hou, X. X., X. P. Yang, F. Zhang, S. Z. Wu, and E. Waclawik. 2008. Stretching-induced orientation to improve mechanical properties of electrospun pan nanocomposites. *International Journal of Modern Physics B* 22 (31–32):5913–5918.

Houweling, D. A., A. J. Lankhorst, W. H. Gispen, P. R. Bär, and E. A. J. Joosten. 1998. Collagen containing neurotrophin-3 (NT-3) attracts regrowing injured corticospinal axons in the adult rat spinal cord and promotes partial functional recovery. *Experimental Neurology* 153 (1):49–59.

Inada, Y., S. Morimoto, K. Moroi, K. Endo, and T. Nakamura. 2005. Surgical relief of causalgia with an artificial nerve guide tube: Successful surgical treatment of causalgia (Complex Regional Pain Syndrome Type II) by *in situ* tissue engineering with a polyglycolic acid-collagen tube. *Pain* 117 (3):251–258.

Inada, Y., S. Morimoto, Y. Takakura, and T. Nakamura. 2004. Regeneration of peripheral nerve gaps with a polyglycolic acid-collagen tube. *Neurosurgery* 55 (3):640–646.

Jacobson, S. and L. Guth. 1965. An electrophysiological study of the early stages of peripheral nerve regeneration. *Experimental Neurology* 11 (1):48–60.

Karimi-Abdolrezaee, S., E. Eftekharpour, J. Wang, C. M. Morshead, and M. G. Fehlings. 2006. Delayed transplantation of adult neural precursor cells promotes remyelination and functional neurological recovery after spinal cord injury. *Journal of Neuroscience* 26 (13):3377–3389.

Kataoka, K., Y. Suzuki, M. Kitada, T. Hashimoto, H. Chou, H. Bai, M. Ohta, S. Wu, K. Suzuki, and C. Ide. 2004. Alginate enhances elongation of early regenerating axons in spinal cord of young rats. *Tissue Engineering* 10 (3–4):493–504.

Kataoka, K., Y. Suzuki, M. Kitada, K. Ohnishi, K. Suzuki, M. Tanihara, C. Ide, K. Endo, and Y. Nishimura. 2001. Alginate, a bioresorbable material derived from brown seaweed, enhances elongation of amputated axons of spinal cord in infant rats. *Journal of Biomedical Materials Research* 54 (3):373–384.

Kauppila, T., E. Jyvasjarvi, T. Huopaniemi, E. Hujanen, and P. Liesi. 1993. A laminin graft replaces neurorrhaphy in the restorative surgery of the rat sciatic nerve. *Experimental Neurology* 123 (2):181–191.

Kim, D. H. and D. C. Martin. 2006. Sustained release of dexamethasone from hydrophilic matrices using PLGA nanoparticles for neural drug delivery. *Biomaterials* 27 (15):3031–3037.

Kim, I. A., S. A. Park, Y. J. Kim, S. H. Kim, H. J. Shin, Y. J. Lee, S. G. Kang, and J. W. Shin. 2006. Effects of mechanical stimuli and microfiber-based substrate on neurite outgrowth and guidance. *Journal of Bioscience and Bioengineering* 101 (2):120–126.

Kim, J. and A. Lee Dellon. 2001. Reconstruction of a painful post-traumatic medial plantar neuroma with a bioabsorbable nerve conduit: A case report. *Journal of Foot and Ankle Surgery* 40 (5):318–323.

Kim, Y. T., V. K. Haftel, S. Kumar, and R. V. Bellamkonda. 2008. The role of aligned polymer fiber-based constructs in the bridging of long peripheral nerve gaps. *Biomaterials* 29 (21):3117–3127.

Koh, H. S., T. Yong, C. K. Chan, and S. Ramakrishna. 2008. Enhancement of neurite outgrowth using nano-structured scaffolds coupled with laminin. *Biomaterials* 29 (26):3574–3582.

Krause, T. L. and G. D. Bittner. 1990. Rapid morphological fusion of severed myelinated axons by polyethylene glycol. *Proceedings of the National Academy of Sciences USA* 87 (4):1471–1475.

Krewson, C. E., M. L. Klarman, and W. M. Saltzman. 1995. Distribution of nerve growth factor following direct delivery to brain interstitium. *Brain Research* 680 (1–2):196–206.

Krewson, C. E. and W. M. Saltzman. 1996. Transport and elimination of recombinant human NGF during long-term delivery to the brain. *Brain Research* 727 (1–2):169–181.

Lee, J. Y., C. A. Bashur, A. S. Goldstein, and C. E. Schmidt. 2009. Polypyrrole-coated electrospun PLGA nanofibers for neural tissue applications. *Biomaterials* 30 (26):4325–4335.

Lee, J. Y., C. A. Bashur, N. Gomez, A. S. Goldstein, and C. E. Schmidt. 2009. Enhanced polarization of embryonic hippocampal neurons on micron scale electrospun fibers. *Journal of Biomedical Materials Research Part A* 92 (4):1398–1406.

Li, M., Y. Guo, Y. Wei, A. G. MacDiarmid, and P. I. Lelkes. 2006. Electrospinning polyaniline-contained gelatin nanofibers for tissue engineering applications. *Biomaterials* 27 (13):2705–2715.

Li, W., Y. Guo, H. Wang, D. Shi, C. Liang, Z. Ye, F. Qing, and J. Gong. 2008. Electrospun nanofibers immobilized with collagen for neural stem cells culture. *Journal of Materials Science: Materials in Medicine* 19 (2):847–854.

Li, W. J., C. T. Laurencin, E. J. Caterson, R. S. Tuan, and F. K. Ko. 2002. Electrospun nanofibrous structure: A novel scaffold for tissue engineering. *Journal of Biomedical Materials Research* 60 (4):613–621.

Li, Y., P. M. Field, and G. Raisman. 1997. Repair of adult rat corticospinal tract by transplants of olfactory ensheathing cells. *Science* 277 (5334):2000–2002.

Liu, S., G. Said, and M. Tadie. 2001. Regrowth of the rostral spinal axons into the caudal ventral roots through a collagen tube implanted into hemisected adult rat spinal cord. *Neurosurgery* 49 (1):143–151.

Lockman, P. R., R. J. Mumper, M. A. Khan, and D. D. Allen. 2002. Nanoparticle technology for drug delivery across the blood–brain barrier. *Drug Development and Industrial Pharmacology* 28 (1):1–13.

Lore, A. B., J. A. Hubbell, D. S. Bobb Jr, M. L. Ballinger, K. L. Loftin, J. W. Smith, M. E. Smyers, H. D. Garcia, and G. D. Bittner. 1999. Rapid induction of functional and morphological continuity between severed ends of mammalian or earthworm myelinated axons. *Journal of Neuroscience* 19 (7):2442–2454.

Lundborg, G. 1988. Nerve injury and repair. *Nerve Injury and Repair*, Churchill Livingstone, New York.

Lundborg, G., L. B. Dahlin, and N. Danielsen. 1991. Ulnar nerve repair by the silicone chamber technique. Case report. *Scandinavian Journal of Plastic and Reconstructive Surgery and Hand Surgery* 25 (1):79–82.

Lundborg, G., L. Dahlin, D. Dohi, M. Kanje, and N. Terada. 1997. A new type of 'bioartificial' nerve graft for bridging extended defects in nerves. *Journal of Hand Surgery* 22 B (3):299–303.

Lundborg, G., B. Rosén, L. Dahlin, J. Holmberg, and I. Rosén. 2004. Tubular repair of the median or ulnar nerve in the human forearm: A 5-year follow-up. *Journal of Hand Surgery* 29 B (2):100–107.

Lundborg, G., B. Rosen, S. O. Abrahamson, L. Dahlin, and N. Danielsen. 1994. Tubular repair of the median nerve in the human forearm: Preliminary findings. *Journal of Hand Surgery* 19 B (3):273–276.

Lundborg, G., B. Rosen, L. Dahlin, N. Danielsen, and J. Holmberg. 1997. Tubular versus conventional repair of median and ulnar nerves in the human forearm: Early results from a prospective, randomized, clinical study. *Journal of Hand Surgery* 22 (1):99–106.

Luo, Y., T. Wang, and H. Fang. 1997. Clinical application of implantation of vascular bundle into silicone tube to bridge the peripheral nerve defect. *Zhongguo xiu fu chong jian wai ke za zhi=Zhongguo xiufu chongjian waike zazhi=Chinese Journal of Reparative and Reconstructive Surgery* 11 (6):340–342.

Ma, Z., M. Kotaki, R. Inai, and S. Ramakrishna. 2005. Potential of nanofiber matrix as tissue-engineering scaffolds. *Tissue Engineering* 11 (1–2):101–109.

Mackinnon, S. E. and A. L. Dellon. 1988. *Surgery of the Peripheral Nerve*. New York: Thieme Med Pub.

Mackinnon, S. E. and A. L. Dellon. 1990. Clinical nerve reconstruction with a bioabsorbable polyglycolic acid tube. *Plastic and Reconstructive Surgery* 85 (3):419–424.

Mahoney, M. J. and W. M. Saltzman. 1999. Millimeter-scale positioning of a nerve-growth-factor source and biological activity in the brain. *Proceedings of the National Academy of Sciences of the United States of America* 96 (8):4536–4539.

McDonald, J. W. and M. J. Howard. 2002. Repairing the damaged spinal cord: A summary of our early success with embryonic stem cell transplantation and remyelination. *Progress in Brain Research* 137:299–309.

McDonald, J. W., X. Z. Liu, Y. Qu, S. Liu, S. K. Mickey, D. Turetsky, D. I. Gottlieb, and D. W. Choi. 1999. Transplanted embryonic stem cells survive, differentiate and promote recovery in injured rat spinal cord. *Nature Medicine* 5 (12):1410–1412.

McRae, A. and A. Dahlström. 1994. Transmitter-loaded polymeric microspheres induce regrowth of dopaminergic nerve terminals in striata of rats with 6-OH-DA induced parkinsonism. *Neurochemistry International* 25 (1):27–33.

Menei, P., J. M. Pean, V. Nerriere-Daguin, C. Jollivet, P. Brachet, and J. P. Benoit. 2000. Intracerebral implantation of NGF-releasing biodegradable microspheres protects striatum against excitotoxic damage. *Experimental Neurology* 161 (1):259–272.

Merle, M., A. L. Dellon, J. N. Campbell, and P. S. Chang. 1989. Complications from silicon-polymer intubulation of nerves. *Microsurgery* 10 (2):130–133.

Millesi, H., J. Gangberger, and A. Berger. 1966. Erfahrungen mit der Mikrochirurgie peripherer. *Chirurgia Plastica* 3:47–55.

Misra, A., S. Ganesh, A. Shahiwala, and S. P. Shah. 2003. Drug delivery to the central nervous system: A review. *Journal of Pharmacy and Pharmaceutical Sciences* 6 (2):252–273.

Molander, H., Y. Olsson, and O. Engkvist. 1982. Regeneration of peripheral nerve through a polyglactin tube. *Muscle and Nerve* 5 (1):54–57.

Mukhopadhyay, G., P. Doherty, F. S. Walsh, P. R. Crocker, and M. T. Filbin. 1994. A novel role for myelin-associated glycoprotein as an inhibitor of axonal regeneration. *Neuron* 13 (3):757–767.

Navissano, M., F. Malan, R. Carnino, and B. Battiston. 2005. Neurotube® for facial nerve repair. *Microsurgery* 25 (4):268–271.

Nisbet, D. R., S. Pattanawong, N. E. Ritchie, W. Shen, D. I. Finkelstein, M. K. Horne, and J. S. Forsythe. 2007. Interaction of embryonic cortical neurons on nanofibrous scaffolds for neural tissue engineering. *Journal of Neural Engineering* 4 (2):35–41.

Nisbet, D. R., A. E. Rodda, M. K. Horne, J. S. Forsythe, and D. I. Finkelstein. 2009. Neurite infiltration and cellular response to electrospun polycaprolactone scaffolds implanted into the brain. *Biomaterials* 30 (27):4573–4580.

Nisbet, D. R., L. M. Y. Yu, T. Zahir, J. S. Forsythe, and M. S. Shoichet. 2008. Characterization of neural stem cells on electrospun poly(Îμ-caprolactone) submicron scaffolds: Evaluating their potential in neural tissue engineering. *Journal of Biomaterials Science, Polymer Edition* 19 (5):623–634.

Orive, G., E. Anitua, J. L. Pedraz, and D. F. Emerich. 2009. Biomaterials for promoting brain protection, repair and regeneration. *Nature Reviews Neuroscience* 10 (9):682–692.

Pardridge, W. M. 2005a. Molecular biology of the blood–brain barrier. *Molecular Biotechnology* 30 (1):57–69.

Pardridge, W. M. 2005b. The blood–brain barrier: Bottleneck in brain drug development. *NeuroRx* 2 (1):3–14.

Pardridge, W. M. 2007. Drug targeting to the brain. *Pharmaceutical Research* 24 (9):1733–1744.

Park, D. H., D. J. Eve, C. V. Borlongan, S. K. Klasko, L. E. Cruz, and P. R. Sanberg. 2009. From the basics to application of cell therapy, a steppingstone to the conquest of neurodegeneration: A meeting report. *Journal of Experimental and International Clinical Research* 15 (2):RA23–RA31.

Parkinson's Disease Foundation. 2008. Fact Sheet about Parkinson's Disease, Retrieved from http://www. pdf.org/en/parkinson_statistics, June 2009.

Patist, C. M., M. B. Mulder, S. E. Gautier, V. Maquet, R. Jérome, and M. Oudega. 2004. Freeze-dried poly(D,L-lactic acid) macroporous guidance scaffolds impregnated with brain-derived neurotrophic factor in the transected adult rat thoracic spinal cord. *Biomaterials* 25 (9):1569–1582.

Pearse, D. D., F. C. Pereira, A. E. Marcillo, M. L. Bates, Y. A. Berrocal, M. T. Filbin, and M. B. Bunge. 2004. cAMP and Schwann cells promote axonal growth and functional recovery after spinal cord injury. *Nature Medicine* 10 (6):610–616.

Pitta, M. C., L. M. Wolford, P. Mehra, and J. Hopkin. 2001. Use of Gore-Tex tubing as a conduit for inferior alveolar and lingual nerve repair: Experience with 6 cases. *Journal of Oral and Maxillofacial Surgery* 59 (5):493–496.

Pogrel, M. A., A. R. McDonald, and L. B. Kaban. 1998. Gore-Tex tubing as a conduit for repair of lingual and inferior alveolar nerve continuity defects: A preliminary report. *Journal of Oral and Maxillofacial Surgery* 56 (3):319–322.

Powell, E. M., M. R. Sobarzo, and W. M. Saltzman. 1990. Controlled release of nerve growth factor from a polymeric implant. *Brain Research* 515 (1–2):309–311.

Powell, S. K. and H. K. Kleinman. 1997. Neuronal laminins and their cellular receptors. *International Journal of Biochemistry and Cell Biology* 29 (3):401–414.

Prabhakaran, M. P., J. R. Venugopal, T. T. Chyan, L. B. Hai, C. K. Chan, A. Y. Lim, and S. Ramakrishna. 2008. Electrospun biocomposite nanofibrous scaffolds for neural tissue engineering. *Tissue Engineering Part A* 14 (11):1787–1797.

Rutishauser, U. 1993. Adhesion molecules of the nervous system. *Current Opinion in Neurobiology* 3 (5):709–715.

Sajadi, A., J. C. Bensadoun, B. L. Schneider, C. Lo Bianco, and P. Aebischer. 2006. Transient striatal delivery of GDNF via encapsulated cells leads to sustained behavioral improvement in a bilateral model of Parkinson disease. *Neurobiology of Disease* 22 (1):119–129.

Samadikuchaksaraei, A. 2007. An overview of tissue engineering approaches for management of spinal cord injuries. *Journal of Neuroengineering and Rehabilitation* 4:15.

Schlosshauer, B., L. Dreesmann, H. E. Schaller, and N. Sinis. 2006. Synthetic nerve guide implants in humans: A comprehensive survey. *Neurosurgery* 59 (4):740–747; discussion 747–748.

Schmidt, C. E. and J. B. Leach. 2003. Neural tissue engineering: Strategies for repair and regeneration. *Annual Review of Biomedical Engineering* 5:293–347.

Schmidt, C. E., V. R. Shastri, J. P. Vacanti, and R. Langer. 1997. Stimulation of neurite outgrowth using an electrically conducting polymer. *Proceedings of the National Academy of Sciences USA* 94 (17):8948–8953.

Schnell, E., K. Klinkhammer, S. Balzer, G. Brook, D. Klee, P. Dalton, and J. Mey. 2007. Guidance of glial cell migration and axonal growth on electrospun nanofibers of poly-epsilon-caprolactone and a collagen/poly-epsilon-caprolactone blend. *Biomaterials* 28 (19):3012–3025.

Schubert, D., R. Dargusch, J. Raitano, and S. W. Chan. 2006. Cerium and yttrium oxide nanoparticles are neuroprotective. *Biochemical and Biophysics Research Communication* 342 (1):86–91.

Schwab, M. E. 2004. Nogo and axon regeneration. *Current Opinion in Neurobiology* 14 (1):118–124.

Schwartz, M., O. Lazarov-Spiegler, O. Rapalino, I. Agranov, G. Velan, and M. Hadani. 1999a. Potential repair of rat spinal cord injuries using stimulated homologous macrophages. *Neurosurgery* 44 (5):1041–1046.

Schwartz, M., G. Moalem, R. Leibowitz-Amit, and I. R. Cohen. 1999b. Innate and adaptive immune responses can be beneficial for CNS repair. *Trends in Neurosciences* 22 (7):295–299.

Seckel, B. R., D. Jones, K. J. Hekimian, K. K. Wang, D. P. Chakalis, and P. D. Costas. 1995. Hyaluronic acid through a new injectable nerve guide delivery system enhances peripheral nerve regeneration in the rat. *Journal of Neuroscience Research* 40 (3):318–324.

Skovronsky, D. M., V. M. Lee, and J. Q. Trojanowski. 2006. Neurodegenerative diseases: New concepts of pathogenesis and their therapeutic implications. *Annual Review of Pathology* 1:151–170.

Stanec, S. and Z. Stanec. 1998a. Reconstruction of upper-extremity peripheral-nerve injuries with ePTFE conduits. *Journal of Reconstructive Microsurgery* 14 (4):227–232.

Stanec, S. and Z. Stanec. 1998b. Ulnar nerve reconstruction with an expanded polytetrafluoroethylene conduit. *British Journal of Plastic Surgery* 51 (8):637–639.

Stoll, G., J. W. Griffin, C. Y. Li, and B. D. Trapp. 1989. Wallerian degeneration in the peripheral nervous system: Participation of both Schwann cells and macrophages in myelin degradation. *Journal of Neurocytology* 18 (5):671–683.

Sundback, C. A., J. Y. Shyu, Y. Wang, W. C. Faquin, R. S. Langer, J. P. Vacanti, and T. A. Hadlock. 2005. Biocompatibility analysis of poly(glycerol sebacate) as a nerve guide material. *Biomaterials* 26 (27):5454–5464.

Suwantong, O., S. Waleetorncheepsawat, N. Sanchavanakit, P. Pavasant, P. Cheepsunthorn, T. Bunaprasert, and P. Supaphol. 2007. *In vitro* biocompatibility of electrospun poly(3-hydroxybutyrate) and poly(3-hydroxybutyrate-*co*-3-hydroxyvalerate) fiber mats. *International Journal of Biological Macromolecules* 40 (3):217–223.

Suzuki, K., Y. Suzuki, K. Ohnishi, K. Endo, M. Tanihara, and Y. Nishimura. 1999. Regeneration of transected spinal cord in young adult rats using freeze- dried alginate gel. *NeuroReport* 10 (14):2891–2894.

Tan, S. A., N. Déglon, A. D. Zurn, E. E. Baetge, B. Bamber, A. C. Kato, and P. Aebischer. 1996. Rescue of motoneurons from axotomy-induced cell death by polymer encapsulated cells genetically engineered to release CNTF. *Cell Transplantation* 5 (5):577–587.

Taylor, G. 1966. The force exerted by an electric field on a long cylindrical conductor. *Proceedings of the Royal Society of London. Series A, Mathematical and Physical Sciences* 291 (1425):145–158.

Teo, W. E. and S. Ramakrishna. 2006. A review on electrospinning design and nanofibre assemblies. *Nanotechnology* 17 (14):R89–R106.

Tian, W. M., S. P. Hou, J. Ma, C. L. Zhang, Q. Y. Xu, I. S. Lee, H. D. Li, M. Spector, and F. Z. Cui. 2005. Hyaluronic acid-poly-D-lysine-based three-dimensional hydrogel for traumatic brain injury. *Tissue Engineering* 11 (3–4):513–525.

Toba, T., T. Nakamura, A. K. Lynn, K. Matsumoto, S. Fukuda, M. Yoshitani, Y. Hori, and Y. Shimizu. 2002. Evaluation of peripheral nerve regeneration across an 80-mm gap using a polyglycolic acid (PGA)-collagen nerve conduit filled with laminin-soaked collagen sponge in dogs. *International Journal of Artificial Organs* 25 (3):230–237.

Tong, X., K. I. Hirai, H. Shimada, Y. Mizutani, T. Izumi, N. Toda, and P. Yu. 1994. Sciatic nerve regeneration navigated by laminin-fibronectin double coated biodegradable collagen grafts in rats. *Brain Research* 663 (1):155–162.

Tortora, G. J. and B. Derrickson. 2009. *Principles of Anatomy and Physiology*. 12th edn. Hoboken, NJ: John Wiley & Sons, Inc.

Tsai, E. C., P. D. Dalton, M. S. Shoichet, and C. H. Tator. 2006. Matrix inclusion within synthetic hydrogel guidance channels improves specific supraspinal and local axonal regeneration after complete spinal cord transection. *Biomaterials* 27 (3):519–533.

Valentini, R. F., T. G. Vargo, J. A. Gardella Jr, and P. Aebischer. 1993. Patterned neuronal attachment and outgrowth on surface modified, electrically charged fluoropolymer substrates. *Journal of Biomaterials Science. Polymer Edition* 5 (1–2):13–36.

Vickers, J. C., A. E. King, A. Woodhouse, M. T. Kirkcaldie, J. A. Staal, G. H. McCormack, C. A. Blizzard et al. 2009. Axonopathy and cytoskeletal disruption in degenerative diseases of the central nervous system. *Brain Research Bulletin* 80 (4–5):217–223.

Wang, H. B., M. E. Mullins, J. M. Cregg, A. Hurtado, M. Oudega, M. T. Trombley, and R. J. Gilbert. 2009. Creation of highly aligned electrospun poly-L-lactic acid fibers for nerve regeneration applications. *Journal of Neural Engineering* 6 (1):016001.

Weber, R. A., W. C. Breidenbach, R. E. Brown, M. E. Jabaley, and D. P. Mass. 2000. A randomized prospective study of polyglycolic acid conduits for digital nerve reconstruction in humans. *Plastic and Reconstructive Surgery* 106 (5):1036–1045.

Weinstein, J. N., R. Blumenthal, S. O. Sharrow, and P. A. Henkart. 1978. Antibody-mediated targeting of liposomes. Binding to lymphocytes does not ensure incorporation of vesicle contents into the cells. *Biochimica et Biophysica Acta* 509 (2):272–288.

Wen, X. and P. A. Tresco. 2006. Effect of filament diameter and extracellular matrix molecule precoating on neurite outgrowth and Schwann cell behavior on multifilament entubulation bridging device *in vitro. Journal of Biomedical Material Research A* 76 (3):626–637.

Whitworth, I. H., R. A. Brown, C. Dore, C. J. Green, and G. Terenghi. 1995. Orientated mats of fibronectin as a conduit material for use in peripheral nerve repair. *Journal of Hand Surgery* 20 B (4):429–436.

Winn, S. R., J. P. Hammang, D. F. Emerich, A. Lee, R. D. Palmiter, and E. E. Baetge. 1994. Polymer-encapsulated cells genetically modified to secrete human nerve growth factor promote the survival of axotomized septal cholinergic neurons. *Proceedings of the National Academy of Sciences of the United States of America* 91 (6):2324–2328.

Xie, J., M. R. MacEwan, X. Li, S. E. Sakiyama-Elbert, and Y. Xia. 2009a. Neurite outgrowth on nanofiber scaffolds with different orders, structures, and surface properties. *ACS Nano* 3 (5):1151–1159.

Xie, J., M. R. MacEwcm, S. M. Willerth, X. Li, D. W. Moran, S. E. Sakiyama-Elbert, and Y. Xia. 2009b. Conductive core-sheath nanofibers and their potential application in neural tissue engineering. *Advanced Functional Materials* 19 (14):2312–2318.

Xie, J., S. M. Willerth, X. Li, M. R. Macewan, A. Rader, S. E. Sakiyama-Elbert, and Y. Xia. 2009c. The differentiation of embryonic stem cells seeded on electrospun nanofibers into neural lineages. *Biomaterials* 30 (3):354–362.

Yamashita, T. and M. Tohyama. 2003. The p75 receptor acts as a displacement factor that releases Rho from Rho-GDI. *Nature Neuroscience* 6 (5):461–467.

Yang, F., R. Murugan, S. Wang, and S. Ramakrishna. 2005. Electrospinning of nano/micro scale poly(L-lactic acid) aligned fibers and their potential in neural tissue engineering. *Biomaterials* 26 (15):2603–2610.

Yao, L., N. O'Brien, A. Windebank, and A. Pandit. 2009. Orienting neurite growth in electrospun fibrous neural conduits. *Journal of Materials Research Part B: Applied Biomaterials* 90 (2):483–491.

Yasuhara, T., T. Shingo, K. Muraoka, K. Kobayashi, A. Takeuchi, A. Yano, Y. Wenji, et al. 2005. Early transplantation of an encapsulated glial cell line-derived neurotrophic factor-producing cell demonstrating strong neuroprotective effects in a rat model of Parkinson disease. *Journal of Neurosurgery* 102 (1):80–89.

Yoshii, S. and M. Oka. 2001. Peripheral nerve regeneration along collagen filaments. *Brain Research* 888 (1):158–162.

Yoshii, S., M. Oka, M. Shima, M. Akagi, and A. Taniguchi. 2003. Bridging a spinal cord defect using collagen filament. *Spine* 28 (20):2346–2351.

Yoshii, S., M. Oka, M. Shima, A. Taniguchi, and M. Akagi. 2002. 30 mm regeneration of rat sciatic nerve along collagen filaments. *Brain Research* 949 (1–2):202–208.

Yoshii, S., M. Oka, M. Shima, A. Taniguchi, Y. Taki, and M. Akagi. 2004. Restoration of function after spinal cord transection using a collagen bridge. *Journal of Biomedical Materials Research–Part A* 70 (4):569–575.

Zeleny, J. 1914. The electrical discharge from liquid points, and a hydrostatic method of measuring the electric intensity at their surfaces. *Physical Review* 3 (2):69.

Zhang, N., H. Yan, and X. Wen. 2005. Tissue-engineering approaches for axonal guidance. *Brain Research and Brain Research Review* 49 (1):48–64.

Zhong, Y. and R. V. Bellamkonda. 2008. Biomaterials for the central nervous system. *Journal of the Royal Society Interface* 5 (26):957–975.

Zurn, A. D., H. Henry, M. Schluep, V. Aubert, L. Winkel, B. Eilers, C. Bachmann, and P. Aebischer. 2000. Evaluation of an intrathecal immune response in amyotrophic lateral sclerosis patients implanted with encapsulated genetically engineered xenogeneic cells. *Cell Transplantation* 9 (4):471–484.

5

Mixed Monolayer System of Mercaptobenzoic Acid and Polyethylene Glycol for pH Sensing: Surface-Enhanced Raman Scattering Studies

Sandra Whaley
Bishnoi
Illinois Institute of
Technology

Robust pH sensors were created by using the pH-dependent surface enhanced Raman scattering (SERS) of mercaptobenzoic acid (MBA) isomers on gold–silica nanoshell (NS) films. All isomers are bound to the NS through the thiol moiety producing nanoscale pH sensors. Using the ratio between the Raman signals from carboxylic acid (COOH, 1712 cm^{-1}) and the carboxylate (COO$^-$, 1416 cm^{-1}) groups, the pK_a's of 2-, 3-, and 4-MBA on NS were found to be between 7.2 and 7.4. In addition, the out-of-plane stretching mode (1568 cm^{-1}) of 3-MBA was found to have a linear response to the local pH and could be used to monitor pH between 5 and 11. To investigate multifunctional sensing, a mixed monolayer system comprised of cysteine-polyethylene glycol (PEG)-fluorescein (Cys-PEG-Fl) and 4-MBA was created and characterized with Raman and fluorescence spectroscopies.

5.1 Introduction

Raman scattering has become an accepted and practical method of chemical sensing since the creation of inexpensive and portable laser sources (Mulvaney and Keating, 2000). Since SERS was discovered more than 20 years ago, the sensitivity and flexibility of SERS as a tool for biological sensing and detection methods has been demonstrated with new detection methods for deoxyribonucleic acid (DNA), ribonucleic acid (RNA) (Cao et al., 2002) and prostate-specific antigen (Grubisha et al., 2003), as well as glucose-sensors (Yonzon et al., 2004) and immunoassays (Xu et al., 2004). Halas et al. recently showed that tremendous SERS enhancements can be obtained on isolated NS by studying the SERS response of *p*-mercaptoaniline (pMA) as a function of the number of NS probed (Jackson and Halas, 2004). They also proved that this response was directly dependent on pMA concentration on the surface of the NS.

Earlier SERS studies of 2- and 4-MBA on silver sols demonstrated that the Raman spectra of the carboxylic acids were dependent on the pH of the sol before imaging (Michota and Bukowska, 2003; Lee et al., 1991). Additionally, infrared spectroscopy studies of 2-, 3-, and 4-MBA on gold thin films demonstrated the pH response of MBA isomers was dependent on the proximity of the carboxylic acid group to the gold surface (Wells et al., 1996). These results have been used to demonstrate a promising pH sensor for *in vitro* applications based on gold colloidal aggregates coated with 4-mercaptobenzoic acid (4-MBA) was demonstrated (Talley et al., 2004). Since NS have been shown to serve as standalone SERS nanosensors, Bishnoi et al. explored the potential of MBA coated NS films as pH sensors (Bishnoi et al., 2006). This proved to be one of the first single nanoparticle pH sensors. Following this result, other groups have used similar strategies to conduct intracellular pH measurements using 4-MBA on gold colloidal structures (Kneipp et al., 2007).

This study compares the performance of the other two isomers of MBA with that of the well-established 4-MBA self-assembled monolayer system (Scheme 5.1).

In addition to monitoring the changes in the protonated versus deprotonated forms of the benzoic acid moieties as has been done by other groups previously, we have found that the ring breathing modes can also be used to determine local pH for the 3-MBA isomer, which may aid in the detection of pH in mixed monolayer systems. In order to allow these particles to have long-term solution stability in buffers or biological media, we also investigated the use of a mixed monolayer system based on 4-MBA and poly(ethylene glycol) to measure local pH.

5.2 Materials and Methods

Gold–silica NSs were fabricated to have maximum absorption at 785 nm in water (core radius of 55 nm and outer shell thickness of 10 nm), making them resonant with the Raman laser source, using previously published techniques (Oldenberg et al., 1998). To fabricate the pH sensing films, NS were immobilized onto 3-aminopropyltriethoxysilane (APTES, Aldrich) coated glass slides (Fisher), previously cleaned with 10% potassium hydroxide in ethanol. NS films were exposed to solutions of MBA (Aldrich, 1 mM) in Milli-Q water (Millipore) for 1 h. Excess MBA was removed and the films were allowed to dry before obtaining SERS spectra in solution.

Cys-PEG-Fl was synthesized by reacting *n*-hydroxysuccinimide-poly(ethylene) glycol-fluorescein (NHS-PEG-Fl, Nektar Therapeutics) with an excess of L-cysteine (Sigma) in phosphate buffered saline (PBS, Sigma, pH 7.4) for 3 h followed by dialysis (MWCO 500, Spectrum Laboratories). To test the formation of a mixed monolayer system, NS films were exposed to 10 mM solutions of Cys-PEG-Fl overnight, excess Cys-PEG-Fl was removed and then a 1 mM solution of 4-MBA was incubated with the films for 1 h before collection of fluorescence and Raman spectra.

Raman spectra were recorded using a Renishaw inVia Raman microscope (Renishaw, UK) equipped with a 785 nm diode laser with a spot size of 100 μm × 3 μm. Backscattered light was collected using a 63× water immersion lens (Leica, Germany) with a NA of 0.90. Laser power was reduced to 55 μW at the sample using motorized neutral density filters. High-resolution spectra were acquired using an integration time of 30 s. In order to measure the pH dependency of MBA monolayers, the NS films were immersed in phosphate buffer whose pH was adjusted using either 1 N hydrochloric acid (HCl, Fisher Chemicals) or 1 N sodium hydroxide (NaOH, Fisher Chemicals). Fluorescence measurements were taken with the inVia Raman microscope using 514.5 nm excitation from an argon–ion laser and backscattered light collected through a 50× long working distance objective for an integration time of 30 s.

5.3 Results and Discussion

5.3.1 2-Mercaptobenzoic Acid

The spectra for 2-MBA monolayers on NS were representative of previously reported spectra on metal colloids (Lee et al., 1991; Michota and Bukowska, 2003). When 2-MBA bound to the gold surface through the thiol group, the carboxylic acid group was in close proximity to the gold surface (Lee et al., 1991). This close proximity can increase the interaction between the carboxylic acid and the surface, leading to deprotonation of the carboxylic acid even at low pH levels and the formation of the v_s (COO$^-$) species indicated by the peak at 1429 cm^{-1} (Figure 5.1a). The most significant changes in the 2-MBA spectra between pH 2.78 and 9.86 were the presence of the v(C-COOH) mode at 800 cm^{-1} for low pH values and the formation of the δ(COO$^-$) mode at 840 cm^{-1} with increasing pH (Figure 5.1a). The relationship between the intensities of these species were used to determine the pK_a of 2-MBA when bound to the gold NS surface. By plotting both species as a function of pH, the pK_a for 2-MBA on NS was found to be ~7.2 (Figure 5.1b).

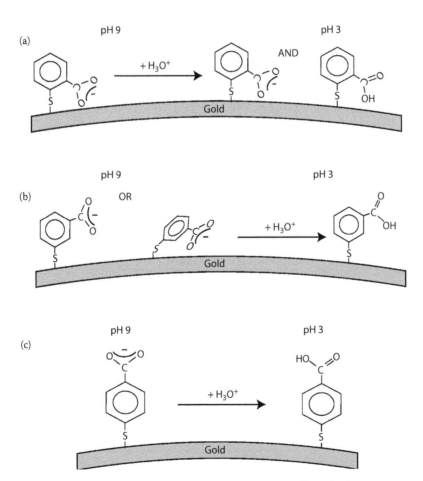

FIGURE 5.1 Illustrative drawing of the three MBA isomers on the surface of gold–silica NSs as a function of pH.

5.3.2 4-Mercaptobenzoic Acid

When monolayers of 4-MBA on NS were studied, the carboxylic acid group was protonated at pH 2.9, as demonstrated by the $\nu(C{=}O)$ species between 1700 and 1715 cm^{-1} (Figure 5.2a). At pH 9, the peak position of the carboxylate species, $\nu_s(COO^-)$, was ~1406 cm^{-1} (Figure 5.2a). The ratio between the intensity of the carboxylic acid and carboxylate ion can be used to create a calibration curve for SERS detection of 4-MBA as a nano-pH sensor (Talley et al., 2004). The error bars in Figure 5.2b were obtained from comparing results from three separate samples. Using the titration curve the pK_a was found to be 7.4 for 4-MBA on NS surface. In order to determine the robustness of a NS pH sensor, the 4-MBA coated NS film was cycled between pH 3 and 9 by exchanging the pH 3 buffer with a pH 9 buffer and then collecting another set of Raman spectra. This process was repeated five times with Raman spectra collected for each cycle (Figure 5.2c). Since the cycling measurements took place over the course of an hour, the data illustrated that the NS pH sensor could be robust and reproducible.

For both the reproducibility studies and the calibration of the nano-pH sensor, there was consistently less error at low pH compared to high pH values. This may be due to the fact that when the carboxylic acid groups were protonated, their affinity for the gold surface was minimal, resulting in a more ordered monolayer. When the pH was raised above 7.4 and the carboxylic acid was deprotonated, the negatively charged carboxylic acid had greater affinity to the gold surface, causing a disruption in the order of the monolayer.

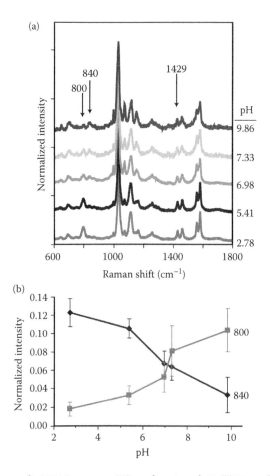

FIGURE 5.2 (a) SERS spectra of 2-MBA isomers on NS as a function of pH. (b) Normalized intensities of 800 cm^{-1} (acidic component) and 840 cm^{-1} (basic component) as a function of pH.

5.3.3 3-Mercaptobenzoic Acid

The interaction between 3-MBA and a gold surface is a balance between the interactions of 2- and 4-MBA on gold (Talley et al., 2004). Since the carboxylate group is further away from the thiol than the case of 2-MBA, more of the 3-MBA molecules remain protonated at low pH compared to 2-MBA. However, since the carboxylate ions are closer to the surface than 4-MBA, 3-MBA bound to the gold surface is sterically hindered in comparison to 4-MBA. This means that 3-MBA cannot pack as densely as 4-MBA on the NS surface, even at very low pH values. Additionally, 3-MBA can interact with the gold surface more freely than 4-MBA.

For 3-MBA bound to NS, the ratio between the COO− and C=O modes followed a similar trend as 4-MBA (Figure 5.3). When the normalized cumulative intensities of the acidic vibrational modes

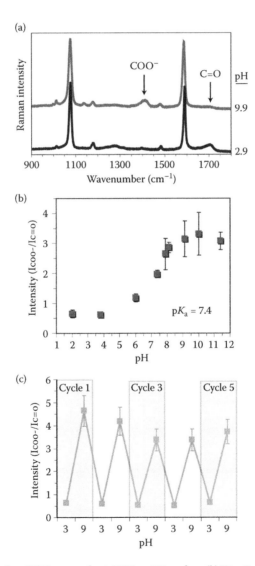

FIGURE 5.3 (a) pH-dependent SERS spectra for 4-MBA on NS surface. (b) Titration curve for 4-MBA pH sensor based on the ratio between basic and acidic carboxylic acid Raman intensities. (c) Reproducibility testing of the Raman pH sensor measured by cycling 4-MBA coated NS between pH 3 and 9, five times. (Modified from Bishnoi, S. W. et al. 2006. *Nano Letters* 6 (8): 1687–1692. With permission. © 2006 American Chemical Society.)

$(840 + 1567 + 1706 \text{ cm}^{-1})$ and basic vibrational modes $(868 + 1145 + 1408 \text{ cm}^{-1})$ were plotted as a function of pH, they could be used to measure the local pH of 3-MBA monolayers on NS (Figure 5.3b). However, 3-MBA has several ring breathing modes whose intensities were also pH sensitive, with the v_{8a} in-plane ring breathing mode (Varsanyi and Szoke, 1969) at 1568 cm^{-1} providing a more sensitive pH measurement than the carboxylic acid groups alone (Figure 5.3). The source of this pH sensitivity was not entirely clear, but was most likely due to a change in the molecule's geometry on the gold surface before and after deprotonation. One possible reason for the decrease in the v_{8a} mode at 1568 cm^{-1} is due to the strong interaction between the carboxylate ion and the NS, which causes a greater tilt in the benzene ring with respect to the surface. The change in the ring's geometry could reduce the polariz-ability of the v_{8a} mode normal to the surface; thus decreasing the intensity of the v_{8a} mode. When the 3-MBA was in the carboxylic acid form, the surface attraction was reduced and the ring was less tilted toward the surface; thus increasing the intensity of the v_{8a} mode.

During the course of these experiments, it was observed that the spectrum of 3-MBA on NS was also greatly dependent on the concentration of the 3-MBA exposed to the NS (Figure 5.4a). Since 4-MBA showed no such dependency (data not shown), we hypothesize that the reason for the concentration and pH dependency is related to the ability of the carboxylate ion to interact with the gold surface. At low concentrations and when at least half of the 3-MBA molecules were in the carboxylate form (pH 7), there was less steric hindrance from other 3-MBA molecules and the carboxylate ion could interact more readily with the NS surface (Figure 5.4b). As the concentration of 3-MBA was increased, more molecules packed onto the NS surface, forcing the carboxylate groups to stand more upright, increasing the intensity of the v_{8a} mode at 1568 cm^{-1} (Figure 5.4b).

5.3.4 Mixed Monolayer System

Since the long-term goal of this project was to produce a multifunctional pH sensor, the formation of a mixed monolayer system (Scheme 5.2) for pH sensing was investigated. 4-MBA pH-sensing molecule was chosen, since its pH sensing ability was independent of surface coverage (data not shown); however, 3-MBA could also be used with proper calibration. Cys-PEG-Fl was a convenient molecule for demonstrating the ability to create a mixed monolayer because Cys molecules selfassemble onto gold surfaces (Cavalleri et al., 2004; Sasaki et al., 1997) and PEG molecules are often used in drug delivery systems (Harris and Zalipsky, 1997) and to prevent biofouling of *in vivo* sensors (Sharma et al., 2003). A fluorescent tag (fluorescein) was incorporated to confirm the formation of a mixed monolayer system (Levin et al., 2006).

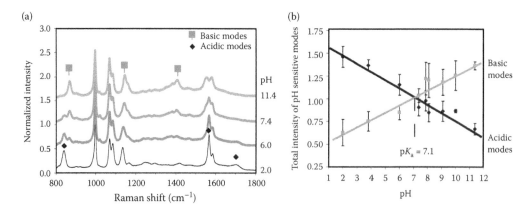

FIGURE 5.4   (a) SERS spectra of 3-MBA coated NS between pH 2 and 11.4. (b) Intensity of the acidic versus basic modes as a function of pH (normalized to the 998 cm^{-1} mode).

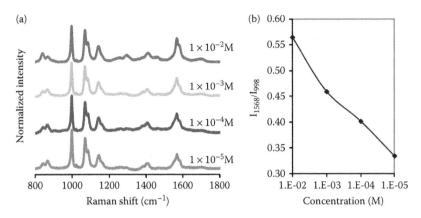

FIGURE 5.5 (a) SERS spectra of 3-MBA monolayers on NS from 10^{-5} to 10^{-2} M concentrations at pH 7. (b) Intensity of 1568 cm^{-1} mode as a function of coverage.

In order to test whether a mixed monolayer system could be made, a monolayer of Cys-PEG-Fl was formed on an NS film and the fluorescence of the film measured (Figure 5.5a). After exposing the Cys-PEG-Fl coated NS to 4-MBA, the fluorescence intensity was reduced (Figure 5.5b), presumably due to the displacement of some of the Cys-PEG-Fl by 4-MBA. The SERS spectrum of the film was measured before and after exposure to 4-MBA, proving that 4-MBA did bind to the NS film along with the Cys-

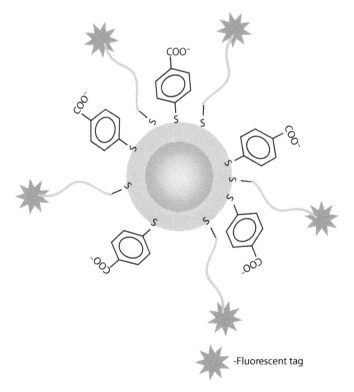

FIGURE 5.6 **(See color insert following page 10-24.)** Multifunctional pH sensor using a mixed monolayer system of 4-MBA and Cys-PEG-Fl.

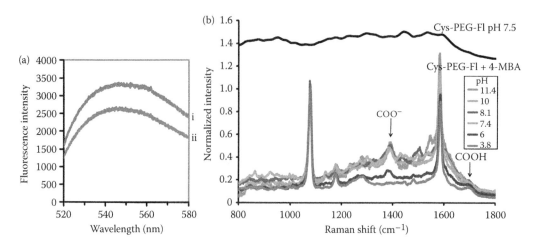

FIGURE 5.7 (a) Fluorescence spectra of mixed monolayer sensor. NS coated with (i) Cys-PEG-Fl and (ii) Cys-PEG-Fl + 4-MBA mixed monolayer. (b) SERS spectra of Cys-PEG-Fl at pH 7.5 and Cys-PEG-Fl and 4-MBA coated NS at various pHs.

PEG-Fl (Figure 5.5b). A pH calibration curve was created using this mixed monolayer film (data not shown) and agreed with the previously tested 4-MBA system alone. A mixed monolayer system with the ability to detect local pH could be useful for *in vitro* studies using targeting molecules such as peptides to direct the uptake of nano-pH sensors into cellular compartments (Figures 5.6 and 5.7).

5.4 Conclusions

By studying the pH response of MBA monolayers on gold NSs, we have demonstrated that nano-sensors can be created to monitor local environmental changes using isolated nanoparticles. In addition, a mixed monolayer system can be created that contains both the pH sensing ability of 4-MBA and the saline stability that is imparted through the incorporation of poly(ethylene glycol) moieties. The ability to use SERS for *in situ* monitoring of pH changes, allows for the creation of robust, sensitive, and real-time sensors based on a molecule's charge and binding geometry on a nanoparticle surface.

Acknowledgment

The author thanks Professor Naomi Halas of Rice University for helpful discussions and access to the Renishaw in Via microscope.

References

Bishnoi, S. W., C. J. Rozell, C. S. Levin, M. K. Gheith, B. R. Johnson, D. H. Johnson, and N. J. Halas. 2006. All-optical nanoscale pH meter. *Nano Letters* 6 (8):1687–1692.

Cao, YunWei Charles, R. Jin, and C. A. Mirkin. 2002. Nanoparticles with Raman spectroscopic fingerprints for DNA and RNA detection. *Science* 297:1536–1540.

Cavalleri, O., G. Gonella, S. Terreni, M. Vignolo, P. Pelori, L. Floreano, A. Morgante, M. Canepa, and R. Rolandi. 2004. High resolution XPS of the S 2p core level region of the L-cysteine/gold interface. *Journal of Physics: Condensed Matter* 16:S2477–S2482.

Grubisha, D. S., R. J. Lipert, H.-Y. Park, J. Driskell, and M. D. Porter. 2003. Femtomolar detection of prostate-specific antigen: An immunoassay based on surface-enhanced Raman scattering and immunogold labels. *Analytical Chemistry* 75:5936–5943.

Harris, J. M. and S. Zalipsky. 1997. *Poly(ethylene glycol): Chemistry and Biological Applications.* Washington, DC: American Chemical Society.

Jackson, J. B. and N. J. Halas. 2004. Surface-enhanced Raman scattering on tunable plasmonic nano-particle substrates. *Proceedings of the National Academy of Science* 101 (52):17930–17935.

Kneipp, J., H. Kneipp, B. Wittig, and K. Kneipp. 2007. One- and two-photon excited optical pH probing for cells using surface-enhanced Raman and hyper-Raman nanosensors. *Nano Letters* 7:2819–2823.

Lee, S. B., K. Kim, and M. S. Kim. 1991. Surface-enhanced Raman-scattering of ortho-mercaptobenzoic acid in silver sol. *Journal of Raman Spectroscopy* 22 (12):811–817.

Levin, C. S., S. W. Bishnoi, N. K. Grady, and N. J. Halas. 2006. Determining the conformation of thiolated poly(ethylene glycol) on Au nanoshells by surface-enhanced Raman scattering spectroscopic assay. *Analytical Chemistry* 78 (10):3277–3281.

Michota, A. and J. Bukowska. 2003. Surface-enhanced Raman scattering (SERS) of 4-mercaptobenzoic acid on silver and gold substrates. *Journal of Raman Spectroscopy* 34:21–25.

Mulvaney, S. P. and C. D. Keating. 2000. Raman spectroscopy. *Analytical Chemistry* 72:145R–157R.

Oldenberg, S. J., R. D. Averitt, S. L. Westcott, and N. J. Halas. 1998. Nanoengineering of optical resonances. *Chemical Physics Letters* 288:243–247.

Sasaki, Y. C., K. Yasuda, Y. Suzuki, T. Ishibashi, I. Satoh, Y. Fujiki, and S. Ishiwata. 1997. Two-dimensional arrangement of a functional protein by cysteine–gold interaction: Enzyme activity and characteriza-tion of a protein monolayer on a gold substrate. *Biophysical Journal* 72:1842–1848.

Sharma, S., R. W. Johnson, and T. A. Desai. 2003. PEG films for silicon-based microdevices: Effect of con-centration on surface uniformity. *Applied Surface Science* 206:218–219.

Talley, C. E., L. Jusinski, C. W. Hollars, S. M. Lane, and T. Huser. 2004. Intracellular pH sensors based on surface-enhanced Raman scattering. *Analytical Chemistry* 76 (23):7064–7068.

Varsanyi, G. and S. Szoke. 1969. *Vibrational Spectra of Benzene Derivatives.* New York: Academic Press.

Wells, M., D. L. Dermody, H. C. Yang, T. Kim, R. M. Crooks, and A. J. Ricco. 1996. Interactions between organized, surface-confined monolayers and vapor-phase probe molecules. 9. Structure/reactivity relationship between three surface-confined isomers of mercaptobenzoic acid and vapor-phase decylamine. *Langmuir* 12:1989–1996.

Xu, S., X. Ji, W. Xu, X. Li, L. Wang, Y. Bai, B. Zhao, and Y. Ozaki. 2004. Immunoassay using probe-labelling immunogold nanoparticles with silver staining enhancement via surface-enhanced Raman scatter-ing. *The Analyst* 129:63–68.

Yonzon, C. R., C. L. Haynes, X. Zhang, Jr. J. T. Walsh, and R. P. Van Duyne. 2004. A glucose biosensor based on surface-enhanced Raman scattering: Improved partition layer, temporal stability, revers-ibility, and resistance to serum protein interference. *Analytical Chemistry* 76:78–85.

6

Nano-enabled Platforms for Metastatic Malignant Melanoma

Sadhana Sharma
The Ohio State University

John Shapiro
The Ohio State University

Robbie J. Walczak
Thermo Fisher Scientific

Piyush M. Sinha
Intel Corporation

6.1 Introduction

Melanoma is the most serious form of skin cancer. In 2009, about 68,720 individuals in the United States were expected to develop melanoma and approximately 8650 were expected to die of it (American Cancer Society, 2009 Facts and Figures). Melanoma is the fifth and sixth most common cancer among men and women, respectively, and is the most prevalent type of cancer in individuals in their second decade of life. Melanoma incidence rates have been increasing for at least 30 years. In most recent times, rapid increases have occurred among young white women (3.8% annual increase since 1995 in those aged 15–34 years) and older white men (8.8% annual increase since 2003 in those 65 and older) (American Cancer Society, 2009 Facts and Figures). Melanoma is a malignant tumor that originates in melanocytes, the cells which produce the pigment melanin that colors our skin, hair, and eyes. The majority of melanomas are black or brown. However, some melanomas are skin colored, pink, red, purple, blue, or white.

Standard care treatment for malignant melanoma requires removal of the primary growth and surrounding normal tissue. Sometimes a sentinel lymph node is biopsied to determine the stage. More extensive lymph node surgery is needed if lymph node metastases are present. Melanomas with deep invasion or that have spread to lymph nodes may be treated with surgery, immunotherapy, chemotherapy, or radiation therapy. Advanced cases of melanoma are treated with palliative surgery, immunotherapy, and/or chemotherapy, and sometimes radiation therapy. If melanoma is recognized and treated early, it is nearly 100% curable. But if it is not, the cancer can advance and spread to other parts of the body, where it becomes hard to treat and can be fatal.

Metastatic melanoma tumors are often unresectable due to their size and/or location near critical structures. These lesions represent a significant challenge for the oncologist as radiotherapy is infrequently successful and chemotherapy induces regressions in less than 20% of cases (Nguyen et al., 2003). Of primary concern is the fact that these lesions disrupt normal organ function, are usually painful, and present a cosmetic dilemma when located in cutaneous sites or in lymph node basins. Thus, new approaches to the treatment of metastatic melanoma are needed. Because melanoma metastases are frequently located in superficial tissues, this cancer represents a model for the development and testing of unique methods to deliver anticancer agents locally.

Immunotherapy has a long history with striking but limited success in patients with melanoma. Till date, interleukin-2 (IL-2) and interferon-alfa2b (IFN-α2b) are the only approved immunotherapeutic agents for melanoma in the United States (Kirkwood, 2008). IFN-α2b is commonly used in the treatment of patients with metastatic melanoma (Belardelli et al., 2002, Ferrantini et al., 2007). Tumor regressions occur at a variety of doses and schedules with an overall response rate of 16.7% (Legha, 1986; Kirkwood et al., 1996; Balch, 1998; Lens and Dawes, 2002). The immunologic effects of IFN-α are a critical part of its antitumor actions. Current treatment regimen requires intravenous or intratumoral injections of free IFN thrice a week. Unfortunately, systemic administration of IFN-α can be toxic, thereby limiting its utility in aged and debilitated patients. The local administration of IFN-α can be quite useful in the control of unresectable lesions (von Wussow et al., 1988; Ikic et al., 1995), but this approach is limited due to the need for frequent clinic visits and the difficulties associated with repeated intratumoral injections.

Over the last three decades considerable advances have marked the field of cancer drug delivery, resulting in many breakthroughs in clinical medicine. However, major unmet needs remain. Among these are board categories of: (1) continuous release of therapeutic agents over extended time periods and in accordance with a predetermined temporal profile (Sershen and West, 2002); (2) local or targeted delivery at a constant rate to the tumor microenvironment, to overcome much of the systemic toxicity and improve antitumor efficacy; (3) improved ease of administration, increasing patient compliance, while minimizing the needed intervention of healthcare personnel and decreasing the length of hospital stays (Boudes, 1998; Lewis and Ferrari, 2003; Ferrari, 2005). Success in addressing some or all these challenges would potentially lead to improvements in efficacy and patient compliance, as well as minimization of side effects. In recent years, a variety of nano-enabled drug delivery modalities have been developed for systemic and local cancer therapy. These are either based on nanoparticles (Davis et al., 2008; Peer et al., 2007) or implantable controlled release technologies (LaVan et al., 2003; Sharma et al., 2006; Staples et al., 2006). Many of these nanotechnologies are applicable to a wide variety of cancer types and drugs, and can be tailored to suit specific needs. In this chapter, we will focus on the available nano-enabled platforms for melanoma therapy, more particularly our nanotechnology platforms, namely silicon-based nanoporous or nanochannel microchips.

6.2 Metastatic Malignant Melanoma: Immunotherapy and Nano-enabled Platforms

6.2.1 Immunotherapy

Current available treatments for patients with melanoma are limited. In patients with metastatic disease chemotherapy, biologic therapy, tumor-infiltrating lymphocytes, lymphokine-activated cells and combination biochemotherapy have yielded low response rates of approximately 20–30% (Kim et al., 2002). Immunotherapy for cancers is based on the principle that the host's immune system is capable of generating immune responses against tumor cells. The potential of cancer immunotherapy was first documented by William Coley in 1890, when bacterial products (Coley's toxins) were administered for advanced inoperable cancers with dramatic responses (Nauts et al., 1953). In the latter part of the twentieth century, studies of chemically induced tumors of inbred mice demonstrated transplantation resistance and spontaneous regression of melanoma fueled speculation that immunological responses contributed to tumor regression (Nathanson, 1976). In the 1980s, lymphocytes activated with lectins or IL-2 was demonstrated to target tumor cells *in vitro* (Strausser et al., 1981; Grimm et al., 1982; Mazumdar et al., 1982). Further studies supported by histological evaluations revealed that this process is mediated by activated lymphocytes (Schneeberger et al., 1995). Consequently, much effort has centered on the development of immune-based treatments for the therapy of advanced disease. Immunotherapy for melanoma includes a number of different strategies with vaccines utilizing whole cell tumors, peptides, cytokine-mediated dendritic cells, deoxyribonucleic acid (DNA) and ribonucleic acid (RNA), and antibodies (Kirkwood, J. M., and M. Ernstoff, 1985; Kirkwood et al., 1985; Kim et al., 2002; Kirkwood et al., 2008). In this chapter, we will focus mainly on developments in cytokine-based therapy.

Cytokine therapy with either IL-2 or IFN-α produces overall response rates of 15–20%, and continues to be a mainstay of therapy in patients with good overall organ function. However, these treatments are administered at high doses and are often poorly tolerated by patients with advanced disease (Atkins et al., 1999; Kirkwood et al., 2002; Lens and Dawes, 2002). In addition, the precise mechanisms underlying the antitumor effects of these treatments are not known, making it difficult to devise improvements or identify patients with a higher likelihood of responding to therapy (Kirkwood, 2002).

While high-dose IL-2 therapy can lead to a dramatic regression of disease in approximately 15% of patients, it can have significant adverse effects upon the cardiac and pulmonary systems and requires hospitalization of the patient in a specialized unit (Kammula et al., 1998). IFN-α can be given on an outpatient basis, but the regimen currently in use calls for a full year of therapy during which nearly 50% patients require treatment delays or dose reductions, due to constitutional, hepatic, or neurologic side effects. IFN-α2b is used in a variety of other malignancies including renal cell carcinoma, hairy cell leukemia, and Kaposi's sarcoma (Kirkwood, 2002; Kirkwood et al., 2002). It is also employed as an adjuvant following the surgical resection of high-risk melanoma lesions. In this setting, it has been shown to reduce the incidence of recurrent disease and improve overall survival (Kirkwood et al., 1996). IFN-α2b exerts direct antiproliferative, proapoptotic, and antiangiogenic effects on tumor cells (Asadullah et al., 2002). Thus, its activity on melanoma cells can be directly measured by monitoring cell growth *in vitro* and *in vivo*. IFN-α2b is also known to have important immunomodulatory properties that influence its antitumor actions. A careful study of the antitumor effects and delivery pattern would lead to rational improvements in IFN-α2b treatment protocols, thus improving efficacy and diminishing potentially life-threatening side effects. In addition to its direct antiproliferative effects, studies have suggested that IFN-α2b, delivered in close proximity to malignant melanoma lesions, might be effective in stimulating tumor reactive immune effectors that have localized in the tumor site (Lesinski et al., 2003).

The results obtained with IFN-α2b in the setting of metastatic melanoma prompted investigators to explore the utility of high-dose IFN-α for patients who had undergone complete surgical excision of their tumor, yet were at high risk for recurrent disease. Kirkwood et al. conducted a phase-III trial in which patients were randomized to receive either high-dose IFN-α (20 MU/m^2 subcutaneously thrice weekly for 48 weeks) or observation. The results of this trial, reported in 1994, revealed increased overall and relapse-free survival in the patients who received IFN-α2b (Kirkwood et al., 1996). Enthusiasm for this treatment has been tempered by the fact that a confirmatory trial comparing the efficacy of high-dose and low-dose IFN-α regimens (3 MU/m^2 subcutaneously thrice weekly ×2 years) in a similar population of surgically treated patients revealed no difference in the overall survival for either schedule of IFN-α2b as compared to observation alone, although increased relapse-free survival was observed in patients receiving the higher dose of IFN-α2b (Kirkwood et al., 2000). Later, an adjuvant trial comparing an antiganglioside vaccine to high-dose IFN-α2b was stopped early after the analysis showed a clear survival advantage to patients in the IFN-α arm (Kirkwood et al., 2001). Despite these conflicting reports, IFN-α2b remains the only commonly used drug for adjuvant treatment of malignant melanoma.

Immunotherapy for cancer has tremendous potential. However, there are several challenges that need to be addressed. To be successful, immunotherapy must overcome a variety of obstacles, including tumor-induced immune suppression. Improvements in our understanding of the immune system, its regulation, and the dynamics of host-tumor interactions, have now led to novel strategies that may stimulate or restore effective antitumor immune responses, such as targeting receptors that modulate the immune response (e.g., CTLA4). These approaches are already being explored in phase-III trials (Kirkwood et al., 2008). These therapeutic strategies may overcome tumor-induced immune suppression and greatly improve the effectiveness of cancer immunotherapy to a wide range of tumor types. In addition, using these strategies, it may be possible to identify more relevant antigens for future vaccine immunotherapy. More so, specifically targeting critical regulatory elements involved in the immune response to tumor may overcome tolerance without inducing autoimmune sequel that mark current cytokine and interferon therapies. Although still early in clinical development, these new approaches demonstrate promising antitumor activity in patients with metastatic melanoma and other tumor types. These approaches, as well as combinatorial immunotherapy, can be expected to be a focus of future work.

6.2.2 Nano-enabled Platforms

Nanotechnology-based platforms offer new capabilities to the existing standard care cancer treatments. Using nanotechnology, it may be possible to achieve (1) improved delivery of poorly water-soluble drugs; (2) targeted delivery of drugs in a cell- or tissue-specific manner; (3) transcytosis of drugs across tight epithelial and endothelial barriers; (4) delivery of large macromolecule drugs to intracellular sites of action; (5) codelivery of two or more drugs or therapeutic modality for combination therapy; (6) targeted and selective radiation-based therapy; (7) visualization of sites of drug delivery by combining therapeutic agents with imaging modalities; and (8) real-time read on the *in vivo* efficacy of a therapeutic agent (Farokhzad and Robert Langer, 2009).

In the setting of malignant melanoma, the development of nanotechnology-enabled modalities or devices capable of delivering drugs or immunomodulating agents such as IFN-α at a constant rate to the tumor microenvironment could avoid the toxicity of systemic administration and inconvenience of frequent clinic visits, and potentially overcome the immunosuppressive nature of the tumor microenvironment. Because of its small size requirements, such a modality/device could be either injected (nanoparticles/nanocarriers) at site or implanted (nanoporous/nanochannel microchips) in proximity to unresectable melanoma lesions using a minimally invasive procedure.

6.2.3 Nanoparticle/Nanocarrier Therapeutics

Particles in the size range 1–100 nm (nanoparticle/nanocarrier) are emerging as a class of therapeutics for cancer. Nanoparticle/nanocarrier therapeutics are typically particles comprised of therapeutic entities, such as small-molecule drugs, peptides, proteins and nucleic acids, and components that assemble with the therapeutic entities, such as lipids and polymers, to form nanoparticles. Such nanoparticles can have enhanced anticancer effects compared with the therapeutic entities they contain. This is owing to more specific localized targeting to tumor tissues via improved pharmacokinetics and pharmacodynamics, and active intracellular delivery. These properties depend on the size and surface properties (including the presence of targeting ligands) of the nanoparticles. Nanoscaled systems for systemic cancer therapy and their latest stage of development are summarized in Table 6.1 (Davis et al., 2008). The family of nanoparticles/nanocarriers includes polymer conjugates, polymeric nanoparticles, lipid-based carriers such as liposomes and micelles, dendrimers, carbon nanotubes, and gold nanoparticles, including nanoshells and nanocages (Figure 6.1) (Peer et al., 2007). These nanoparticles/nanocarriers have been explored for a variety of applications such as drug delivery, imaging, photothermal ablation of tumors, radiation sensitizers, detection of apoptosis, and sentinel lymphnode mapping (LaVan et al., 2003; Ferrari, 2005; Duncan, 2006). Till date, at least 12 polymer-drug conjugates have entered Phase-I and II clinical trials and are especially useful for targeting blood vessels in tumors. Examples include antiendothelial immunoconjugates, fusion proteins, and caplostatin, the first polymer-angiogenesis inhibitor conjugates (Peer et al.,

TABLE 6.1 Nanoscaled Systems for Systemic Cancer Therapy

Platform	Latest Stage of Development	Examples
Liposomes	Approved	DaunoXome, Doxil
Albumin-based particles	Approved	Abraxane
PEGylated proteins	Approved	Oncospar, PEG-Intron, PEGASYS, Neulasta
Biodegradable polymer–drug composites	Clinical trials	Doxorubicin Transdrug
Polymeric micelles	Clinical trials	Genexol-PM[a], SP1049C, NK911, NK012, NK105, NC-6004
Polymer–drug conjugated-based particles	Clinical trials	XYOTAX (CT-2130), CT-2106, IT-101, AP5280, AP5346, FCE28068 (PK1), FCE28069 (PK2), PNU166148, PNU166945, MAG-CPT, DE-310, Pegamotecan, NKTR-102, EZN-2208
Dendrimers	Preclinical	Polyamidoamine (PAMAM)
Inorganic or other solid particles	Preclinical (except for gold nanoparticle that is clinical)	Carbon nanotubes, silica particles, gold particles (CYT-6091)

Source: Reprinted by permission from Macmillan Publishers LTD: Davis, M. E., Z. Chen, and D. M. Shin, 2008. *Nat. Rev. Drug Discov.* 7:771–782. Copyright 2008.

[a] Approved in South Korea, PEG, polyethylene glycol.

2007). Notably, several review articles have recently been published that cover different aspects or types of nanoparticles/nanocarriers in detail (Duncan, 2006; Nishiyama and Kataoka, 2006; Peer et al., 2007; Davis et al., 2008; Ganta et al., 2008; Jabr-Milane et al., 2008). While all these nanoparticle/nanocarrier technologies have potential applications for melanoma, here we will focus on the nanoparticles/nanocarriers that have been designed, developed, and tested specifically for melanoma.

Piddubnyak et al. (2004) synthesized nanoparticles using oligo-3 hydroxybutyrates and used them to deliver doxorubicin to a melanoma cell line. These naturally occurring high molecular weight polymers first discovered in *Bacillus megaterium*, are biodegradable and nontoxic. Using a tailor-made polymer of oligo-[R,S]-3-hydroxybutyrate, it was shown that conjugation of doxorubicin to the polymer resulted in uptake and localization of the drug to the cytoplasm in this cell line. This is in contrast to the normal localization of doxorubicin to the cell nucleus when the drug is dosed in the free form. Kester et al. (2008) designed nanoparticles (20–30 nm diameter) comprised of a calcium phosphate matrix described as calcium phosphate nanocomposite particles (CPNPs) designed to encapsulate and to target anti-neoplastic agents such as ceramide directly to cancerous lesions. Delivery of ceramide to the UACC 903 melanoma cell line using CPNPs resulted in a 10-fold increase in apoptotic effects over direct delivery of the drug at the same concentration.

Several nanoscaled therapeutics based on polyethylene glycol conjugated (PEGylated) proteins have been approved or are in clinical trials for cancer therapy. PEGylation has been applied to various proteins including enzymes, cytokines, and monoclonal antibody Fab fragments. For a valid cytokine immunotherapy of malignancies, a slow release of cytokines is required, because their short half-life *in vivo* ruins therapeutic efficacy while causing severe systemic toxic effects.

PEGylation provides a means to increase protein solubility, reduce immunogenicity, prevent rapid renal clearance (due to the increased size of conjugates), and prolong plasma half-life (Harris and Chess, 2003). Two PEGylated IFN-α conjugates, PEGASYS (Roche) for IFN-α2a and PEGINTRON (Schering) for IFN-α2b, have already demonstrated clinically superior antiviral activity compared with free IFN-α and approved for hepatitis C therapy (Wang et al., 2002). They have also been shown to be effective for the treatment of melanoma (Wang et al., 2002; Fiaherty et al., 2005) and are currently being tested in other solid tumors (Bukowski et al., 2002). Because of the prolonged half-lives of PEG–IFN-α conjugates, they can be given by subcutaneous injection once every 12 weeks instead of thrice a week for free IFNs.

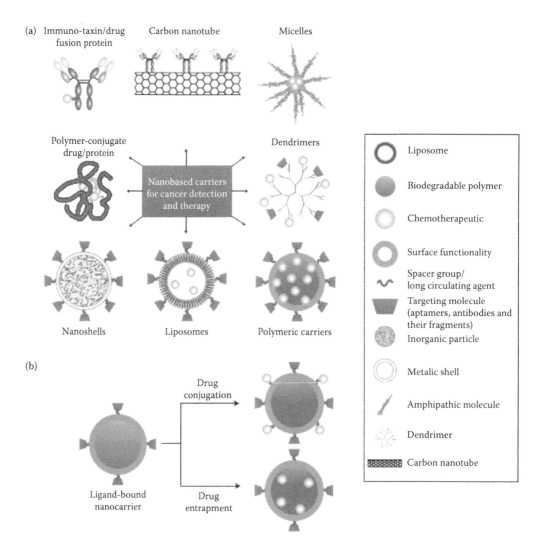

FIGURE 6.1 **(See color insert following page 10-24.)** Examples of nanoparticles/nanocarriers for targeting cancer. (a) A whole range of delivery agents are possible but the main components typically include a nanoparticle/nanocarrier, a targeting moiety conjugated to the nanoparticle/nanocarrier, and a cargo (such as the desired chemotherapeutic drugs). (b) Schematic diagram of the drug conjugation and entrapment processes. The chemotherapeutics could be bound to the nanoparticle/nanocarrier, as in the use of polymer–drug conjugates, dendrimers and some particulate carriers, or they could be entrapped inside the nanoparticle/nanocarrier. (Reprinted by permission from Macmillan Publishers LTD: Peer, D. et al., 2007. *Nat. Nanotechnol.* 2:751–760. Copyright 2007.)

Shimizu et al. (2008) developed a nanogel-based drug delivery system (Nanogel DDS) for a sustained release of cytokines for tumor immunotherapy. This was based on their previously developed cholesterol-bearing pullulan (CHP)-based hydrogel nanoparticles or nanogels. They applied Nanogel DDS to *in vivo* administration of recombinant murine IL-12 (rmIL-12) that was successfully incorporated into CHP nanogel simply by incubating with CHP at room temperature. After subcutaneously injected into mice, the CHP/rmIL-12 complex led to a prolonged elevation in IL-12 concentration in the sera. Repetitive administrations of the CHP/rmIL-12, but not rmIL-12 alone, induced drastic growth retardation of pre-established subcutaneous fibrosarcoma without causing any serious toxic event. Nanogel DDS can be used for systematic or localized cytokine delivery to melanoma lesions.

Protein cage architectures such as virus capsids and ferritins are versatile nanoscale platforms amenable to both genetic and chemical modification. The incorporation of multiple functionalities within these nanometer-sized protein architectures demonstrate their potential to serve as functional nanomaterials with applications in medical imaging and therapy. Uchida et al. (2006) synthesized an iron oxide (magnetite) nanoparticle within the interior cavity of a genetically engineered human H-chain ferritin (HFn). A cell-specific targeting peptide, RGD-4C which binds $\alpha_v\beta_3$ integrins upregulated on tumor vasculature, was genetically incorporated on the exterior surface of HFn. Both magnetite-containing and fluorescently labeled RGD4C-Fn cages bound C32 melanoma cells *in vitro*. Together these results demonstrated the capability of genetically modified protein cage architecture to serve as a multifunctional nanoscale container for simultaneous iron oxide loading and cell-specific targeting. Flenniken et al. (2006) used the ability of monomers of heat shock proteins (HSPs) to self-assemble into protein cages and used these cages to demonstrate an ability to target the C32 melanoma cell line. The cages assembled from 24 identical subunits from the hyperthermophilic archaeon bacteria-*Methanococcus jannaschii* into an empty sphere of diameter 12 nm. The subunits could either have targeting moieties covalently bound with a linking molecule (such as an antibody) or the heat-shock gene could be genetically engineered to express binding moieties such as the RGD-4C peptide. Although no drug was delivered in the empty sphere, the study demonstrated good binding capability of the protein cages using both the RGD-4C and an antibody to the membrane receptor CD-4. Additionally, the cages were able to be labeled with a dual system that included either of the two targeting moieties as well as flourescein. This gives the protein cages the capability to both target and be used as an imaging agent as well.

Hyperthermia is a promising approach to cancer therapy (van der Zee, 2002). The rationale underlying hyperthermia is the fact that temperatures over 42.5°C are cytotoxic for tumor cells (Dewey et al., 1977), especially in an environment with a low pO_2 and low pH conditions that are typically found in tumor tissue due to insufficient blood perfusion. A major technical problem with hyperthermia is the difficulty of heating the local tumor region to the intended temperature without damaging the normal tissue. Recent developments in nanotechnology and lasers have renewed interest in hyperthermia-based cancer therapy. Kobayashi and coworkers (Ito et al., 2006) developed an intracellular hyperthermia system using magnetite nanoparticles (magnetite cationic liposomes, MCLs). This novel hyperthermia system could induce necrotic cell death via HSP expression, which induces antitumor immunity. They tested the efficacy of this platform in animals with several types of tumors, such as the B16 mouse melanoma (Suzuki et al., 2003). Their research suggested that HSP70 is an important modulator of tumor cell immunogenicity during hyperthermia. In 2002, a vaccine consisting of the autologous tumor-derived HSP gp96–peptide complexes (HSPPC-96, Oncophage; Antigenics, Woburn, MA, USA) entered clinical trials, and the feasibility of treatment in metastatic melanoma patients was demonstrated (Belli et al., 2002). Since the HSP–peptide complexes have to be extracted from tumors in the body, surgery is required in this therapeutic protocol. The surgery and extraction will be unnecessary if the hyperthermia is induced by MCLs. Ito et al. (2005) also demonstrated that hyperthermia can be combined with cytokines to improve the effectiveness of cancer therapy. In fact, combinations with cytokines (IL-2 and GM-CSF), heat-inducible TNF-α gene therapy, recombinant HSP70, HSP70 gene therapy, and dendritic cell therapy, were performed and significantly improved results were obtained.

Noble metal nanoparticles such as gold nanoparticles have become very useful as agents for photothermal therapy on account of their enhanced absorption cross-sections, which are four to five orders of magnitude larger than those offered by conventional photoabsorbing dyes. This strong absorption ensures effective laser therapy at relatively lower energies rendering the therapy method minimally invasive. Additionally, metal nanostructures have higher photostability, and they do not suffer from photobleaching. Currently, gold nanospheres, gold nanorods, gold nanoshells, gold nanocages, and carbon nanotubes are the chief nanostructures that have been demonstrated in photothermal therapeutics due to their strongly enhanced absorption in the visible and near-infrared regions on account of their surface plasmon resonance (SPR) oscillations (Huang et al., 2008). Of these structures, the first three nanostructures are especially promising because of their ease of preparation, ready multifunctionalization, and tunable optical properties. Several studies have explored the use of gold nanostructures for cancer photothermal ablation, including nanorods (Huang et al., 2006), nanocages (Skrabalak et al., 2007), and "core/shell" structures (Hirsch et al., 2003; Loo et al., 2004; O'Neal et al., 2004; Gobin et al., 2007; Ji et al., 2007). However, a major and challenging requirement for successful biomedical applications of nanomaterials is efficient *in vivo* delivery to the target sites after systemic administration.

Schwartzberg et al. (2006) fabricated a second-generation nanostructure based on hollow gold nanospheres (HAuNS). These gold nanostructures had the unique combination of small size (outer diameter, 30–60 nm), spherical shape, hollow interior, and strong and tunable (520–950 nm) absorption band as a result of their highly uniform structure. Lu et al. (2009) developed HAuNS for selective photothermal ablation in melanoma. Using peptides as the targeting ligand, they showed receptor-mediated active targeting and efficient photothermal ablation of melanoma in a murine tumor model. HAuNS were stabilized with polyethylene glycol (PEG) coating and attached with α-melanocyte-stimulating hormone (MSH) analog, [Nle⁴,D-Phe⁷]α-MSH (NDP-MSH), which is a potent agonist of melanocortin type-1 receptor overexpressed in melanoma. The nanoparticles were specifically taken up by melanoma cells, which initiated the recruitment of β-arrestins, the adapters to link the activated G-protein-coupled receptors to clathrin, indicating the involvement of receptor-mediated endocytosis. This resulted in enhanced extravasation of NDP-MSH-PEG-HAuNS from tumor blood vessels and their dispersion into tumor matrix compared with nonspecific PEGylated HAuNS. The successful selective photothermal ablation of B16/F10 melanoma with targeted HAuNS was confirmed by histologic and [18F] fluorodeoxyglucose positron emission tomography evaluation at 24 h post near-IR-region laser irradiation at a low-dose energy of 30 J/cm². Although promising, more detailed preclinical studies with regard to excretion/clearance, safety, and efficacy of targeted HAuNS are needed for further translation of this technology to clinic.

Encapsulation of tumor-associated antigens (TAA) in polymer nanoparticles is a promising approach to increasing the efficiency of antigen (Ag) delivery for antitumor vaccines. Solbrig et al. (2007) optimized a polymer preparation method to deliver both defined tumor-associated proteins and the complex mixtures of tumor Ags present in tumors. Tumor Ags were encapsulated in a biodegradable, 50:50 poly(D,L-lactide *co*-glycolide) copolymer (PLGA) by emulsification and solvent extraction. Two particular Ags were studied, gp100 (a melanoma-associated antigen) and ovalbumin (OVA), as well as mixtures of proteins and lysates of tumor cells. They used the B16 melanoma cell line, because this highly aggressive and poorly immunogenic melanoma tumor cell line has been used in C57BL/6 mice as the model of choice for developing vaccination protocols useful in immunotherapy of human melanoma. They found that gp100 encapsulation in nanoparticles led to superior cytokine production for both cytokines that were tested (IL-2, 10-fold increased stimulation; IFNγ, 3-fold increase), indicating nanoparticle encapsulation was associated with an increased level of production of the CTL- or Th1-associated cytokines crucial to antitumor immunity. They were also able to produce an *in vivo* resistance to the growth of B16 melanoma in mice. Mice vaccinated with nanoparticle–tumor conjugates had the smallest tumors and the longest tumor free durations when challenged with B16 melanoma cells.

Liposomes (~100 nm and larger) carrying chemotherapeutic small-molecule drugs have been approved for cancer since the mid-1990s, and are mainly used to solubilize drugs, leading to biodistributions that favor higher uptake by the tumor than the free drug (Zamboni, 2005). However, liposomes do not provide control for the time of drug release, and in most cases do not achieve effective intracellular delivery of the drug molecules (Zamboni, 2005), therefore limiting their potential to be useful against multidrug-resistant cancers. Recently, a unique nanoliposomal-ultrasound-mediated approach has been developed for delivering small interfering RNA (siRNA) specifically targeting ^{V600E}B-Raf and Akt3 into melanocytic tumors present in skin to retard melanoma development (Tran et al., 2008). These novel cationic nanoliposomes stably encapsulate siRNA targeting ^{V600E}B-Raf or Akt3, providing protection from degradation and facilitating entry into melanoma cells to decrease the expression of these proteins. Low-frequency ultrasound using a lightweight four-cymbal transducer array enabled the penetration of nanoliposomal–siRNA complex throughout the epidermal and dermal layers of laboratory-generated or animal skin. Nanoliposomal-mediated siRNA targeting of [V600E]B-Raf and Akt3 led to a cooperatively acting ~65% decrease in early or invasive cutaneous melanoma compared with inhibition of each singly with negligible associated systemic toxicity.

6.2.4 Nanoporous or Nanochannel Microchips for Controlled Drug Delivery

The importance of controlled-release drug delivery systems may be argued with reference to the goal of achieving a continuous drug release profile consistent with zero-order kinetics, wherein blood levels of drugs would remain constant throughout the delivery period. By contrast, injected drugs follow first-order kinetics, with initial high blood levels of the drug after initial administration, followed by an exponential fall in blood concentration (Stoelting, 1999). Toxicity often occurs when blood levels peak, while efficacy of the drug diminishes as the drug levels fall below the therapeutic range (Figure 6.2). The potential therapeutic advantages of continuous-release drug delivery systems are thus significant, and encompass: *In vivo* predictability of release rates on the basis of *in vitro* data, minimized peak plasma levels and thereby reduced risk of adverse reactions, predictable and extended duration of action, reduced inconvenience of frequent dosing, and thereby improved patient compliance (Breimer, 1999; Klausner et al., 2003).

The development of drug delivery systems encompasses broad categories, such as implantable devices with percutaneous components, fully implantable devices, polymer-based systems, microchips, and osmotic pumps (Cao et al., 2001; Krulevitch and Wang, 2001; Yasukawa et al., 2001; Megeed et al., 2002; Sershen and West, 2002). Infection is a major concern with clinically available implantable drug delivery pumps, as are catheter-related complications, such as kinking, dislodgements, disconnections, tears, and occlusions (Follet and Naumann, 2000). Poor patient compliance is a significant obstacle that often leads to suboptimal treatment and inferior outcomes (Dew et al., 1999; Baines et al., 2002). These problems could potentially be ameliorated though the use of appropriate implantable drug delivery systems. Implants with degradable polymers suffer from two major drawbacks. Polymer depots exhibit an initial "burst effect" prior to sustained drug release, and typically are not as efficient in controlling the release rates of small molecules (Narasimhan and Langer, 1997). Polymer MicroChips developed by Santini, Cima, and Langer (Santini et al., 1999, 2000, 2003) employ the electrochemical dissolution of the cover of a number of reservoirs to obtain the controlled release of their contents and may yield a desired, and potentially variable, release profile. Recently, these microchips have been demonstrated for the

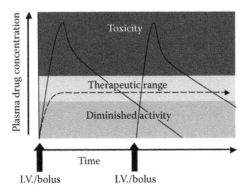

FIGURE 6.2 (See color insert following page 10-24.) Concept of controlled drug delivery. Plasma concentration versus time curve for intravenous drug administration showing first-order kinetics (——). Plasma concentration versus time curve for sustained release profile of zero-order kinetics (- - - -).

controlled pulsatile release of the polypeptide leuprolide from microchip implants over 6 months in dogs (Prescott et al., 2006). However, this device has not been proven capable of providing the zero-order release of the immunomodulating molecules such as interferon.

Ferrari and coworkers introduced the surface and bulk silicon nanomachining protocols for the fabrication of nanopore/nanochannel with exquisite control over pore/channel dimensions and surface composition (Chu et al., 1996; Chu and Ferrari, 1996; Keller and Ferrari, 1997, 1999a, 1999b, 2000; Chu and Ferrari, 1998, 1999a, 1999b, 2000; Chu et al., 1999; Tu and Ferrari, 1999; Tu et al., 1999; Desai et al., 2001). These nanofeatured devices are based on constrained diffusion and controllable electrokinetic transport, and therefore do not lead to any build up of pressure (unlike osmotic pumps) during its use. It is possible to design nanopore/nanochannel substrates, which achieve almost constant rate of drug delivery, avoiding the "burst effect." Therefore, these devices are ideally suited for drug delivery applications, including controlled diffusion and sustained release. By precisely controlling the pore size, pore length, and pore density, the nanoporous membrane fitted with a drug reservoir suitable for subcutaneous implantation can serve as a diffusion barrier for a variety of biological drugs (Desai et al., 1999). Also, these devices do not require the development of novel formulations for the delivery of functionally active molecules (Lesinski et al., 2005). A variety of progressively improved designs of silicon-based nanoporous/nanochannel systems have been developed, patented, and investigated for a range of applications, including bioseparation, immunoisolation, and controlled drug delivery (Desai et al., 2000a, 2000b; Leoni et al., 2002; Sinha et al., 2004; Lesinski et al., 2005; Martin et al., 2005; Walczak et al., 2005; Ferrari et al., 2006).

Recently electrochemically engineered nanopores/nanotube materials such as nanoporous alumina and nanotubular titania have also been explored for drug delivery applications (Losic and Simovic, 2009). Commercially available nanoporous alumina (Anopore) was proposed for the administration of antiangiogenic and antioxidant drugs, with potential clinical application in the treatment of proliferative diabetic retinopathy (PDR) and age-related macular degeneration (AMD) (Orosz et al., 2004). Gong et al. (2003) fabricated nanoporous alumina capsules by anodization of an aluminum tube and tested them for potential drug delivery applications using fluorescein isothiocyanate and dextran conjugates of varying molecular weight. Popat et al. (2004) developed a poly(ethylene) glycol-based surface modification protocol to enhance the biocompatibility of nanoporous alumina that was later tested for immunoisolation applications (La Flamme et al., 2007). Desai and coworkers investigated the efficacy of titania nanotubes as drug-eluting coatings for implantable devices. The nanotubes could be loaded with various amounts of drugs and their release controlled by varying the tube length, diameter, and wall thickness. By varying the amount of proteins loaded into the nanotubes, they were able to control the release rates of bovine serum albumin (BSA) and lysozyme model proteins (Popat et al., 2007). Later they demonstrated the usefulness of titania nanotube platforms of various dimensions for long-term (days-to-weeks) delivery of common small molecule drugs such as sirolimus and paclitaxel (Peng et al., 2009). Vasilev et al. (2010) developed a flexible and facile method for surface modification of titania nanotubes to tailor new interfacial properties important in many biomedical applications. Plasma surface modification using allylamine (AA) as a precursor was applied to generate a thin and chemically reactive polymer (AAPP) film rich in amine groups on top of the titania nanotube surface. This initial polymer film was used for further surface functionalization by the attachment of desired molecules.

6.3 Nanoporous and Nanochannel Microchips for Metastatic Melanoma

The nanoporous/nanochannel silicon microchips, with highly uniform pores in the nanometer range, were first fabricated using standard microfabrication techniques of photolithography, thin film deposition, and selective etching (Desai et al., 1999). Nanopores were generated by a key process step, based on the use of thermally grown sacrificial silicon oxide layer, sandwiched between two structural layers—a process termed "sacrificial oxide nanopore formation" (Chu and Ferrari, 1996; Keller and Ferrari, 1997; Desai et al., 1999; Tu and Ferrari, 1999; Desai et al., 2000b). Over the years, nanopore/ nanochannel technology has undergone continued improvements. Nevertheless, the basic structure and fabrication protocol for the nanopores has remained the same. The membrane area is made of thin layers of polysilicon, silicon dioxide, and/or single crystalline silicon depending on the design employed. The other main part of the membrane is the anisotropically backside etched wafer. Since photolithography in general has a lower limit of resolution of 0.25–1 μm, strategies using sacrificial layers were utilized to achieve desired pore size down to the tens of nanometers. The strategies were initially based on the use of a sacrificial oxide layer, sandwiched between two structural layers, for the definition of the pore pathways. However, all designs of the microfabricated membrane consisted of a surface micromachined membrane on top of an anisotropically etched silicon wafer, which provides mechanical support. Changes in the pore size, density, and geometry as well as path length were the main features changed while optimizing the membrane design.

The first design of nanoporous membranes consisted of a bilayer of polysilicon with L-shaped pore paths. The flow path of fluids and particles through the membrane is shown in Figure 6.3a (Desai et al., 2000a). As shown, fluid enters the pores through openings in the top polysilicon layer, travels laterally through the pores, makes a 90° turn, and exits the pores through the bottom of the pore where both the top and bottom polysilicon layers lay on the etch stop layer. While this design performed well for preventing the diffusion of the larger, unwanted immune system molecules, its L-shaped path slowed down and, in some cases, prevented the diffusion of the smaller molecules of interest. The pores in this design were fairly long, which led to the slow diffusion of the desired molecules. Also, because of the large area per pore, it was difficult to increase the pore density and thus the diffusion rate. The next design had an improvement in the production of short, straight, vertical pores through a single crystal base layer. This design had the advantage of direct flow paths (Figure 6.3b) (Desai et al., 2000a). This

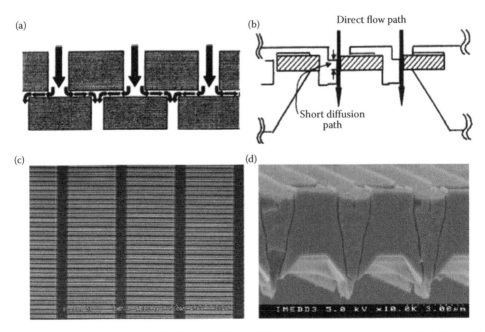

FIGURE 6.3 (a) Flow path through M1 filters, with lateral diffusion through the nanopores defined by sacrificial oxide. (b) Cross-section of M2 design showing direct flow path. Scanning electron micrographs of microfabricated nanoporous membrane; (c) top-view detail; (d) side-view detail. (With kind permission from Springer Science+Business Media: Leoni, L., A. Boiarski, and T. A. Desai, 2002. *Biomed. Microdevices* 4(2):131–139. Copyright 2002.)

direct path allows the smaller molecules of interest to diffuse much quicker through the membrane, while still size-separating the larger molecules. To further improve the reliability of the nanoporous membranes, several basic changes were made in the fabrication protocol from the previous membrane design to eliminate problems with the diffused etch stop layer (Leoni et al., 2002). This design also incorporated a shorter diffusion path length, based on the thicknesses of the two structural layers. The design of a new membrane fabrication protocol incorporated several desired improvements: a well-defined etch stop layer, precise control of pore dimensions, and a lower stress state in the membrane (Figure 6.3c and d). The new protocol also increased the exposed pore area of the membranes. Next generation nanochannel delivery systems (nDS) are based on bulk micromachining and encapsulated-filter design. It consists of two bonded silicon wafers, the micromachined filtration structural wafer, and the cap wafer, providing more mechanical and structural strength to the device (Sinha et al., 2004). Additionally, nDS platform has the capabilities for electronics integration required for preprogrammed- and remote-activated delivery of drugs.

Most recent designs of nanopore/nanochannel technology are: (1) silicon NanoGATE microchips (by iMedd Inc.) and (2) Nanochannel Microchips called Nanochannel Delivery Systems (nDS) will be discussed in detail here with special reference to interferon delivery for melanoma.

6.3.1 NanoGATE Microchips

Improvements in the microfabrication protocols have enabled the development of robust and reproducible method for the mass production of silicon nanoporous microchips of various pores sizes and pore areas of precise dimensions (Figure 6.4a). These nanoporous microchips were especially designed by iMEDD Inc. for their NanoGATE subcutaneously implantable drug delivery device (Martin et al., 2005). The NanoGATE implant is designed to slowly release the encapsulated drug at an optimal rate to mimic a slow infusion, so that the patient will have therapeutic levels of the drug in his/her body for the entire course of therapy. The drug reservoir of the NanoGATE implant contains a highly concentrated form of the drug either as a dry powder or concentrated suspension to minimize the size of the device required to hold the cumulative dose required for an extended period of treatment (e.g., 3–6 months) (Figure 6.4b). NanoGATE technology has been developed to deliver IFN-α for the treatment of metastatic melanoma or chronic hepatitis C (Walczak et al., 2005).

6.3.1.1 Fabrication

Silicon NanoGATE microchips were fabricated using top-down microfabrication methods to create nanopore membranes consisting of arrays of parallel rectangular channels which, in their smallest aspect, range from 7 to 50 nm. The original method pioneered by Ferrari and colleagues (Chu et al., 1999) consists of two basic steps: (1) surface micromachining of nanochannels in a thin film on the top of a silicon wafer, and (2) forming the nanopore membrane by etching away bulk of the silicon wafer underneath the thin-film structure. The overall fabrication process is shown schematically in Figure 6.5.

The first major fabrication process step involves etching channels in the silicon substrate over its entire surface to define the overall shape of the pores (Figure 6.5a). The etched channels are 2 μm wide separated by 2 μm and they are 5 μm deep. These channels are formed using a plasma-etch procedure with a thermally grown oxide layer as an etch-mask. The next major step involves growing a sacrificial oxide layer over the entire wafer surface including the surface area of the channels (Figure 6.5b). The sacrificial-oxide layer thickness defines the channel width in the final membrane. Proper selection of the time and temperature of this thermal oxidation step allows control of the sacrificial layer thickness to tolerances less than 0.5 nm across the entire wafer. Anchor points are created within the channels to define the pore length (45 μm distance). These anchor points are 10 μm long and are formed between each 45-μm long pore region. The anchors provide rigidity to the membrane structure, because there are no pores in the anchor regions. The anchor points are formed across the entire wafer by selectively etching through the sacrificial layer in a series of 10-μm wide strips perpendicular to the channel

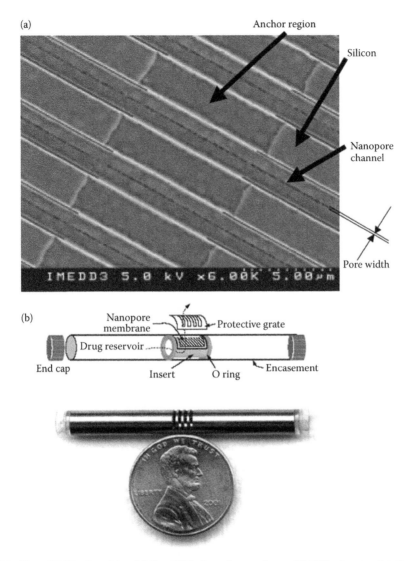

FIGURE 6.4 NanoGATE microchips. (a) Top SEM view of a membrane (6000X), showing details of pore and anchor structures. (b) Implant device fitted with nanoporous microchip. (Top) Drawing illustrating key features of the device. The dashed arrow represents a possible diffusion path of a drug molecule held within the device reservoir. (Bottom) Photograph of prototype implant to scale. (With kind permission from Springer Science+Business Media: Walczak, R. et al., 2005. *Nanobiotechnology* 1(1):35–42. Copyright 2005.)

direction. The next fabrication step involves filling the channels using a polysilicon deposition process (Figure 6.5c). This filling step forms the membrane structure by providing silicon material on each side of the sacrificial oxide layers. The deposition also provides solid silicon–polysilicon areas in the anchor regions to stabilize the membrane. The deposited polysilicon layer is then "planarized" (Figure 6.5d) using a plasma-etch process leaving a smooth surface structure with the pores exposed. Following planarization, a boron-doping step is performed where boron ions are diffused into the surface of the silicon–polysilicon material to a depth of 3 μm (see dashed line in Figure 6.5e). Boron-doped silicon etches in KOH at a much lower rate than un-doped silicon so the boron doping provides an etch-stop that will later define the membrane thickness.

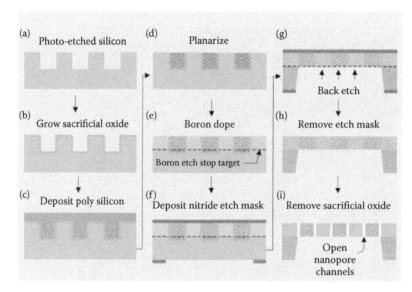

FIGURE 6.5   **(See color insert following page 10-24.)** Schematic of key steps in the silicon nanopore membrane fabrication process. (From Martin, F. et al., 2005. *J. Control. Release* 102:123–133. With permission.)

A protective nitride mask layer is then deposited on the wafer completely covering both sides. This layer is impervious to the KOH chemical etch that will be used to form the membranes out of the silicon substrate. On the back of the wafer, windows are plasma-etched in the nitride layer to define the membrane dimensions. These windows in the protective nitride layer expose the silicon wafer to KOH etchant in the desired regions (Figure 6.5f). The wafer is then placed in a 55°C KOH bath to etch the unprotected silicon through the windows in the nitride and up to the boron etch-stop to form the membrane (Figure 6.5g). After the silicon is removed, the protective nitride etch mask (Figure 6.5h) and sacrificial oxide (Figure 6.5i) are removed using an HF etchant. This final etching step opens the pores and provides the desired nanopore membrane structure.

6.3.1.2 Diffusion Studies

Diffusion kinetics of solutes from a region of higher concentration to a region of lower concentration through a thin, semipermeable membrane generally follows Fick's laws. However, as the sizes of the membrane pores approach that of the solute, unexpected effects can occur, which deviate substantially from those predicted by Fick's laws. Diffusion studies through early design nanoporous membranes indicated that the diffusion rates were slower than predicted from Fick's law for smaller pore sizes membranes (Desai, 2002). To better understand this phenomenon, the relationship between diffusion rates of various solutes (interferon and BSA) and the width of nanoporous membranes was systematically investigated (Martin et al., 2005). A detailed analysis of the diffusion characteristics of various biological molecules revealed that these NanoGATE microchips had the capability of generating a sustained release of drugs for long durations.

6.3.1.2.1 Interferon Release Data

The interferon release profile is shown in Figure 6.6a, the membrane used in the experiment has 20 nm pore size, the initial concentration in the donor well is 4.68 mg/mL, and the Stokes radius of interferon is about 2.3 nm. The solid line has been obtained by simply combining the first Fick's law with the mass conservation principle, and multiplying the mass flux times the total nominal pores area; the resulting diffusion profile, as well known, results to be exponential. The steady-state value is close to 100% of the

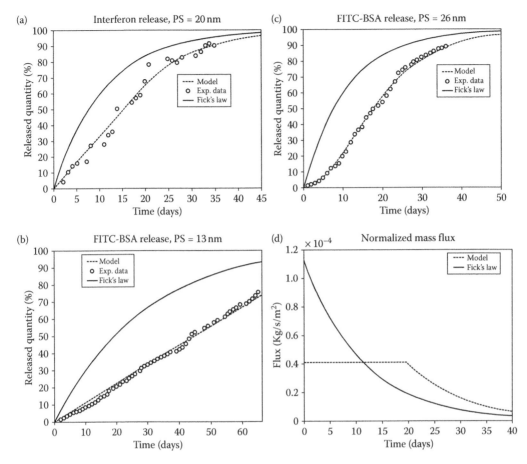

FIGURE 6.6 *In vitro* diffusion kinetics of (a) interferon-α through 20 nm pore size, (b) fluorescein isothiocyanate (FITC) labeled-bovine serum albumin through (b) 13 nm pore size and (c) 26 nm pore size. Experimental data (o), Fick's law prediction (-): experimental data (o), Fick's law prediction. (d) Simulated interferon mass flux through a 20 nm pore size membrane (based on data in Figure 5a): Fick's law prediction (-), model based simulation (- -). (From Martin, F. et al., 2005. *J. Control. Release* 102:123–133. With permission.)

amount of drug loaded into the donor well, because the acceptor well volume is much larger than the donor well; therefore, in order to make the concentration homogeneous on both sides of the membrane, only a little amount of drug has to be retained in the donor well. Looking at the experimental measurements (circle markers), it is fairly clear that, even changing the parameter values with respect to the nominal ones, the experimental diffusion profile could not be explained by Fick's law, because it is not exponential. On the contrary, the release rate keeps constant (zero order kinetics) for a long period (about 25 days), until 75% of the total amount has been released (Martin et al., 2005).

6.3.1.2.2 Bovine Serum Albumin Release Data

Studies on the long-term albumin release from the prototype implant for different amounts (1.4–2.0 mg) of albumin (concentration: 5 mg/mL) were performed using different pore sizes. Virtually, no BSA diffusion was seen through nanopore membranes of 7 nm (data not shown), which would be expected since the hydrodynamic diameter of BSA is about 8 nm. The albumin released through the two nanopore membrane sizes (13 and 26 nm) as a function of time is shown in Figure 6.6b and c. The mass flux was constant in the 13 nm case (Figure 6.6b), and zero-order kinetics was maintained for the whole experiment duration, while the 26 nm test data (Figure 6.6c) showed an exponential release profile. As one would intuitively expect, even with pore sizes greater than 26 nm, BSA diffusion remains Fickian (data not shown). These data indicated that flux could be controlled by porosity and kinetic rate by channel width. Similar profiles were obtained for various model biomolecules and drugs (having MW in the range of 0–200 kDa) such as glucose, lysozyme, and so on (data not shown).

6.3.1.2.3 Modeling and Data Fitting

Strikingly, these data showed that the diffusion from NanoGATE microchips does not follow Fick's law of diffusion for semipermeable membranes. Rather, as the size of the nanopore approaches the molecular dimensions of the diffusant, zero-order kinetics predominate. Thus, by tailoring the nanopore dimension to the physical characteristics of the biological molecule of interest, silicon NanoGATE microchips constrict the ability of the molecule to freely diffuse in all dimensions. Such non-Fickian behavior of diffusant molecules has also been observed in other microporous media such as zeolites and is considered to be a result of phenomena such as traffic control, called single file diffusion (SFD) (Wei et al., 2000; Lin et al., 2000). In order to achieve further insights into the mechanisms involved in nanopore/nanochannel diffusion and to predict drug release without exhaustive experimentation with desired molecules, a dynamical model was developed to analyze the experimental phenomenon in mathematical terms (Cosentino et al., 2005). The main core of the model is constituted by first Fick's law combined with the mass conservation principle. The main hypothesis the model relies upon is that the membrane effect can be mathematically described by means of saturation on the mass flux, where the threshold is intuitively dependent on the nanochannel width and molecular dimensions. The simulated mass flux (using Intereon release data in Figure 6.6a) is depicted in Figure 6.6d, along with the same quantity obtained from a simulation of the free (Fickian) diffusion case, with the same parameters values. Clearly, the flux at the beginning assumes the highest value, because the concentration gradient is maximum. Assuming a saturation level below this maximum value, results in a constant flux for a certain time interval. The switch from a constant to an exponentially decreasing profile occurs when the concentration gradient becomes so low that the flux value is less than or equal to the fixed threshold (drag effect). This model makes it possible to simulate the release profiles for a particular drug molecule for a particular microchip pore size. A detailed investigation and description of this model is presented elsewhere (Cosentino et al., 2005). Whether a consequence of SFD-like phenomena or potential drag effects (or a combination of both), the NanoGATE microchip is diffusion rate-limiting and, if properly tuned, restricts solute mobility. Thus, by strictly controlling the oxide deposition during the fabrication process of the nanoporous microchip, it is possible to custom generate an exact pore size that will permit zero-order release for virtually any molecule of interest.

6.3.1.3 *In Vivo* Bioavailability Testing

In order to capitalize on the constrained diffusion feature offered by these nanoporous membranes, their utility as a means of controlling the bioavailability of a protein *in vivo* was also tested (Martin et al., 2005). Devices fitted with 13 nm membranes and filled with 300 μL of a solution containing 0.15 mg of 125I-BSA were implanted subcutaneously on the backs of three rats. The devices were adjusted to have an *in vitro* output rate of 15 μg/day and thus were designed to release the albumin for about 100 days. The pharmacokinetics of the labeled BSA in blood was measured and compared to a dose of BSA delivered by a standard subcutaneous bolus injection. Figure 6.7 shows the mean values for blood levels over a period of 45 days after implantation. In the case of the NanoGATE implant group, following an initial period of rapid decline (during the first 9 days), the rate of clearance of BSA from the central compartment slowed, maintaining measurable levels for the ensuing 4 weeks. The initial decline is attributed to the equilibration of the radiolabeled BSA appearing in blood with the albumin pool in the interstitial fluid volume. This equilibration has been reported to have a half-life of about 3–7 days, which is in line

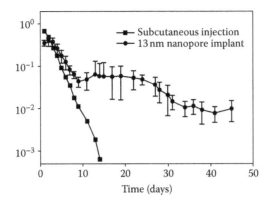

FIGURE 6.7 Pharmacokinetics of ^{125}I-BSA in rats given as a single bolus subcutaneous injection (■) or following implantation of nanopore devices with an *in vitro* output rate of 15 μg/day (▲). Mean values for three implants and standard deviation are plotted. (From Martin, F. et al., 2005. *J. Control. Release* 102:123–133. With permission.)

with the results (Spiess et al., 1996). In comparison to the standard subcutaneous injection, BSA delivered in the nanopore device was detectable for a substantially longer period. As expected, when the devices were recovered from experimental animals, they were encapsulated in a fibrous capsule, but upon visual inspection the nanopore membrane itself was free of any tissue intrusion. The encapsulation response did not appear to retard the bioavailability of the albumin released from the device; about half the labeled albumin was recovered from the nanopore device, which conforms to the expectation that half the drug was released during the 7-week implantation period.

6.3.1.4 Long-Term Biofouling and Biocompatibility Studies

The material–tissue interaction that results from the device implantation is one of the major obstacles in developing viable, long-term implantable drug delivery systems. Membrane biofouling is a process that starts immediately upon contact of a device with the body when cells, proteins, and other biological components adhere to the surface, and in some cases, impregnate the pores of the material (Wisniewski et al., 2001). Not only does biofouling of the membrane impede drug diffusion (i.e., release) from the implant causing reduced therapeutic levels of drug in the patient's blood stream, it is believed that the adhering proteins are one of the main factors that modulate the longer term cellular and/or fibrous encapsulation response (Ratner et al., 1996).

The site and the extent of injury created in the implantation, biomaterial chemical composition, surface free energy, surface charge, porosity, roughness, and implant size and shape, all govern the degree of fibrosis and vascularization (Babensee et al., 1998). A thin fibrous tissue reaction may have a negligible diffusion resistance relative to the membrane itself. In contrast, a granular tissue reaction would include vascular structures to facilitate the delivery of therapeutic products. A thin tissue of high vascularity can be induced with membranes of particular porosities or architectures, or with membranes coated with biocompatible polymers.

Polymeric membranes commonly used for drug delivery applications do not have all the desired "ideal" membrane properties such as stability, biocompatibility, and well-controlled permselectivity. Moreover, these membranes do not allow the passage of desired biomolecules without biological fouling over a period of time. The straight pore architecture of micromachined nanoporous membranes as opposed to the tortuous-path associated with polymeric membranes offers better antifouling behavior (Desai et al., 2000b). In addition, the silicon surface chemistry itself does not promote mineralization associated with other membrane materials (Desai et al., 1995). Furthermore, the silicon membranes can be coupled with protein-resistant molecules to improve biocompatibility (Sharma et al., 2002).

A key component of NanoGATE implant is a microfabricated silicon nanopore membrane engineered to the exact size and requirements of the individual molecule. Therefore, long-term biocompatibility of NanoGATE implant in terms of the biofouling of the nanopore membrane and the extent of formation of a fibrotic tissue capsule around the implant was systematically investigated.

6.3.1.5 Long-Term Lysozyme Diffusion Studies

In vivo and *in vitro* release of a model drug, lysozyme (MW = 14.4 kDa), from a NanoGATE implant was systematically investigated (Walczak et al., 2005). The goal was to determine whether a correlation existed between *in vivo* and *in vitro* drug diffusion kinetics from similar implant populations. Establishing such a correlation would be useful for determining the effects of fibrotic tissue capsule on drug release kinetics. The choice of lysozyme as a model drug was prompted by the fact that its molecular weight is very close to the molecular weight to IFN-α (MW = 19.2 kDa), a drug of interest for NanoGATE implant therapy.

A solution of ^{125}I-labeled lysozyme was loaded into several NanoGATE implants at a concentration of 5 mg/mL and investigated *in vivo* using a rat model. This concentration resulted in an initial delivery of 20 μg per day of ^{125}I-labeled lysozyme using a 13 nm silicon nanopore membrane. The implants were analyzed for lysozyme release rates for several days prior to surgical implantation. The blood concentration level of lysozyme released from NanoGATE implants is shown in Figure 6.8a. In each case, a single-phase pattern existed for lysozyme levels as represented by a distinct zone of slowly decreasing plasma concentration with time after implantation. In contrast, blood samples from

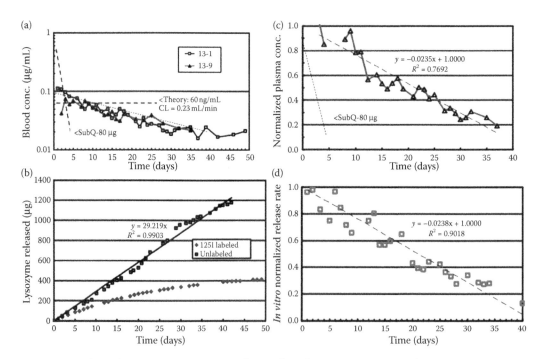

FIGURE 6.8 (a) ^{125}I-lysozyme concentration in plasma of rats for two NanoGATE implants (13–1 and 13–9) initially releasing 20 μg/day (*in vivo*), (b) *in vitro* diffusion of ^{125}I-lysozyme and unlabeled lysozyme, (c) ^{125}I-lysozyme *in vivo* normailized plasma concentration as a function of time, (d) ^{125}I-lysozyme *in vitro* normalize d release rate as a function of time. (With kind permission from Springer Science+Business Media: Walczak, R. et al., 2005. *Nanobiotechnology* 1(1): 35–42. Copyright 2005.)

control rats administered with a bolus subcutaneous dose (80 µg) showed radiolabeled lysozyme levels declining rapidly with time (Figure 6.8a). The initial lysozyme plasma concentration of 100 ng/mL agreed well with the predicted value of 60 ng/mL calculated using a clearance, CL, value of 0.23 mL/min. This CL value was calculated from the subcutaneous injection data using standard pharmacokinetic modeling techniques (Lave et al., 1995). Ideally, the plasma levels of the drug should remain constant at the predicted level for the entire duration of the experiment. Nevertheless, as shown in Figure 6.8, the plasma levels did not stay at the predicted level, and fell to ~20 ng/mL after 40 days *in vivo*. This slow decrease in lysozyme level in the bloodstream could have been associated with fibrotic capsule formation and biofouling, but further investigations indicated that this was not the case.

A long-term *in vitro* diffusion study was carried out using ^{125}I-labeled and unlabeled lysozyme in order to compare the *in vivo* lysozyme plasma levels to *in vitro* release data (Figure 6.8b). Data in Figure 6.7b show that the initial rate of *in vitro* diffusion of ^{125}I-labeled lysozyme was 20 µg/day, but the rate decreased with time, suggesting that ^{125}I-labeled lysozyme did not diffuse from the implant with zero-order kinetics. In contrast, unlabeled lysozyme diffused from NanoGATE implants containing 13 nm pore at a constant rate of 29 µg/day consistent with zero-order kinetics. These *in vitro* results suggest that the radiolabeled lysozyme undergoes some sort of structural rearrangement during the course of experiment, possibly forming aggregates (dimers, trimers) with higher molecular weight than the original, monomeric lysozyme. This inference was further supported by size-exclusion chromatography (data not shown). This established that the time-dependent aggregation of radiolabeled lysozyme reduced the diffusion rate over a period of time resulting in lower than expected levels of ^{125}I-lysozyme detected in the rat plasma.

In order to derive a correlation between the *in vivo* plasma levels of ^{125}I-lysozyme (Figure 6.8a) and the *in vitro* release rate of the radiolabeled material (Figure 6.8b), calculations were performed to determine how the slope of the two plots changed with time. The average plasma concentration, C, from the two implanted devices (Figure 6.8a) was divided by the initial plasma concentration, C_0, at time zero, and these normalized concentrations are shown in Figure 6.8c. The daily *in vitro* ^{125}I-lysozyme release rates (µg/day) were derived from total released amounts shown in Figure 6.8b, that is, the profile shows the normalized release rates (i.e., the ratio of the daily rate, Rate, divided by the initial rate, $Rate_0$) of 20 µg/day. The slopes in Figures 6.8c and d are nearly identical indicating that there exists a good *in vitro/in vivo* correlation for the ^{125}I-labeled lysozyme diffusion from a NanoGATE implant. This also implies that the tissue capsule surrounding the implant surface does not have any deleterious effects on lysozyme diffusion from the implant for a period of 40 days.

6.3.1.6 *In Vivo* Biocompatibility Evaluation

In vivo membrane biocompatibility was evaluated using glucose as a model molecule. Glucose being relatively small molecule (180 Da) can be used for a broad range of pore sizes (7–50 nm) and analyzed using very quick, already established, and easy to perform assay procedures. *In vivo* NanoGATE microchip biocompatibility data demonstrated that even after 6-month implantation, the glucose release rates through these microchips remain unchanged, illustrating that these microchips did not foul over the implantation duration (Figure 6.9a) (Walczak et al., 2005). Figure 6.9b shows a photograph of the implant site after 30 days of implantation in a rodent model. As it can be seen, only a thin vascular capsule forms around the implant as opposed to the avascular fibrous capsule a major problem for any subcutaneously implanted device. Thus, the lack of any diffusion retardation along with the ability to minimize fibrous encapsulation at the site of implantation suggested that the NanoGATE device is highly impervious to diffusion fouling events *in vivo*, permitting long-term biocompatibility for delivery of small molecules like glucose. Further, postimplantation diffusion studies were performed using two model biomolecules, namely bovine serum albumin (MW = 66 kDa) and hen egg white lysozyme (MW = 14.4 kDa) (Figure 6.9c). These data indicated that for large biomolecules like

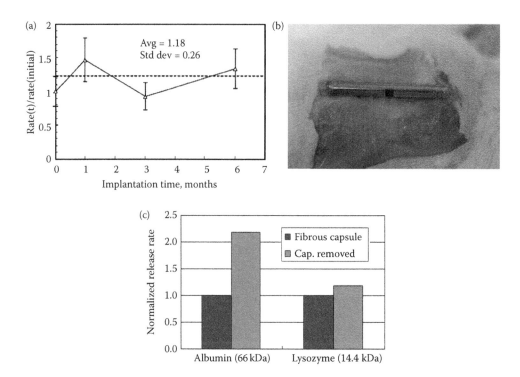

FIGURE 6.9 (See color insert following page 10-24.) (a) Ratio of pre- and postimplantation glucose diffusion rates from the NanoGATE device. (b) *Ex vivo* analysis of implanted devices after the sacrifice of a rat. Note the lack of tissue attachment to both the Ti shell, Si device, and polymethyl methacrylate plugs in device. (c) Postimplantation diffusion testing (with and without tissue capsule). The normalized release rates were obtained by dividing the biomolecular release rates from the implant before and after the tissue capsule was removed from the implant surface after explantation. (With kind permission from Springer Science+Business Media: Walczak, R. et al., 2005. *Nanobiotechnology* 1(1): 35–42. Copyright 2005.)

albumin, the diffusion rate doubles once the tissue capsule is removed, indicating that the presence of the fibrotic capsule resulted in lower diffusion rates for albumin. However, for a smaller biomolecule like lysozyme, there was only a 10% increase in diffusion rate from the implant once the tissue capsule is removed, suggesting that the presence of fibrotic capsule has only a small effect on lysozyme diffusion. These results clearly indicated that the fibrotic tissue capsule surrounding the implant should not impede the diffusion of IFN-α (MW = 19.2 kDa) from the NanoGATE implant (Walczak et al., 2005). Previously it was demonstrated that nanostructured PEG thin films could enhance the biocompatibility and biofouling resistance properties of silicon nanoporous membranes (Sharma, 2002; Sharma et al., 2002, 2004). This suggests that this surface modification strategy could further augment the long-term biocompatibility of NanoGATE implants enabling better release rates for larger biomolecules.

The NanoGATE microchips described here are advantageous for a wide variety of drugs classes as potential therapeutic candidates where a long-term sustained release is desired. Peptides and protein drugs are excellent choices for use in the current system, due to both the nonfouling nature of the membrane as well as its immunoisolation properties. By increasing pore area, small, potent bioactive molecules can also be used within the NanoGATE system. Finally, by increasing pore size, nucleic acid derivative become likely therapeutic candidates. Nevertheless, this design lacks the capabilities for the development of microchips for preprogrammed- and remote-activated delivery of drugs for drug-on demand.

6.3.2 Nanochannel (nDS) Microchips

Most recently, nDS microchips with improved mechanical stability were developed by Ferrari and coworkers (Sinha et al., 2004). These devices are based on bulk micromachining and sandwich encapsulated filter design (Tu et al., 1999; Sinha et al., 2004). The nDS device consists of two bonded wafers: the micromachined filtration structural wafer and the cap wafer (Figure 6.10a and b). Fluids enter through the hole etched in the cap wafer, then flow horizontally through the filtration channel as defined by the gap between the cap wafer and the machined features on the structural wafer, and then out the hole etched in the structural wafer. Since the flow is between two directly bonded wafers, the filter has more mechanical support and is thus structurally stronger. The features on the structural wafer are shown in Figure 6.9a and b and are fabricated using bulk micromachining (Sinha et al., 2004). To achieve high throughputs, interdigitated finger geometry was used. With the use of a silicon dioxide sacrificial layer, pore sizes as small as 20 nm were fabricated with size variations less than 4%. It was already established in the case of other types of silicon nanoporous microchips that the diffusion of molecules though nanopores is constant, and therefore, the sandwich design filter could also be used for sustained drug delivery applications. The first device in this proposed sequence of nDS is the passive release device called nDS1. Other embodiments of nDS microchips have the capability of integration of electronics on board, and are being developed for preprogrammed- (electroosmotically driven, nDS2) and remote-activated (drug on demand, nDS3) delivery of drugs. An applied electrical current across the electrodes controls the electrokinetic flow of molecules of interest through this device. The connected external circuit can be a preprogrammable circuit, a wireless circuit or a feedback control circuit for a biological sensor, to achieve preferred control of drug release.

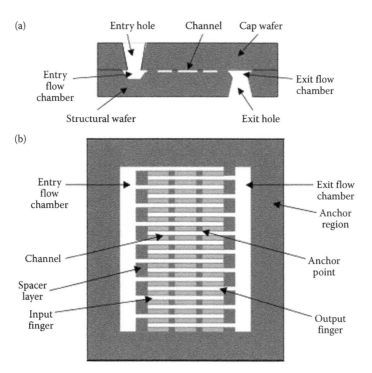

FIGURE 6.10 Nanochannel microchips. (a) Cross-sectional view of the nDS; (b) Top and cross-sectional view of nDS structure on the structural wafer. (Reprinted with permission from IOP Publishing Ltd.: Sinha, P. et al., 2004. *Nanotechnology* 15:S585–S589. Copyright 2004.)

6.3.2.1 Fabrication

6.3.2.1.1 Nanochannel Delivery System

Passive release device (nDS1). Nanochannels were formed between the two silicon substrates by growing and subsequently etching an oxide layer (called sacrificial oxide) in nDS1. Detailed fabrication protocol for nDS device is described elsewhere (Sinha et al., 2004). Briefly, the overall fabrication process can be divided into three major steps: (1) bottom substrate processing, (2) top substrate processing, and (3) wafer bonding and packaging. Double-side polished <100> single-crystal 4 silicon wafers were used for fabrication. Figure 6.11 shows the process for bottom substrate fabrication. In the first step, the entry flow chamber, exit flow chamber, and the fingers were photolithographically defined and etched into silicon using 0.5 μm thick oxide as a mask for the etching. The oxide mask layer was then removed using a concentrated hydrofluoric acid (HF) solution. Photolithography was also used to define nanochannel regions. Low stress low pressure chemical vapor deposition (LPCVD) silicon nitride was used as a mask. The nanochannel regions in the mask layer were photolithographically defined and selectively etched. The unetched regions protected by the nitride became the anchor points and the spacer regions. Next, a sacrificial layer with thickness T was grown using a thermal oxidation process that consumed substrate silicon from the channel region. This oxide was etched at the end of the bottom substrate fabrication. This resulted in lowering of the surface of the channel region with respect to the surface of the rest of the channel ridge, including the anchor points, thereby defining the height of the channel (H). The height H is related to the thickness T of the sacrificial oxide by the relationship: $H = 0.46 \times T$. The dry oxidation process provides a sacrificial oxide with a precisely controlled thickness. The exit port was formed on the back of the bottom substrate. A second layer of low stress LPCVD nitride was deposited to protect the sacrificial oxide. An opening in the nitride on the back was photolithographically defined and

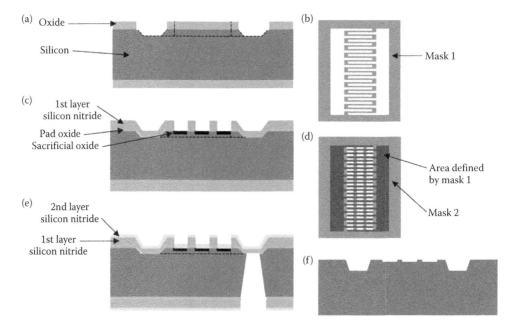

FIGURE 6.11   (See color insert following page 10-24.) Nanochannel microchip fabrication: (a) Cross-sectional view demonstrating steps in the fabrication process. (b) Plan of mask 1, defining flow chambers and fingers. (c) Nanochannels and anchor points. (d) Plan of mask 2, defining nanochannels and anchor points. (e) Nanochannels protected by second layer of nitride and exit port (deep etch). (f) Complete bottom substrate fabrication. (With kind permission from Springer Science+Business Media: Lesinski, G. B. et al., 2005. *Biomed. Microdevices* 7(1): 71–79. Copyright 2005.)

etched. The exit port was deeply etched, in 45 wt% KOH:H_2O solution heated at 80°C, through the silicon substrate to reach the exit flow chamber. The nitride mask and sacrificial oxide were then removed using concentrated HF solution. The entry port was formed in the top silicon substrate. Low stress LPCVD silicon nitride was used as a mask for the deep etch process. An opening was photolithographically defined and etched in the mask. The silicon was then etched completely through to form the entry port. The mask layer was stripped afterwards in concentrated HF. The processed top substrate was then bonded to the processed bottom substrate using silicon–silicon fusion bonding. The wafers were annealed in nitrogen ambient at 1050°C for 4 h to strengthen the bond. Using this method, the thickness can be controlled within ±1 nm. The overall device dimensions were chosen to be 4 mm × 3 mm × 1 mm (Figure 6.12a). Prior to bonding, the nanochannels were characterized using AFM and determined the step height from the channel to the anchor point (size of the nanochannel once the bottom substrate is bonded to the top substrate) to be 100 nm (Figure 6.12b) (Lesinski et al., 2005). Figure 6.12c shows an infrared (IR) image of the bonded wafers, illustrating the entry port, exit port, and features in between the two. It is not possible to resolve all the features at this magnification; however, these features include the input finger, output finger, nanochannels, and anchor points. Figure 6.12d shows an scanning electron microscopy (SEM) image of the top surface of the bottom substrate, showing the fingers, the nanochannel regions, and the spacer region. The image was taken at ×6k magnification. The nanochannels are between two fingers (input finger and output finger), and each finger is blocked by a spacer

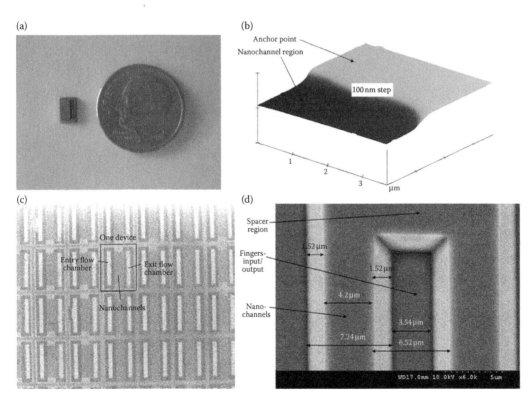

FIGURE 6.12 (a) Photograph of the nDS1 device, (b) AFM image of a 100 nm step in bottom substrate (scan size: 3.679 μm; scan rate: 1.001 Hz). (c) IR image of bonded silicon wafers. One device is outlined showing the entry port, exit port, and the features in between. This includes input fingers, output fingers, anchor points, and nanochannels, (d) scanning electron microscope (SEM) image of top surface of the bottom substrate showing input/output fingers, nanochannel regions, and spacer layer. The image was taken at ×6k magnification. (Reprinted with permission from IOP Publishing Ltd.: Sinha, P. et al., 2004. *Nanotechnology* 15:S585–S589. Copyright 2004.)

region at the end. The wall slope in the finger region is a result of the crystallographically selective nature of the KOH etch (Sinha et al., 2004).

6.3.2.1.2 Nanochannel Delivery System—Passive Release Device-Glass Top (nDS1g)

Further design improvements in nDS1 device included replacing silicon cap wafer with a glass wafer (nDS1g) (Figure 6.13a). With a transparent glass top, one can visually check defects, void bonding, or blocked channels, that is, they allow a good quality control. This also simplified the fabrication process as anodic bonding of silicon–glass cap is much easier and efficient as compared to silicon–silicon cap direct bonding. The design and fabrication details of this device are described elsewhere (Sinha, 2005). These devices also facilitate nano-fluidics study by means of fluorescent microscopy. Figure 6.13b shows a photo micrograph of a bonded nDS1g device. Anchor points, input/output fingers, and nanochannels can be seen through the glass top substrate. In order to see the wetting through the nanochannels iso-propyl-alcohol (IPA) was flowed through the 100 nm channel and the fluid front was photographed (Figure 6.13c). Such visual inspection of features and fluid flow inside an nDS-glass top device enables real-time monitoring of drug diffusion processes through nanochannels.

6.3.2.1.3 Nanochannel Delivery System—Manipulable Release Device (nDS2)

The nDS2 device was conceptualized to achieve a manipulable release profile in drug therapy. An electrode was integrated into this device. An applied current across the electrodes controls the

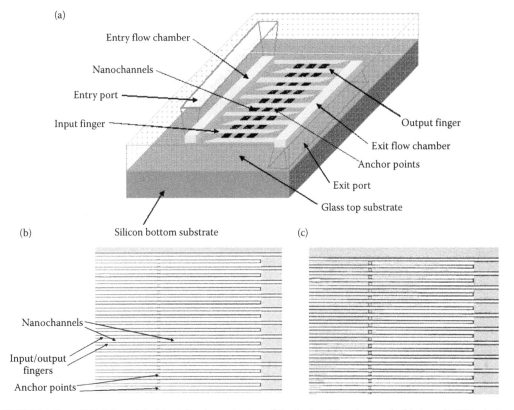

FIGURE 6.13 nDS1g Microchip: (a) a 3-D schematic view of the device, (b) a picture of a fabricated nDS1g device showing anchor points, input/output fingers, and nanochannels. These features can be seen through the glass-top substrate, (c) a fluid front showing Iso-propyl-alcohol (IPA) flow through an nDS1g device. The color shadow in the nanochannels is the moving fluid front. (Reprinted from Sinha, P. M. 2005. Nanoengineered implantable devices for controlled drug delivery, Ph.D. Thesis, The Ohio State University. With permission.)

electrokinetic flow of molecules of interest through this device. These electrodes could be connected to an external circuit that can be a pre-programmable circuit, a wireless circuit, or a feedback control circuit for a biological response (Sinha, 2005). A schematic diagram of an nDS2 device is shown in Figure 6.14a. These devices are made up of a bottom silicon substrate and a top glass substrate. The bottom substrate has many similar features to the nDS1 device. In addition to the advantages mentioned earlier, use of a top glass substrate in nDS2 provides insulation. Electrodes are integrated in the top glass substrate, and the insulating properties of glass prevents any short-circuit between the two electrodes. As with nDS1 and nDS1g the nanochannels exist between the two bonded wafer surfaces. A top view of the device is shown in Figure 6.14b. Locations of three cross sections are marked as A, B, and C in this figure. Cross-sectional views at these locations are shown in Figure 6.14c. Cross-section A shows the internal features including entry/exit flow chambers, input/output fingers, nanochannels, anchor points, anchor regions, and spacer regions. Cross-section B shows the glass seal around the electrodes to prevent fluid leaking from the entry/exit flow chambers to the contact pad regions. Cross-section C shows the bonding pad regions. The top substrate has electrode contact chambers that are fabricated to expose the electrodes to the fluid. These chambers are aligned with the entry and exit flow chambers on the bottom silicon substrate. The top glass substrate also has an entry port that is etched all the way through the wafer, and aligns with one of the electrode contact chambers. The bottom substrate contains the rest of the features. The nanochannel height and applied current between the electrodes define the delivery rate. The design and fabrication details of this device are described elsewhere (Sinha, 2005).

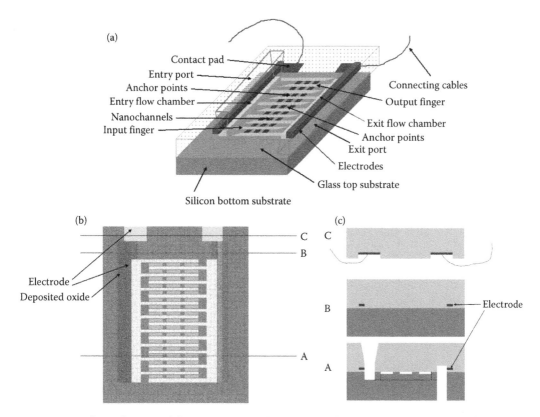

FIGURE 6.14 **(See color insert following page 10-24.)** nDS2 Microchip: (a) a 3-D schematic view of the device, (b) a top view of the device. There are three cross-section locations marked as A, B, and C in this figure, cross-sectional views at these locations are shown in (c). (Reprinted from Sinha, P. M. 2005. Nanoengineered implantable devices for controlled drug delivery, Ph.D. Thesis, The Ohio State University. With permission.)

6.3.2.2 Diffusion Studies

Diffusion characteristics of nDS1 were initially investigated using glucose as a model molecule. These studies suggested that these devices (60 nm and 100 nm channel size) permit the release of glucose in a linear fashion, in accordance with "zero-order" kinetics for the period investigated (Sinha et al., 2004; Lesinski et al., 2005). Figure 6.15a shows glucose release profile from a 100 nm device. Next, it was tested whether the pore size (100 nm) of the nDS devices would permit the diffusion of functionally active IFN-α. For this, diffusion chambers containing the nDS were mounted on individual wells of a Costar Transwell plate, to which a solution containing 19 μg/mL IFN-α (equivalent to 5.94×1011 μM) was added. Plates were incubated at room temperature with gentle shaking. Aliquots from the bottom chamber of the Costar Transwell plate were removed daily (days 0–7), snap frozen and stored at $-80°C$ until they were analyzed for IFN-α content by commercial ELISA (R&D Systems, Inc.). Release profile for IFN-α also demonstrated sustained release for the period investigated (Figure 6.15b). Further studies using phosphorylated STAT1 (P-STAT1) as a marker of IFN-α activity in viable PBMCs and tumor cells confirmed that functionally active IFN-α could diffuse through the nDS1 microchip. By way of comparison, subcutaneous administration of IFN-α-2b (3 M IU/m^2) to a melanoma patient resulted in an Fsp of 1.56 in PBMCs harvested 1 h posttherapy (Figure 6.16). This suggested that nDS microchips used in this study were capable of administering physiologically relevant doses of IFN-α directly to

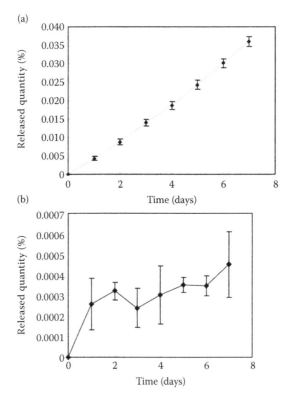

FIGURE 6.15 (a) Release profiles from nDS mounted in Costar diffusion chambers mounted on the wells of a transwell plate. Glucose release (depicted as percent released) was measured on a daily basis using the Glucose-SL assay (Diagnostic Chemicals Limited) for 7 days. Data shown were derived from experiments utilizing three independent devices; (b) IFN-α release from the nDS. The release profile was measured as explained above and quantitated by a commercially available IFN-α ELISA (R & D Systems). Data shown were derived from experiments using three independent devices. (With kind permission from Springer Science+Business Media: Lesinski, G. B. et al., 2005. *Biomed. Microdevices* 7(1): 71–79. Copyright 2005.)

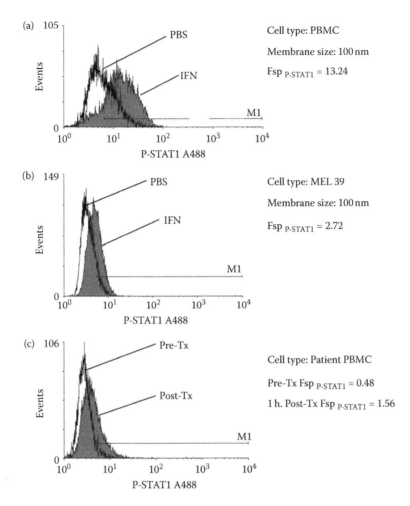

FIGURE 6.16 IFN-α diffuses through nDS and exhibits functional activity. (a, b) The functional ability of IFN-α released from the nDS was confirmed by measuring P-STAT1 in PBMCs or MEL 39 tumor cells in the bottom well of transwell plates mounted with Costar diffusion chambers containing the nDS (as shown in Figure 16.5). Clear histograms represent PBS-treated PBMCs and shaded histograms represent PBMCs responding to IFN-α diffusing through the nDS. (c) P-STAT1 levels in PBMCs of a patient with malignant melanoma harvested immediately before and 1 hour after subcutaneous administration of 3 M IU/m² of IFN-α2b. The M1 marker denotes the measured region, which was set based on a background staining from an isotype control antibody. All data were derived from at least 10,000 events gated on the lymphocyte population. (With kind permission from Springer Science+Business Media: Lesinski, G. B. et al., 2005. *Biomed. Microdevices* 7(1): 71–79. Copyright 2005.)

the tumor microenvironment, and therefore, could be used to develop alternative strategies for the treatment of unresectable tumors (Lesinski et al., 2005). It is also important to mention here that IFN-α used for these studies was the same that is used for IV injections in clinical practice.

Nanochannel microchips described here have the capability of integration of electronics on board and, therefore, can be used for pre-programmed and remote-activated (drug on demand) delivery of drugs. Further, this technology offers advantages in the scalability of the manufacturing process and exquisite device reproducibility. Additionally, these systems do not require the development of novel formulations for drugs. Therefore, already approved FDA formulations can be used in these devices potentially resulting in faster clinic translation of this technology. Commercial development of this technology for therapeutic use is currently being done by NanoMedical Systems (Houston, TX).

6.4 Concluding Remarks

Metastatic melanoma has remained refractory to systemic treatment for decades. A single agent or combination chemotherapy or new agents or biologic response modifiers alone have not resulted in response rates of durable remissions that are high enough to affect median survival (Mouawad, 2009). Despite encouraging data from phase-II trials, no agent or regimen has yet shown improvement in overall survival in phase-III trials. There is an urgent need to develop new innovative treatment options that utilize the recent advancements in nanotechnology and controlled drug delivery. Nanoparticle-based therapeutics enhance anticancer effects compared with the therapeutic entities they contain due to more specific targeting to tumor tissues, via improved pharmacokinetics and pharmacodynamics, and active intracellular delivery. Nanoporous/nanochannel microchips provide an invaluable platform for controlled local or systemic delivery of drugs/immunomodulators, either alone or in combination. nDS microchips have the capability of integration of electronics on board and, therefore, can be used for preprogrammed- and remote-activated (drug on demand) delivery of drugs. Additionally, these platforms could use the already available FDA-approved formulations. Such simplification could help in the transition of this technology to clinic. Furthermore, these microchips can also be combined with nanoparticles/nanocarriers to achieve even better therapeutic benefits. We anticipate that the use of these nano-enabled platforms in standard clinical practice would have significant impact on metastatic malignant melanoma treatment and cure.

References

American Cancer Society. *Cancer Facts and Figures 2009.* American Cancer Society, Atlanta, GA.

Asadullah, K., W., Sterry, and U. Trefzer, 2002. Cytokines: Interleukin and interferon therapy in dermatology. *Clin. Exp. Dermatol.* 27(7):578–584.

Atkins, M. B., M. T. Lotze, J. P. Dutcher, R .I. Fisher, G. Weiss, K. Margolin, J. Abrams, et al., 1999. High-dose recombinant interleukin 2 therapy for patients with metastatic melanoma: Analysis of 270 patients treated between 1985 and 1993. *J. Clin. Oncol.* 17:2105–2116.

Babensee, J. E., J. M. Anderson, L.V. McIntire, and A. G. Mikos, 1998. Host response to tissue engineered devices. *Adv. Drug Deliv. Rev.* 33:111–139.

Baines, L. S., J. T. Joseph, and R. M. Jindal, 2002. Compliance and late acute rejection after kidney transplantation: A psychomedical perspective. *Clin. Transpl.* 16:69–73.

Balch, C. M., 1998. *Biologic Therap.* Quality Medical Publishing, St. Louis, p. 419.

Belardelli, F., M. Ferrantini, E. Proietti, and J. M. Kirkwood, 2002. Interferon-alpha in tumor immunity and immunotherapy. *Cytokine Growth Factor Rev.* 13:119–134.

Belli, F., A. Testori, L. Rivoltini, M. Maio, G. Andreola, M. R. Sertoli, G. Gallino, et al., 2002. Vaccination of metastatic melanoma patients with autologous tumor-derived heat shock protein gp96–peptide complexes: Clinical and immunologic findings. *J. Clin. Oncol.* 20:4169–4180.

Boudes, P., 1998. Drug compliance in therapeutic trials: A review. *Controlled Clinical Trials* 19: 257–268.

Breimer, D. D., 1999. Future challenges for drug delivery. *J. Controlled Release* 62(1–2): 3–6.

Bukowski, R., M. S. Ernstoff, M. E. Gore, J. J. Nemunaitis, R. Amato, S. K. Gupta, and C. L. Tendler, 2002. Pegylated interferon a-2b treatment for patients with solid tumors: A phase I/II study. *J. Clin. Oncol.* 20:3841–3849.

Cao, X., S. Lai, and L. J. Lee, 2001. Design of a self-regulated drug delivery device. *Biomed. Microdev.* 3(2):109–118.

Chu, W. H., R. Chin, T. Huen, and M. Ferrari, 1999. Silicon membrane nanofilters from sacrificial oxide removal. *Journal of Microelectromech. Systems* 8:34–42.

Chu, W. H. and M. Ferrari, 1996. Micromachined capsules having porous membranes and bulk supports. US Patent No. 5,770,076.

Chu, W. H. and M. Ferrari, 1998. Microfabricated filter with specially constructed channel walls, and containment well and capsule constructed with such filters, US Patent No. 5,798,042.

Chu, W. H. and M. Ferrari, 1999a. Method for forming a filter, U.S. Patent No. 5,985,164.

Chu, W. H. and M. Ferrari, 1999b. Micromachined porous membranes with bulk support, US Patent No. 5,985,328.

Chu, W. H. and M. Ferrari, 2000. Microfabricated filter with specially constructed channel walls, and containment well and capsule constructed with such filters, U.S. Patent No. 6,044,981.

Chu, W., T. Huen, J. Tu, and M. Ferrari, 1996. Silicon-micromachined direct pore filters for ultrafiltration. *Proceedings of the SPIE* 2978:111–122.

Cosentino, C., F. Amato, A. Boiarski, R. Walczak, and M. Ferrari, 2005. A dynamic model of biomolecules diffusion through two-dimensional nanochannels. *J. Phys. Chem. B.* 109(15):7358–7364.

Davis, M. E., Z. Chen, and D. M. Shin, 2008. Nanoparticle therapeutics: An emerging treatment modality for cancer. *Nat. Rev. Drug Discov.* 7:771–782.

Desai, T. A., D. J. Hansford, and M. Ferrari, 2000a. Micromachined interfaces: New approaches in cell immunoisolation and biomolecular separation. *Biomol. Eng.* 17:23–36.

Desai, T. A., D. J. Hansford, L. Kulinsky, A. H. Nashat, G. Rasi, J. Tu, Y. Wang, M. Zhang, and M. Ferrari, 1999. Nanopore technology for biomedical applications. *Biomed. Microdev.* 2(1):11–40.

Desai, T. A., D. J. Hansford, L. Leoni, M. Essenpreis, and M. Ferrari, 2000b. Nanoporous anti-fouling silicon membranes for biosensor applications. *Biosens. Bioelectron.*15:453–462.

Desai, T. A., M. Ferrari, and D. Hansford, 2001. Implantable analyte sensor, International Patent No. PCT/ EP01/03027.

Desai, T. A., M. Ferrari, and G. Mazzoni, 1995. Silicon microimplants: Fabrication and biocompatibility. *Materials and Design Technology*, Kozik, T. (ed.) ASME, NewYork, pp. 97–103.

Desai, T. A., 2002. Microfabrication technology for pancreatic cell encapsulation. *Expert Opin. Biol. Therap.* 2:633–646.

Dew, M. A., R. L. Kormos, L. H. Roth, S. Murali, A. DiMartini, and B. P. Griffith, 1999. Early post-transplant medical compliance and mental health predict physical morbidity and mortality one to three years after heart transplantation. *J. Heart Lung Transpl.* 18(6):549–562.

Dewey, W. C., L. E. Hopwood, L. A. Sapareto, and L.E. Gerweck, 1977. Cellular responses to combinations of hyperthermia and radiation. *Radiology* 123:463–474.

Duncan, R. 2006. Polymer conjugates as anticancer nanomedicines. *Nat. Rev. Cancer* 6: 688–701.

Farokhzad, O. C. and R. Langer, 2009. Impact of nanotechnology on drug delivery. *ACS Nano* 3(1): 16–20.

Ferrantini, M., I. Capone, and F. Belardelli, 2007. Interferon-α and cancer: Mechanisms of action and new perspectives of clinical use. *Biochimie* 89(6–7):884–893.

Ferrari, M., XLiu, P. M. Sinha, B. Smith, and S. Sharma, 2006. Diffusion delivery systems and methods of fabrication. (PCT/US2006/012699), WO/2006/108053.

Ferrari, M., 2005. Cancer nanotechnology: Opportunities and challenges. *Nat. Rev. Cancer* 5:161–171.

Fiaherty, L., L. Heilbrun, C. Marsack, and U. N. Vaishampayan, 2005. Phase II trial of pegylated interferon (Peg-Intron) and thalidomide (Thal) in pretreated metatastic malignant melanomal. *J. Clin. Oncol.* 23 (Meeting Abstracts, Suppl. 16):7562.

Flenniken, M. L., D. A. Willits, A. L. Harmsen, L. O. Liepold, A. G. Harmsen, M. J. Young, and T. Douglas, 2006. Melanoma and lymphocyte cell-specific targeting incorporated into heat shock rotein cage architecture. *Chem. Biol.* 13:161–170.

Follet, K. A. and C. P. Naumann, 2000. A prospective study of catheter-related complications of intrathecal drug delivery systems. *J. Pain Symptom Manage.* 19(3):209–215.

Ganta, S., H. Devalapally, A. Shahiwala, and M. Amiji, 2008. A review of stimuli-responsive nanocarriers for drug and gene delivery. *J. Control. Release* 126:187–204.

Gobin, A. M., M. H. Lee, N. J. Halas, W. D. James, R. A. Drezek, and J. L. West, 2007. Near-infrared resonant nanoshells for combined optical imaging and photothermal cancer therapy. *Nano Lett.* 7:1929–1934.

Gong, D., V. Yadavalli, M. Paulose, M. Pishko, and C. A. Grimes, 2003. Controlled molecular release using nanoporous alumina capsules. *Biomed. Microdev.* 5(1):75–80.

Grimm, E. A., A. Mazumder, H. Z. Zhang, and S. A. Rosenberg, 1982. Lymphokine-activated killer cell phenomenon: Lysis of natural killer-resistant fresh solid tumor cells by interleukin 2-activated autologous human peripheral blood lymphocytes. *J. Exp. Med.* 155:1823–1841.

Harris, J. M. and R. B. Chess, 2003. Effect of peglyation on pharmaceuticals. *Nat. Rev. Drug Discov.* 2:214–221.

Hirsch, L. R., R. J. Stafford, J. A. Bankson, S. R. Sershen, B. Rivera, R. E. Price, J. D. Hazle, N. J. Halas, and J. L. West, 2003. Nanoshell mediated near-infrared thermal therapy of tumors under magnetic resonance guidance. *Proc. Natl. Acad. Sci. USA* 100:13549–13554.

Huang, X., I. H. El-Sayed, W. Qian, and M. A. El-Sayed, 2006. Cancer cell imaging and photothermal therapy in the near-infrared region by using gold. *J. Am. Chem. Soc.* 128(6):2115–2120.

Ikic, D., S. Spaventi, I. Padovan, Z. Kusic, V. Cajkovac, D. Ivankovic, N. Dakovic, and P. Nola, 1995. Local interferon therapy for melanoma patients. *Int. J. Dermatol* 34:872–874.

Ito, A., H. Honda, and T. Kobayashi, 2006. Cancer immunotherapy based on intracellular hyperthermia using magnetite nanoparticles: A novel concept of "heat-controlled necrosis" with heat shock protein expression. *Cancer Immunol. Immunother.* 55:320–328.

Ito, A., M. Shinkai, H. Hiroyuki, and T. Kobayashi, 2005. Medical application of functionalized magnetic nanoparticles. *J. Biosci. Bioeng.* 100(1):1–11.

Jabr-Milane, L., L. van Vlerken, H. Devalapally, D. Shenoy, S. Komareddy, M. Bhavsar, and M. Amiji, 2008. Multi-functional nanocarriers for targeted delivery of drugs and genes. *J. Control. Release* 130:121–128.

Jain, P. K., I. H. El-Sayed, and M. A. El-Sayed, 2008. Plasmonic photothermal therapy (PPTT) using gold nanoparticles. *Lasers Med. Sci.* 23:217–228.

Ji, X., R. Shao, A. M. Elliott, R. J. Stafford, E. Esparza-Coss, J. A. Bankson, G. Liang, et al., 2007. Bifunctional gold nanoshells with a superparamagnetic iron oxide-silica core suitable for both MR imaging and photothermal therapy. *J. Phys. Chem. C* 111:6245–6251.

Kammula, U. S., D. E. White, and S. A. Rosenberg, 1998. Trends in the safety of high dose bolus interleukin-2 administration in patients with metastatic cancer. *Cancer* 83:797–805.

Keller, C. G. and M. Ferrari, 1997. Microfabricated particle filter. US Patent No. 5,651,900.

Keller, C. G. and M. Ferrari, 1999a. Microfabricated capsules for immunological isolation of cell transplants. US Patent No. 5,893,974.

Keller, C. G. and M. Ferrari, 2000. High vertical aspect ratio thin film structures. U.S. Patent No. 6,015,559.

Keller, C. G. and M. Ferrari, 1999b. Microfabricated particle thin film filter and method of making it. U.S. Patent No. 5948255, September 7.

Kester, M., Y. Heakal, T. Fox, A. Sharma, G. P. Robertson, T. T. Morgan, E. I. Altinoglu, et al., 2008. Calcium phosphate nanocomposite particles for *in vitro* imaging and encapsulated chemotherapeutic drug delivery to cancer cells. *Nano Lett.* 8(12): 4116–4121.

Kim, C. J., S. Dessureault, D. Gabrilovich, D. S. Reintgen, and C. L. Slingluff, Jr, 2002. Immunotherapy for melanoma. *Cancer Control* 9:22–30.

Kirkwood, J., 2002. Cancer immunotherapy: The interferon-alpha experience. *Semin. Oncol.* 29:18–26.

Kirkwood, J. M., C. Bender, S. Agarwala, A. Tarhini, J. Shipe-Spotloe, B. Smelko, S. Donnelly, and L. Stover, 2002. Mechanisms and management of toxicities associated with high-dose interferon alfa-2b therapy. *J. Clin. Oncol.* 20:3703–3718.

Kirkwood, J. M., M. S. Ernstoff, and C. A. Davis, 1985. Comparison of intramuscular and intravenous recombinant alpha-2 interferon in melanoma and other cancers. *Ann. Intern. Med.* 103:32–36.

Kirkwood, J. M. and M. Ernstoff, 1985. Melanoma: Therapeutic options with recombinant interferons. *Semin. Oncol.* 12:7–12.

Kirkwood, J. M., J. G. Ibrahim, J. Richards, L. E. Flaherty, M. S. Ernstoff, T. J. Smith, U. Rao, M. Steele, and R. H. Blum, 2000. High- and low-dose interferon alfa-2b in high-risk melanoma: First analysis of intergroup trial E1690/S9111/C9190. *J. Clin. Oncol.* 18:2444–2458.

Kirkwood, J. M., J. G. Ibrahim, J. A. Sosman, V. K. Sondak, S. S. Agarwala, M. S. Ernstoff, and U. Rao, 2001. High-dose interferon alfa-2b significantly prolongs relapse-free and overall survival compared with the GM2-KLH/QS-21 vaccine in patients with resected stage IIB-III melanoma: Results of intergroup trial E1694/S9512/C509801. *J. Clin. Oncol.* 19:2370–2380.

Kirkwood, J. M., M. H. Strawderman, M. S. Ernstoff, T. J. Smith, E. C. Borden, and R. H. Blum, 1996. Interferon alpha-2b adjuvant therapy of high-risk resected cutaneous melanoma: The Eastern Cooperative Oncology Group Trial EST 1684. *J. Clin. Oncol.* 14:7–17.

Klausner, E. A., S. Eyal, E. Lavy, M. Friedman, and A. Hoffman, 2003. Novel levodopa gastroretentive dosage form: *In-vivo* evaluation in dogs. *J. Control. Release* 88:117–126.

Krulevitch, P. A. and A. W. Wang, 2001. Microfabricated injectable drug delivery system. US Patent Appl. Publ. No. 2001044620.

La Flamme, K. E., K. C. Popat, L. Leoni, E. Markiewicz, T. J. La Tempa, B. B. Roman, C. A. Grimes, and T. A. Desai, 2007. Biocompatibility of nanoporous alumina membranes for immunoisolation. *Biomaterials* 28(16):2638–2645.

LaVan, D. A., T. McGuire, and R. Langer, 2003. Small-scale systems for *in vivo* drug delivery. *Nat. Biotechnol.* 21:1184–1191.

Lave, T., B. Levet-Trafit, A. Schmitt-Hoffmann, B. Morgenroth, W. Richter, and R. C. Chou, 1995. Interspecies scaling of interferon disposition and comparison of allometric scaling with concentration–time transformations. *J. Pharm. Sci.* 84(11):1285–1290.

Legha, S. S., 1986. Interferons in the treatment of malignant melanoma: A review of recenttrials. *Cancer* 57:1675–1677.

Lens, M. B. and M. Dawes, 2002. Interferon alfa therapy for malignant melanoma: A systematic review of randomized controlled trials. *J. Clin. Oncol.* 20:1818–1825.

Leoni, L., A. Boiarski, and T. A. Desai, 2002. Characterization of nanoporous membranes for immunoisolation: Diffusion properties and tissue effects. *Biomed. Microdevices* 4(2):131–139.

Lesinski, G. B., S. Sharma, K. Varker, P. Sinha, M. Ferrari, and W. E. Carson, 2005. Release of biologically functional interferon-alpha from a nanochannel delivery system. *Biomed. Microdevices* 7(1):71–79.

Lesinski, G. B., M. Anghelina, J. Zimmerer, T. Bakalakos, B. Badgwell, R. Parihar, Y. Hu, et al., 2003. The anti-tumor effects of interferon-alpha are abrogated in a STAT1-deficient mouse. *J. Clin. Invest.* 112(2):170–180.

Lewis, J. R. and M. Ferrari, 2003. BioMEMS for drug delivery applications. In: *Lab-on-a-chip: Miniaturized systems for (Bio)chemical analysis and synthesis*, E. Oosterbroek and A. van den Berg (eds) pp. 373–395, Elsevier.

Lin, B., J. Yu, and S. Rice, 2000. Direct measurements of constrained brownian motion of an isolated sphere between two walls. *Phys. Rev. E Stat. Phys. Plasmas Fluids Relat. Interdiscip. Top.* 62(3 Pt B):3909–3919.

Loo, C., A. Lin, L. Hirsch, M. H. Lee, J. Barton, N. Halas, J. West, and R. Drezek, 2004. Nanoshell-enabled photonics-based imaging and therapy of cancer. *Technol. Cancer Res. Treat.* 3:33–40.

Losic, D. and S. Simovic, 2009. Self-ordered nanopore and nanotube platforms for drug delivery applications. *Expert Opin. Drug Deliv.* Oct 27. [Epub ahead of print].

Martin, F., R. Walczak, A. Boiarski, M. Cohen, T. West, C. Cosentino, J. Shapiro, and M. Ferrari, 2005. Tailoring width of microfabricated nano-channels to solute size can be used to control diffusion kinetics. *J. Control. Release* 102:123–133.

Mazumder, A., E. A. Grimm, H. Z. Zhang, and S. A. Rosenberg, 1982. Lysis of fresh human solid tumors by autologous lymphocytes activated *in vitro* with lectins. *Cancer Res.* 42:913–918.

Megeed, Z., J. Cappello, and J. Ghandehari, 2002. Genetically engineered silk-elastin-like protein polymers for controlled drug delivery. *Adv. Drug Deliv. Rev.* 54(8):1075–1091.

Mouawad, R., M. Sebert, J. Michels, J. Bloch, J. P. Spano, and D. Khayat, Sep 23, 2009. Treatment for metastatic malignant melanoma: Old drugs and new strategies. *Crit. Rev. Oncol. Hematol.* [Epub ahead of print].

Narasimhan, B. and R. Langer, 1997. Zero-order release of micro- and macromolecules from polymeric devices: The role of the burst effect. *J. Control. Release* 47(1):13–20.

Nathanson, L., 1976. Spontaneous regression of malignant melanoma: A review of the literature on incidence, clinical features, and possible mechanisms. *Natl. Cancer Inst. Monogr.* 44:67–76.

Nauts, H. C., G. A. Fowler, and F. H. Bogatko, 1953. A review of the influence of bacterial infection and of bacterial products (Coley's toxins) on malignant tumors in man: A critical analysis of 30 inoperable cases treated by Coley's mixed toxins, in which diagnosis was confirmed by microscopic examination selected for special study. *Acta Med. Scand. (Suppl)* 276:1–103.

Nguyen, N. P., B. Levinson, S. Dutta, U. Karlsson, A. Alfieri, C. Childress, and S. Sallah, 2003. Concurrent interferon-[alpha] and radiation for head and neck melanoma. *Melanoma Res.* 13:67–71.

Nishiyama, N. and K. Kataoka, 2006. Current state, achievements, and future prospects of polymeric micelles as nanocarriers for drug and gene delivery. *Pharmacol. Therap.* 112:630–648.

O'Neal, D. P., L. R. Hirsch, N. J. Halas, J. D. Payne, and J. L. West, 2004. Photo-thermal tumor ablation in mice using near infrared-absorbing nanoparticles. *Cancer Lett.* 209:171–176.

Orosz, K. E., S. Gupta, M. Hassink, M. Abdel-Rahman, L. Moldovan, F. H. Davidorf, and N. I. Moldovan, 2004. Delivery of antiangiogenic and antioxidant drugs of ophthalmic interest through a nano-porous inorganic filter. *Mol. Vis.* 18(10):555–565.

Peer, D., J. M. Karp, S. Hong, O. C. Farokhzad, R. Margalit, and R. Langer, 2007. Nanocarriers as an emerging platform for cancer therapy. *Nat. Nanotechnol.* 2:751–760.

Peng, L., A. D. Mendelsohn, T. J. LaTempa, S. Yoriya, C. A. Grimes, and T. A. Desai, 2009. Long-term small molecule and protein elution from TiO_2 nanotubes. *Nano Lett.* 9(5):1932–1936.

Piddubnyak, V., P. Kurcok, A. Matuszowicz, M. Glowala, A. Fiszer-Kierzkowska, Z. Jedlinski, M. Juzwa, and Z. Krawczyk, 2004. Oligo-3-hydroxybutyrates as potential carriers for drug delivery. *Biomaterials* 25:5271–5279.

Popat, K. C., G. Mor, C. A. Grimes, and T. A. Desai (2004). Surface modification of nanoporous alumina surfaces with poly(ethylene glycol). *Langmuir* 20(19):8035–8041.

Popat, K. C., M. Eltgroth, T. J. LaTempa, C. A. Grimes, and T. A. Desai, 2007. Titania nanotubes: A novel platform for drug-eluting coatings for medical implants? *Small* 3(11):1878–1881.

Prescott, J. H., S. Lipka, S. Baldwin, N. F. Sheppard Jr, J. M. Maloney, J. Coppeta, B. Yomtov, M. A. Staples, and J. T. Santini Jr., 2006. Chronic, programmed polypeptide delivery from an implanted, multi-reservoir microchip device. *Nat. Biotechnol.* 24(4):437–438.

Ratner, B. D., A. S. Hoffman, F. J. Schoen, and J. E. Lemons (Eds.), 1996. *Biomaterials Science. An Introduction to Materials in Medicine.* Academic Press, San Diego, CA.

Santini, J. T., A. C. Richards, R. Scheidt, M. J. Cima, and R. Langer, 2000. Microchips as controlled drug-delivery devices. *Angewandte Chemie, International Edition* 39:2396–2407.

Santini, J. T., M. J. Cima, and R. Langer, 1999. A controlled-release microchip. *Nature* 397:335–338.

Santini, J. T., M. J. Cima, and S. A. Uhland, 2003. Thermally-activated microchip chemical delivery devices. *PCT Int. Appl* (US2003/6527762).

Schneeberger, A., F. Koszik, and G. Stingl, 1995. Immunologic host defense in melanoma: Delineation of effector mechanisms involved and of strategies for the augmentation of their efficacy. *J. Invest. Dermatol.* 105:110S–116S.

Schwartzberg, A. M., T. Y. Olson, C. E. Talley, and J. Z. Zhang, 2006. Synthesis, characterization, and tunable optical properties of hollow gold nanospheres. *J. Phys. Chem. B* 110:19935–19944.

Sershen, S. and J. West, 2002. Implantable, polymeric systems for modulated drug delivery. *Adv. Drug Deliv. Rev.* 54:1225–1235.

Sharma, S., A. J. Nijdam, P. M. Sinha, R. J. Walczak, X. Liu, M. M. Cheng, and M. Ferrari, 2006. Controlled-release microchips. *Expert Opin. Drug Deliv.* 3(3):379–394.

Sharma, S., 2002. Nanostructured poly(ethylene glycol) (PEG) thin films for silicon-based bio-microsystems. Ph.D. Thesis, University of Illinois at Chicago.

Sharma, S., K. C. Popat, and T. A. Desai, 2002. Controlling non-specific protein interactions in silicon bio-microsystems with poly(ethylene glycol) films. *Langmuir* 18(23):8728–8731.

Sharma, S., R. W. Johnson, and T. A. Desai, 2004. Evaluation of the stability of nonfouling ultrathin poly(ethylene glycol) films for silicon-based microdevices. *Langmuir* 20(2):348–356.

Shimizu, T., T. Kishida, U. Hasegawa, Y. Ueda, J. Imanishi, H. Yamagishi, K. Akiyoshi, E. Otsuji, and O. Mazda, 2008. Nanogel DDS enables sustained release of IL-12 for tumor immunotherapy. *Biochem. BiophyRes Commun.* 367:330–335.

Sinha, P., G. Valco, S. Sharma, X. Liu, and M. Ferrari, 2004. Nanoengineered device for drug delivery application. *Nanotechnology* 15:S585–S589.

Sinha, P. M., 2005. Nanoengineered implantable devices for controlled drug delivery. Ph.D. Thesis, The Ohio State University.

Skrabalak, S. E., L. Au, X. Lu, X. Li, and Y. Xia, 2007. Gold nanocages for cancer detection and treatment. *Nanomed* 2:657–668.

Solbrig, C. M., J. K. Saucier-Sawyer, V. Cody, W. M. Saltzman, and D. J. Hanlon, 2007. Polymer nanoparticles for immunotherapy from encapsulated tumor-associated antigens and whole tumor cells. *Mol. Pharm.* 4(1):47–57.

Spiess, A., V. Mikalunas, S. Carlson, M. Zimmer, and R. M. Craig, 1996. Albumin kinetics in hypoalbuminemic patients receiving total parenteral nutrition. *J. Parenteral Enteral Nutr.* 20: 424–428.

Staples, M., K. Daniel, M. J. Cima, and R. Langer, 2006. Application of micro- and nano-electromechanical devices to drug delivery. *Pharm. Res.* 23(5):847–863.

Stoelting, R. K. (ed.), 1999. Pharmacokinetics and pharmacodynamics of injected and inhaled drugs. In *Pharmacology and Physiology in Anesthetic Practice*, pp. 3–35. Lippincott-Raven, New York.

Strausser, J. L., A. Mazumder, and E. A. Grimm, 1981. Lysis of human solid tumors by autologous cells sensitized *in vitro* to alloantigens. *J. Immunol.* 127:266–271.

Suzuki, M., M. Shinkai, H. Honda, and T. Kobayashi, 2003. Anticancer effect and immune induction by hyperthermia of malignant melanoma using magnetite cationic liposomes. *Melanoma Res.* 13:129–135.

Tran, M. A., R. Gowda, A. Sharma, E.-J. Park, J. Adair, M. Kester, N. B. Smith, and G. P. Robertson, 2006. Targeting [V600E]B-Raf and Akt3 using nanoliposomal-small interfering RNA inhibits cutaneous melanocytic lesion development. *Cancer Res.* 68(18):7638–7649.

Tu, J. K. and M. Ferrari, 1999. Microfabricated filter and capsule using a substrate sandwich. U.S. Patent No. 5,938,923.

Tu, J. K., T. Huen, R. Szema, and M. Ferrari, 1999. Filtration of sub-100 nm particles using a bulk-micromachined, direct-bonded silicon filter. *Biomed. Microdevices* 1(2):113–120.

Uchida, M., M. L. Flenniken, M. Allen, D. A. Willits, B. E. Crowley, S. Brumfield, A. F. Willis, et al. 2006. Targeting of cancer cells with ferrimagnetic ferritin cage nanoparticles. *J. Am. Chem. Soc.* 128(51):16626–16633.

van der Zee, J., 2002. Heating the patient: A promising approach? *Ann Oncol* 13:1173–1184.

Vasilev, K., Z. Poh, K. Kant, J. Chan, A. Michelmore, and D. Losic, 2010. Tailoring the surface functionalities of titania nanotube arrays. *Biomaterials* 31(3):532–540.

Von Wussow, P., B. Block, F. Hartmann, and H. Deicher, 1988. Intralesional interferon-alpha therapy in advanced malignant melanoma. *Cancer* 61:1071–1074.

Walczak, R., A. Boiarski, T. West, J. Shapiro, S. Sharma, and M. Ferrari, 2005. Long-term biocompatibility of NanoGATE drug delivery implant. *Nanobiotechnology* 1(1):35–42.

Wang, Y. S., S. Youngster, M. Grace, J. Bausch, R. Bordens, and D. F. Wyss, 2002. Structural and biological characterisation of pegylated recombinant interferon a2b and its therapeutic implications. *Adv. Drug Del. Rev.* 54:547–570.

Wei, Q., C. Bechinger, and P. Leiderer, 2000. Single-file diffusion of colloids in one dimensional channels. *Science* 287:625–627.

Wisniewski, N., B. Klitzman, B. Miller, and W. M. Reichert, 2001. Decreased analyte transport through implanted membranes: Differentiation of biofouling from tissue effects. *J. Biomed. Mater. Res.* 57:513–521.

Yasukawa, T., H. Kimura, Y. Tabata, and Y. Ogura, 2001. Biodegradable scleral plugs for vitreoretinal drug delivery. *Adv. Drug Deliv. Reviews* 52:25–36.

Zamboni, W. C., 2005. Liposomal, nanoparticle, and conjugated formulation of anticancer agents. *Clin. Cancer Res.* 11:8230–8234.

7

Immune Response to Implanted Nanostructured Materials

Kristy M. Ainslie
The Ohio State University

Rahul G. Thakar
University of California, San Francisco

Daniel A. Bernards
University of California, San Francisco

Tejal A. Desai
University of California, San Francisco

Nanostructured materials are used *in vivo* for dynamic therapies, such as drug delivery, tissue engineering, biosensing, and imaging. Nanowires and other nonparticulate nanostructured materials have been proposed to alter cellular attachment and motility, detect analytes *in vivo*, simulate tissue organization, and serve as an alternative stent topography. The interaction between nanostructured materials and elements of the body can be beneficial but can also lead to a variety of adverse immune responses ranging from bacterial infection to tumorigenesis. A primary concern with increased use of nanomaterials is safety, with regard to possible toxicity. Numerous studies have linked inhaled nanoparticles to airway injury or diseases such as coronary diseases. The reported toxicity of nanoparticles brings into question the immunogenicity of nonparticulate nanomaterials. Numerous studies have focused on the inflammation response to particulate nanomaterials such as nanoparticles and carbon nanotubes, but little attention has been focused on the immune response to nanostructured materials, such as nanowires, nanoporous membranes, and nanotubular surfaces. Recently, an increasing number of studies have characterized the inflammation response of nanostructured materials both *in vitro* and *in vivo*. To understand the immune response to nanostructured materials, first the response to flat and nanoparticulate materials will be reviewed.

7.1 Inflammation Response to Biomaterials

The innate immune system is considered the primary response to a sterile foreign implanted material. In contrast to the adaptive immune system that responds to pathogen fragments presented on the surface of antigen presenting cells, the innate immune system responds through specific signal (or pattern) recognition. The cells of the innate and adaptive immune system function cooperatively: one system can initiate the response to the other. For the purposes of this chapter, however, innate functions will be highlighted since cells of that system are fundamental to the body's response to implants.

The immune system response to implanted biomaterials is depicted by the flow chart in Figure 7.1. Phagocytic cells, such as macrophages and neutrophils, comprise the primary response to the innate immune system. Upon implantation, proteins from the existing extracellular matrix and blood

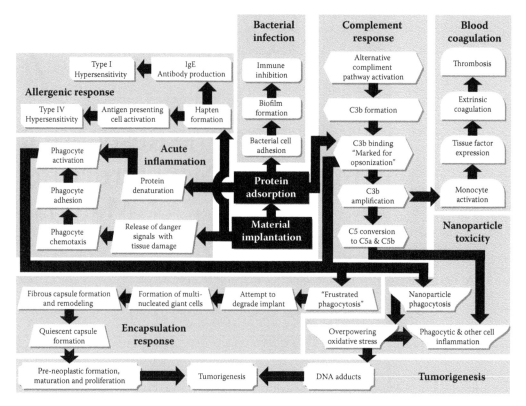

FIGURE 7.1 Schematic of potential immune responses to implanted materials. A cascade of possible immuno-logical responses are depicted as initiated by material implantation and protein adsorption, represented in the middle of the flow chart. Normal arrows (➡) indicate responses that have been well characterized; an incomplete arrow (➡) represents a tentative immune response that is not yet well established.

immediately adhere to the surface of the implant. Inherent tissue damage caused by surgical implanta-tion as well as protein adsorption and misfolded protein conformations at the material surface can lead to further immune response. Tissue damage activates an immune response through release of "danger signals." Danger signals are proteins (released by cells that die through necrosis, viral infection, or stress) that act as biochemical alarms to activate the immune system. According to the danger model, apoptotic cells do not release danger signals or promote an immune response. Danger signals activate immune cells and promote immune-cell proliferation and chemotaxis (directed cellular migration induced by a cytokine concentration gradient). Chemotaxis, activation, and proliferation of immune cells results in the body's inflammation response to implanted biomaterials.

Several cell types have functional roles in the inflammation response, as listed in Table 7.1. Damage to fibroblasts, endothelial cells, and mast cells results in the release of danger signals initiating an inflam-mation response. These signals can cue other cells to migrate to the area of implantation through chemotaxis or activate immune cells to further propagate the signal.

Immune cell chemotaxis primarily involves phagocytic cells. Initially neutrophils migrate to the site of inflammation, and as the short-lived cells die off, they are replaced by monocytes that can differen-tiate into macrophages or antigen-presenting dendritic cells. Dendritic cells stimulate T-cells by pre-senting antigens as part of the adaptive immune response. Cytokine signals from neutrophils and macrophages upregulate adhesion molecules at the endothelial cell surface. These adhesion molecules (I-CAM for phagocytes and selectins for endothelial cell surfaces) facilitate the extravasation of additional phagocytes to the implant site. Once phagocytes arrive at the implant site, they adhere to the

TABLE 7.1 Role of Immune Cells in the Acute Inflammation and Encapsulation Response to Implanted Materials

Effector Cell	Role	Chemokines	Affected Cell			
			Macrophages	Monocytes	Neutrophils	Endothelial Cells
Fibroblasts	Part of danger signal cascade in response to implantation	MCP-1, CXCL10, MIP-1α, IL-8	A	C	A & C	—
Macrophages	Phagocytic cell that can release degrading species or form giant cells	MCP-1, TNF-α, IL-6, GM-CSF, MIP-1α and β, IL-8	A & F	C	A	—
Mast cells	Part of danger signal cascade in response to implantation	TNF-α, MIP-1α	A & U	C	—	—
Monocytes	Differentiate into macrophages or dendritic cells upon chemical stimulation	CX3CL1, IL-6, MCP-1, TGF-β, CXCL10	A & F	A	—	U
Neutrophils	Initial phagocyte to implanted material and characterizes acute inflammation	MIP-1β	—	C	—	—
Vascular endothelial cells	Part of danger signal cascade in response to implantation	CX3CL1	—	C	A & C	U

The effect of the cell on other cells important to inflammation are indicated as follows: activation (A), chemoattractant (C), fusion of cells into multinucleated cells (F), and upregulation (U) of adhesion molecules.

material surface. For objects larger than a few microns, phagocytes are incapable of engulfing them and undergo "frustrated phagocytosis." Frustrated phagocytosis is due to the inability of the phagocytes to engulf a foreign object larger than itself. When the phagocyte cannot remove the foreign object by engulfment, it attempts to degrade the material surface and form a capsule to separate the implant from the tissue surrounding it. In order to form a continuous capsule, phagocytic cells fuse into multinucleated giant cells. These cells combine with extracellular matrix components and fibroblasts to form a cellular capsule. Within a month after implantation, a cell capsule can encase the implant with a thickness that ranges from tens to hundreds of microns. Once the implant is successfully surrounded, the capsule generally reaches a quiescent phase.

The wound healing response is characterized by three steps: inflammation, proliferation, and remodeling. Inflammation recruits monocytes and other phagocytic cells to the implant site in an attempt to dilute and clear damaged tissues and cells. Once the area is clear of such debris, the body can begin to repair itself through cell proliferation and tissue remodeling. Proliferation of endothelial cells promotes vascularization at the implant site to augment damaged capillaries. For tissue surrounding the implant that cannot be correctly reinstated, fibroblastic tissue can turn into scar tissue. Also, multinucleated giant cells, formed as a result of frustrated phagocytosis, become surrounded by a fibrous capsule, further encapsulating the implant. The fibrous capsule is formed from extracellular matrix components such as collagen, proteoglycans, and fibroblasts.

The body's inflammation response to biomaterials has an acute short-term phase and a chronic long-term phase. Initially, acute inflammation is observed when phagocytic cells adhere to the foreign surface and become activated. Neutrophils migrate to the material surface in response to the release of danger signals associated with tissue damage. These short-lived cells then induce trafficking (chemotaxis) of other monocytes to the surface. Monocytes can then differentiate into macrophages or dendritic cells. Activation of macrophages through denatured protein or cytokine-signaling characterizes the acute response of the innate system to an implanted material surface. Histological observations, such as edema and redness of tissue, are seen clinically with acute inflammation. Without excision of the implanted biomaterial, acute inflammation may progress to chronic inflammation.

Chronic inflammation takes many forms (Figure 7.1) and has been observed with both nonstructured surfaces and nanoparticles, such as metal particles and carbon nanotubes. The toxicity of nanoparticles and carbon nanotubes has been linked to activation of phagocytic cells and resulting nanoparticle engulfment. Concentrations of nanoparticles of 1 mg/mL or greater can adversely affect tissues. When exposed to toxic levels of nanoparticles, phagocytic cells produce reactive oxygen species that may cause either cell death or tumorigenesis. While nanoparticles can be engulfed by phagocytic cells, planar materials induce frustrated phagocytosis. With frustrated phagocytosis, cells initiate an encapsulation response, where the implant is walled off from surrounding tissue. Additionally, activated macrophages release products, such as reactive oxygen species, in an attempt to degrade the material surface. Macrophages then fuse together to wall off the implant from the surrounding tissue. An encapsulation response rarely results in tumorigenesis.

In addition to the encapsulation response, some of the immune responses are shown in Figure 7.1 are less common but can still occur at the implant surface. A link between nanoparticle feature size and complement (C3b) binding has been reported, indicating the potential importance of C3b in nanostructured implants. Another critical immune response is tumorigenesis. This response was observed in case of chronic nanoparticle inhalation and mammoplasty. With concentrated chronic nanoparticle inhalation, oxidative stress overwhelms the cells the nanoparticles are in contact with; the resulting DNA damage can lead to tumorigenic cell formation, similar to clinical examples following asbestos exposure and mesothelioma formation.

7.2 Acute Inflammation and Encapsulation in Response to Nanostructured Biomaterials

A nanostructured device is defined as a planar-based material with at least one feature less than 100 nm in dimension. Materials such as nanowires, nanoporous metal oxides, nanotubular surfaces, and some microfabricated surfaces are all nanostructured surfaces. Nanoparticles fail to satisfy this definition since they lack a planar base and are introduced in a suspension. Additionally, the biocompatibility of nanoparticles has been thoroughly reviewed.

7.2.1 *In Vitro* Studies

The inflammation response studied *in vitro* typically investigates the interaction of a single cell type (Table 7.1) with a nanostructured surface. The release of inflammatory cytokines and changes in cellular properties, such as morphology, proliferation, and viability, are indicative of the inflammation response these surfaces might generate *in vivo*. There is considerable evidence both *in vitro* and *in vivo* (presented in Tables 7.2 and 7.3) that nanostructures can alter the inflammation response relative to conventional surfaces. Most of the research regarding the inflammation response to nanostructured materials concludes that structured surfaces are equally or less inflammatory than a conventional surface of the same material, with one exception where toxic nanowires increased inflammation.

Titania nanotubes significantly reduced the amount of inflammatory cytokines released from human monocytes adhered to the material surface. The nanotube surface was significantly less inflammatory, resulting in an increased rate of apoptosis of adherent monocytes due to lack of activation. In the same monocyte study, long (27 μm in length) PCL nanowires and short (6–8 μm in length) silica nanowires were significantly less inflammatory than their conventional counterparts. Both nanostructured materials induced significantly downregulated inflammatory cytokine expression from adherent human monocytes compared to a conventional surface of the same material. In the Ainslie et al. study, short PCL and long silica nanowires were also studied. Interestingly, the length of the nanowires led to

TABLE 7.2 *In Vivo* Acute and Chronic Inflammation Response to Nanomaterials

Reference	Material	Dimensions	Conclusion	Cell	Cytokine Panel	ROS	SO	Cell Morphology	Cell Viability	Microarray	Other
								Method			
Ainslie et al.	Nanoporous silicon	2–50 nm diameter pores	The nanoporous silicon surface was not significantly more inflammatory than silicon	Human monocyte	10	X	X	X	X		
Ainslie et al.	Nanochanneled silicon	Channels of 100 nm	The nanochanneled silicon surface was considered equally inflammatory to silicon	Human monocyte	10	X	X	X	X		
	Short PCL nanowires	196 nm in diameter and 2.6 μm in length	Cytokine expression was less on the nanowire surface compared to flat PCL, but the overall inflammation response was not significantly less								
Ainslie et al.	Long PCL nanowires	196 nm in diameter and 27 μm in length	Cytokines IL-10, IFN-γ, and TNF-α were significantly less on the nanowire surface compared to PCL and considered significantly less inflammatory than PCL	RAW macrophages and BAEC	18			X	X		
	Titania nanotubes	79 nm in diameter, 0.4 μm in length	Cytokines IL-6, IL-10, TNF-α, IL-12, MIP-1α & β were significantly different comparing the tubular surface over flat titanium, with IL-1β significantly more. The nanotubular surface was considered significantly less inflammatory than the flat titanium surface								
	Short silicon oxide nanowires	40 nm in diameter and 6–8 μm in length	On average the expression of all 10 cytokines were less for the monocytes on the nanowire surface than the flat glass surface with TNF-α and MIP-1β significantly less. The short nanowires were considered significantly less inflammatory than glass								

continued

TABLE 7.2 (continued) *In Vivo* Acute and Chronic Inflammation Response to Nanomaterials

Reference	Material	Dimensions	Conclusion	Cell	Method Cytokine Panel	ROS	SO	Cell Morphology	Cell Viability	Microarray	Other
	Long silicon oxide nanowires	40 nm in diameter and 30–40 μm in length	IFN-γ expression with the long nanowire surface was significantly less than glass. The long nanowires were not less inflammatory than glass								
	Nanofibrous PTFE	20–30 nm in width and 3–4 mm in length	The nanofibrous PTFE surface is not immunogenic and might attenuate foreign body giant cell formation *in vivo*								
Ainslie et al.	Ni–Co–Fe nanowire	75 nm in diameter and 10 μm in length	Cells grown on the nanowire surface, compared to a flat surface of the same material, were smaller and less viable. The nanowire surface was considered more inflammatory	RAW macrophages	18			X	X		
Dalby et al.	Nanopitted PMMA	120 nm diameter pits with a depth of 100 nm	Chemokines and complement activation involved in inflammation downregulated compared to flat PMMA	Human fibroblasts						X	
Cool et al.	Nanocolumnar PMMA	10 nm high nanocolumns	Chemokines and complement activation involved in inflammation downregulated compared to flat PMMA	RAW macrophages							nF-k B gene expression
	PHBV with hydroxyapatite (HA)	HA crystals 60 × 20 nm²	Had the lowest expression of pro-inflammatory signaling compared to poly(3-hydroxybutyrate-co-3-valerate) (PHBV), PHBV with HA and PHBV with βTP								
Karlsson et al.	PHBV with calcined HA	HA crystals 80 × 25 nm² and 100–400 nm	PHBV and HA had lower pro-inflammatory signaling than PHBV	Human neutrophils		X		X			Elastase activity

Reference	Material	Dimensions	Findings	Cell type				
	PHBV with β-tricalcium phosphate (βTP)	βTP crystals 80 × 25 nm² and 100–400 nm	b-TCP + PHBV had lower pro-inflammatory signaling than PHBV					
	Nanoporous alumina	20 and 200 nm in diameter	Pore-size in the nano-range has very little influence on neutrophil activation when the membrane is coated with a single protein or with serum					
Giavaresi et al.	Nanopits of 3-hydroxybutyrate-co-3-hydroxyvalerate	Pillars 100 nm in depth, 120 nm in diameter, and 300 nm in pitch	Pro-inflammatory cytokine release was decreased on nanotopography compared to flat surface of the same polymer	Fibroblasts	3		X	
Karlsson et al.	PCL nanocylinders	160 nm in height, 100 nm in diameter	Pro-inflammatory cytokine release was decreased on nanotopography compared to flat surface of the same polymer. IL-1b was upregulate on all PCL surfaces including nanocylinders	Human neutrophils		X	X	
	Nanoporous alumina	20 and 200 nm in diameter	Higher Initial ROS levels were seen on the non-coated 20 nm pore-size membrane than on the 200 nm membrane, where the activation time was longer and the reduction of ROS started decreasing later					
Dalby et al.	Polystyrene co-poly(4-bromostyrene) nanohills	95 nm in height	No differences were noted between the nanohills and their controls	Human platelets and mononuclear cells			X	
Wojciak-Stothard et al.	Silicon nanogroves	2 and 10 μm in width and 30–282 nm deep	Macrophages grown in nanochannels increased phagocytic activity	Macrophages				Phagocytosis of PS beads

Note: *In vivo* studies reported here were performed by murine subcutaneous implantation. BAEC—bovine aortic endothelial cells, ROS—reactive oxygen species, SO—superoxide.

TABLE 7.3 *In Vivo* Acute and Chronic Inflammation Response to Nanomaterials

Reference	Material	Dimensions	Conclusion	Method
Peng et al.	Titania nanoparticles in gelatin	20–60 nm in diameter nanoparticles	TNF-α and IL-6 serum levels were similar at day 7 and 14 compared to control. The wound healing response observed for the nanostructured matrix at 12 was superior to that of the control and complete healing was observed only in with the nanostructured matrix at day 18	Murine dermal damage and skin replacement with matrix. IL-6 and TNF-α blood plasma levels at 0, 7, and 14 days
Popat et al.	Titania nanotubes	79 nm in diameter, 0.4 μm in length.	Lack of fibrous scar formation after 4 weeks implantation	Subcutaneous implantation and fibrous capsule formation
Giavaresi et al.	Nanopits of 3-hydroxybutyrate-*co*-3-hydroxyvalerate	Pillars 100 nm in depth, 120 nm in diameter, and 300 nm in pitch	Nanopits lead to an increased fibrous capsule formation compared to PCL nanocylinders, but the capsule formation was not significantly different from the flat polymer surface capsule formation	Subcutaneous implantation and fibrous capsule formation
Giavaresi et al.	PCL nanocylinders	160 nm in height, 100 nm in diameter, and had an average center-to-center distance of 200 nm	Nanocylinders displayed increased cellularity of the fibrous capsule and the vascular density, compared to nanopits	Subcutaneous implantation and fibrous capsule formation
Areva et al.	Nanopourous titania	150 nm	After 7 and 12 days, the number of layers of fibroblasts on the implant surface were signficantly less on the nanopourous surface compared to flat titanium	Subcutaneous implantation and fibrous capsule formation

Note: In vivo studies reported here were performed by murine subcutaneous implantation.

different results in silicon oxide and PCL: the short nanowires were least inflammatory in the silicon oxide series (compared to the long nanowires) and vice versa for the PCL substrates. This disparity displays that material plays a significant role in determining how aspect ratio affects inflammation response *in vitro*. Compared to nanowires, a reduced inflammation response was also reported for several nanostructured materials with decreased aspect ratios. While the aforementioned nanowires have aspect ratios on the order of 100, PMMA and PCL nanocolumns (cylinders) had aspect ratios on the order of 1. The inflammation response to PMMA and PCL nanocolumns was less for the nano-structured surface than the conventional control. For a surface with nanopits of the same aspect ratio, the inflammation response was also reduced compared to the nonstructured control. Furthermore, when low-aspect ratio crystals were embedded in a matrix to form a composite, a reduced inflammation response was observed. Nanosized crystals of three different materials (hydroxyapatite, calcined hydroxyapatite, and tricalcium phosphate) embedded in poly(3-hydroxybutyrate-*co*-3-valerate) (PHBV) induced a reduced inflammatory signaling compared to neat PHBV.

The inconsistent dependence of the inflammation response on the aspect ratio of the nanostructured material would indicate that material properties (e.g., surface energy and surface charge) play a role in the inflammation response. Indeed, it has been hypothesized that increased hydrophilicity, as a result of increased surface roughness, leads to decreased protein adsorption on Ni–Co–Fe nanowires. By altering protein adsorption, subsequent cell adherence is certainly modulated and thus the cell-based inflam-mation response is influenced. Additionally, surface charge may play a role. Among nanoparticles, cationic particles are more likely to induce inflammatory reactions than anionic particles and neutral species; however, due to difficulty in measuring surface charge of nanostructured materials, no data are available for the charge effects on these nanostructured surfaces.

A smaller subset of nanostructured materials induces an inflammation response that is similar to that of the respective conventional material. A comparison of nanoporous silicon and alumina to their respective conventional surfaces reported that the activation of immune cells was similar. Similarly, the immune response to nanochanneled silicon was similar to that induced by silicon. The inflammation response induced by short PCL and long silicon oxide nanowires was similar to that observed on conventional PCL and silicon, respectively. Additionally, nanohills of polystyrene-*co*-poly(4-bromostyrene) induced a similar inflammation response compared to a conventional surface of the same co-polymer. Macrophages did not significantly upregulate their inflammation response when chemically inert and biocompatible polytetrafluoroethylene (PTFE) was investigated as a nanofibrous mat. The results presented here conclude that nanostructured materials have the attractive property of being equal or less inflammatory with the addition of nanoarchitecture.

In contrast to the aforementioned studies that show equivalent or decreased inflammation response to nanostructured materials one study to date found that nanostructures led to increased inflammation. Nanowires of magnetostrictive and cytotoxic Ni–Co–Fe proved to be more inflammatory than a conventional surface of the same material. Two of the three alloy metals, nickel and cobalt, are considered cytotoxic. In contrast to nanostructures created from relatively inert materials, nanostructures of these toxic elements (Ni and Co), led to an increased inflammation response. Nanostructures fabricated using typically noninflammatory materials produce noninflammatory surfaces; in contrast when toxic elements are used to generate nanostructured materials, the inflammation response increases. Increased interfacial surface area may result in increased release of toxic ions, such as Co and Ni, which induce elevated activation of inflammatory cells.

Another study explored the phagocytic activity of macrophages on inert silicon structured into nanogrooves. Evaluation of the phagocytic activity alone is inconclusive for increased macrophage activation, but it can be indicative of an increased inflammation response. It was shown that increased phagocytic activity can be induced by the topography of material surfaces. This study might indicate that inert materials with nanostructure may induce inflammation signals, but further study would need to be performed to completely elucidate a complete conclusion with regard to inflammation, based on this work.

7.2.2 *In Vivo* Studies

Of the few *in vivo* studies performed on the inflammatory and wound healing response to nanomaterial implants, most report the thickness of the fibrotic capsule to indicate degree of immune activation (Table 7.3). Similar to observations made in the *in vitro* studies, the *in vivo* studies reported that nanostructures led to a decreased inflammation response compared to a conventional surface. Murine peritoneal implantation of a nanotubular titania surface lacked fibrous scar formation at the implant site. When nanoporous titania was implanted subcutaneously in a murine model, the number of layers of fibroblasts that was observed around the nanostructured implant (an indication of capsule thickness) was significantly less compared to conventional titanium at the same time scale. When nanocylindrical PCL, was implanted subcutaneously in a murine model, increased number of fibroblasts and increased vascular density were observed. PCL nanopits induced increased fibrous capsule formation but the inflammation response was similar to that observed with conventional PCL. The wound healing response was enhanced with PCL nanocylinders compared to the inverted nanopit structures. This response was also observed in fibroblasts grown on an array of silicone micropegs, where proliferation was decreased. Here, it was observed that this effect relied on altered adhesive and micromechanical interactions between individual cells and micropegs. In addition to the marked decreased in proliferation, fibroblasts adhering to a/the micropeg(s) showed an accompanying and distinct elongation in cell and nuclear shape. Furthermore, when fibroblast contractility was pharmacologically attenuated through low-dose inhibition of either Rho-associated kinase or myosin light chain kinase, the potency with which micropeg adhesion suppressed cell proliferation was significantly reduced. These results support a model where cell fate decisions may be directly manipulated within tissue engineering scaffolds by the inclusion of microtopographical structures that alter cellular mechanics.

An improved wound-healing response in a subcutaneous murine model was also observed in a composite material of titania nanoparticles in gelatin. Wound healing was accelerated by the nanostructured composite compared to a conventional control of the same material.

In summary, *in vivo* studies indicated that not only was the inflammation response attenuated in the presence of nanostructured materials, but that the wound healing process was accelerated. For applications such as biosensing, drug delivery, and tissue engineering, which require close proximity of the vasculature for analyte sensing, therapeutics delivery, and delivery of nutrients to newly formed tissue, accelerated wound healing and angiogenesis are most beneficial.

Nanostructured surfaces induce an immune response distinct from that of nanoparticles. Champion et al. have concluded that, when the particle volume is greater than a typical cell (~15 μm in diameter) macrophages do not engulf such particles. The largest nanostructured dimensions of the materials listed in Tables 7.2 and 7.3 are well under 15 μm, but since cells can not engulf the continuous material, frustrated phagocytosis results. In addition, nanoparticles with a volume larger than the typical cell dimension induce macrophage spreading while nanostructured surfaces have the opposite effect. Besides phagocytosis of foreign materials and cell spreading, activated macrophages also generate reactive oxygen species (ROS) when exposed to concentrated nanoparticles. ROS formation, however, was not significant when monocytes were incubated with nanostructured materials.

Ainslie et al. reported that monocytes in contact with a variety of nanostructured materials did not produce either ROS or superoxides. Lack of engulfment, cell spreading, and ROS formation indicates that nanostructured materials, like conventional biomaterials, induce frustrated phagocytosis *in vitro*. *In vivo* data (Table 7.3) provide additional evidence that nanostructured materials, like conventional materials, induce frustrated phagocytosis that can result in a limited fibrous capsule formation. Both *in vitro* and *in vivo* research has indicated that nanostructured materials do not provoke an immune response similar to that induced by nanoparticles, but rather induce a frustrated phagocytosis response similar to that associated with conventional biomaterial implants.

7.3 Conclusions

Nanotechnology is becoming intricately linked with the study of the cell in its microenvironment. Nanomaterials, like nanofibers and self-assembled peptides, are emerging as promising alternatives for three-dimensional *in vivo*-like microenvironments. Surfaces with nanostructured features, such as wires, tubes, and pits, provide contact guidance and enable design and fabrication of novel implantable tissue-engineered scaffolds. Such technologies pave the way for future discoveries as well as the continual merging of medicine, biology, and engineering.

Nanostructured surfaces both attenuate the acute inflammation response of immune cells to implanted materials and affect the encapsulation response. Some general conclusions can be ascertained from the studies reported in the literature:

- The inflammation response around nanostructured materials is primarily an innate system immune response.
- The immune response is not dependent on the nanostructure aspect ratio.
- Nanostructures induce decreased inflammation, perhaps due to their increased surface energy affecting protein adsorption and therefore cell adhesion.
- Nanomaterials that release toxic substances interact adversely with surrounding tissue *in vivo*.
- The time course of wound healing is decreased in the presence of nanostructures.

- Whereas nanoparticles may induce toxicity, nanostructured materials induce "frustrated phago-cytosis" responses by macrophages. This response can lead to an altered encapsulation response.

Like other aspects of biocompatibility, further studies are needed on a per-material-basis to properly evaluate the inflammation potential of new prospective nanomaterials. In addition to understanding how nanostructured materials interact with the human body, insight into these materials and their interactions with the immune system may aid in developments like novel vaccines and tolerance therapies.

Bibliography

Ainslie, K. M., E. M. Bachelder, S. Borkar, A. S. Zahr, A. Sen, J. V. Badding, and M. V. Pishko. 2007. Cell adhesion on nanofibrous polytetrafluoroethylene (Nptfe). *Langmuir* 23, no. 2: 747–54.

Ainslie, K. M., E. M. Bachelder, G. Sharma, C. Grimes, and M. V. Pishko. 2007. Macrophage cell adhesion and inflammation cytokines on magnetostrictive nanowires. *Nanotoxicology* 1, no. 4: 279–90.

Ainslie, K. M., G. Sharma, M. A. Dyer, C. A. Grimes, and M. V. Pishko. 2005. Attenuation of protein adsorption on static and oscillating magnetostrictive nanowires. *Nano Letters* 5, no. 9: 1852–56.

Ainslie, K. M., S. L. Tao, K. C. Popat, and T. A. Desai. 2008. *In vitro* immunogenicity of silicon based micro- and nano-structured surfaces. *ACS Nano* 2, no. 5: 1076–84.

Ainslie, K. M., S. L. Tao, K. C. Popat, and T. A. Desai. 2009. *In vitro* inflammatory response of nano-structured titania, silicon oxide, and polycaprolactone. *J. Biomed. Mater. Research* 91, no. 3: 647–55.

Anderson, J. M. 1998. Soft tissue response. In *Handbook of Biomaterial Properties*, eds. J. Black and G. Hastings. New York: Chapman & Hall.

Anderson, J. M., G. Cook, B. Costerton, S. R. Hanson, A. Hensten-Pettersen, N. Jacobsen, R. J. Johnson, et al. 2004. Host reactions to biomaterials and their evalulation. In *Biomaterials Science*, eds. B. D. Ratner, A. S. Hoffmann, F. J. Schoen, and J. E. Lemons. San Francisco: Elsevier Academic Press.

Anderson, J. M., K. Defife, A. McNally, T. Collier, and C. Jenney. 1999. Monocyte, macrophage and foreign body giant cell interactions with molecularly engineered surfaces. *J. Mater. Sci. Mater. Med.* 10, no. 10/11: 579–88.

Areva, S., H. Paldan, T. Peltola, T. Narhi, M. Jokinen, and M. Linden. 2004. Use of sol-gel-derived titania coating for direct soft tissue attachment. *J. Biomed. Mater. Res. A* 70, no. 2: 169–78.

Barlow, P. G., A. Clouter-Baker, K. Donaldson, J. Maccallum, and V. Stone. 2005. Carbon black nanopar-ticles induce type Ii epithelial cells to release chemotaxins for alveolar macrophages. *Part Fibre Toxicol.* 2: 11.

BeruBe, K., D. Balharry, K. Sexton, L. Koshy, and T. Jones. 2007. Combustion-derived nanoparticles: Mechanisms of pulmonary toxicity. *Clin. Exp. Pharmacol. Physiol.* 34, no. 10: 1044–50.

Bico, J., C. Tordeux, and D. Quere. 2001. Rough wetting. *Europhys. Lett.* 55, no. 2: 214–20.

Buzea, C., Pacheco, II, and K. Robbie. 2007. Nanomaterials and nanoparticles: Sources and toxicity. *Biointerphases* 2, no. 4: MR17–MR71.

Champion, J. A., Y. K. Katare, and S. Mitragotri. 2007. Particle shape: A new design parameter for micro- and nanoscale drug delivery carriers. *J. Control Release* 121, no. 1–2: 3–9.

Champion, J. A. and S. Mitragotri. 2006. Role of target geometry in phagocytosis. *Proc. Natl. Acad. Sci. USA* 103, no. 13: 4930–4.

Cool, S. M., B. Kenny, A. Wu, V. Nurcombe, M. Trau, A. I. Cassady, and L. Grondahl. 2007. Poly(3-hydroxybutyrate-*co*-3-hydroxyvalerate) composite biomaterials for bone tissue regeneration: *In vitro* performance assessed by osteoblast proliferation, osteoclast adhesion and resorption, and mac-rophage proinflammatory response. *J. Biomed. Mater. Res. A* 82, no. 3: 599–610.

Cui, Y., Q. Wei, H. Park, and C. M. Lieber. 2001. Nanowire nanosensors for highly sensitive and selective detection of biological and chemical species. *Science* 293, no. 5533: 1289–92.

Curtis, A. S., N. Gadegaard, M. J. Dalby, M. O. Riehle, C. D. Wilkinson, and G. Aitchison. 2004. Cells react to nanoscale order and symmetry in their surroundings. *IEEE Trans. Nanobiosci.* 3, no. 1: 61–5.

Dalby, M. J., N. Gadegaard, P. Herzyk, H. Agheli, D. S. Sutherland, and C. D. Wilkinson. 2007. Group analysis of regulation of fibroblast genome on low-adhesion nanostructures. *Biomaterials* 28, no. 10: 1761–19.

Dalby, M. J., G. E. Marshall, H. J. Johnstone, S. Affrossman, and M. O. Riehle. 2002. Interactions of human blood and tissue cell types with 95-Nm-High nanotopography. *IEEE Trans. Nanobiosci.* 1, no. 1: 18–23.

Dalby, M. J., M. O. Riehle, D. S. Sutherland, H. Agheli, and A. S. Curtis. 2004. Changes in fibroblast morphology in response to nano-columns produced by colloidal lithography. *Biomaterials* 25, no. 23: 5415–22.

Davoren, M., E. Herzog, A. Casey, B. Cottineau, G. Chambers, H. J. Byrne, and F. M. Lyng. 2007. *In vitro* toxicity evaluation of single walled carbon nanotubes on human A549 lung cells. *Toxicol In Vitro* 21, no. 3: 438–48.

Dobrovolskaia, M. A. and S. E. McNeil. 2007. Immunological properties of engineered nanomaterials. *Nat. Nanotechnol.* 2, no. 8: 469–78.

Gallagher, J. O., K. F. McGhee, C. D. Wilkinson, and M. O. Riehle. 2002. Interaction of animal cells with ordered nanotopography. *IEEE Trans. Nanobiosci.* 1, no. 1: 24–8.

Gallucci, S., M. Lolkema, and P. Matzinger. 1999. Natural adjuvants: Endogenous activators of dendritic cells. *Nat. Med.* 5, no. 11: 1249–55.

Giavaresi, G., M. Tschon, J. H. Daly, J. J. Liggat, D. S. Sutherland, H. Agheli, M. Fini, P. Torricelli, and R. Giardino. 2006. *In vitro* and *in vivo* response to nanotopographically-modified surfaces of poly(3-hydroxybutyrate-*co*-3-hydroxyvalerate) and polycaprolactone. *J. Biomater. Sci. Polym. Ed.* 17, no. 12: 1405–23.

Huang, N. F., S. Patel, R. G. Thakar, J. Wu, B. S. Hsiao, B. Chu, R. J. Lee, and S. Li. 2006. Myotube assembly on nanofibrous and micropatterned polymers. *Nano Lett* 6, no. 3: 537–42.

Inoue, K., H. Takano, R. Yanagisawa, M. Sakurai, T. Ichinose, K. Sadakane, and T. Yoshikawa. 2005. Effects of nano particles on antigen-related airway inflammation in mice. *Resp. Res.* 16, no. 6: 106.

Janeway, C. A., P. Travers, M. Walport, and M. Shlomchik. 2001. *Immunobiology.* 5 ed. New York: Garland Science.

Karlsson, M. and L. Tang. 2006. Surface morphology and adsorbed proteins affect phagocyte responses to nano-porous alumina. *J. Mater. Sci. Mater. Med.* 17, no. 11: 1101–11.

Kim, D. H., P. Kim, K. Y. Suh, S. K. Choi, S. H. Lee, and B. Kim. 2005. Modulation of adhesion and growth of cardiac myocytes by surface nanotopography. *27th Annual International Conference of the Engineering in Medicine and Biology Society.* 4091–94.

Lam, C. W., J. T. James, R. McCluskey, S. Arepalli, and R. L. Hunter. 2006. A review of carbon nanotube toxicity and assessment of potential occupational and environmental health risks. *Crit. Rev. Toxicol.* 36, no. 3: 189–217.

Lemaire, I., H. Yang, V. Lafont, J. Dornand, T. Commes, and M. F. Cantin. 1996. Differential effects of macrophage- and granulocyte–macrophage colony-stimulating factors on cytokine gene expression during rat alveolar macrophage differentiation into multinucleated giant cells (Mgc): Role for Il-6 in type 2 Mgc formation. *J. Immunol.* 157, no. 11: 5118–25.

Lin, H. and R. H. Datar. 2006. Medical applications of nanotechnology. *Natl. Med. J. India* 19, no. 1: 27–32.

Little, M. C., D. J. Gawkrodger, and S. MacNeil. 1996. Chromium- and nickel-induced cytotoxicity in normal and transformed human keratinocytes: An investigation of pharmacological approaches to the prevention of Cr(Vi)-induced cytotoxicity. *Br. J. Dermatol.* 134, no. 2: 199–207.

McNally, A. K. and J. M. Anderson. 2003. Foreign body-type multinucleated giant cell formation is potently induced by alpha-tocopherol and prevented by the diacylglycerol kinase inhibitor R59022. *Am. J. Pathol.* 163, no. 3: 1147–56.

Mitchell, R. N. 2004. Innate and adaptive immunity: The immune response to foreign material. In *Biomaterials Science: An Introduction to Materials in Medicine* eds. B. D. Ratner, A. S. Hoffmann, F. J. Schoen, and J. E. Lemons. San Francisco: Elsevier.

Nel, A., T. Xia, L. Madler, and N. Li. 2006. Toxic potential of materials at the nanolevel. *Science* 311, no. 5761: 622–27.

Padera, R. F. and C. K. Colton. 1996. Time course of membrane microarchitecture-driven neovascularization. *Biomaterials* 17, no. 3: 277–84.

Paul, W. E. 1994. *Fundamental Immunology*, 4th ed. New York: Raven Press.

Peng, C. C., M. H. Yang, W. T. Chiu, C. H. Chiu, C. S. Yang, Y. W. Chen, K. C. Chen, and R. Y. Peng. 2008. Composite nano-titanium oxide-chitosan artificial skin exhibits strong wound-healing effect-an approach with anti-inflammatory and bactericidal kinetics. *Macromol. Biosci.* 8, no. 4: 316–27.

Popat, K. C., L. Leoni, C. A. Grimes, and T. A. Desai. 2007. Influence of engineered titania nanotubular surfaces on bone cells. *Biomaterials* 28, no. 21: 3188–97.

Sayes, C. M., R. Wahi, P. A. Kurian, Y. P. Liu, J. L. West, K. D. Ausman, D. B. Warheit, and V. L. Colvin. 2006. Correlating nanoscale titania structure with toxicity: A cytotoxicity and inflammatory response study with human dermal fibroblasts and human lung epithelial cells. *Toxicol. Sci.* 92, no. 1: 174–85.

Schindler, M., E. Kamal, A. Nur, I. Ahmed, J. Kamal, H. Y. Liu, N. Amor, et al. 2006. Living in three dimensions: 3d nanostructured environments for cell culture and regenerative medicine. *Cell Biochem. Biophys.* 45, no. 2: 215–27.

Tanaka, Y., I. Morishima, and K. Kikuchi. 2008. Invasive micropapillary carcinomas arising 42 years after augmentation mammoplasty: A case report and literature review. *World J. Surg. Oncol.* 6: 33.

Tang, L. and J. W. Eaton. 1999. Natural responses to unnatural materials: A molecular mechanism for foreign body reactions. *Mol. Med.* 5, no. 6: 351–8.

Thakar, R. G., M. G. Chown, A. Patel, L. Peng, S. Kumar, and T. A. Desai. 2008. Contractility-dependent modulation of cell proliferation and adhesion by microscale topographical cues. *Small* 4, no. 9: 1416–24.

Tsuji, J. S., A. D. Maynard, P. C. Howard, J. T. James, C. W. Lam, D. B. Warheit, and A. B. Santamaria. 2006. Research strategies for safety evaluation of nanomaterials, part Iv: Risk assessment of nanoparticles. *Toxicol. Sci.* 89, no. 1: 42–50.

Williams, D. F.. 1998 General concepts of biocompatibility. In *Handbook of Biomaterial Properties*, eds. J. Black and G. Hastings. New York: Chapman & Hall.

Wojciak-Stothard, B., A. Curtis, W. Monaghan, K. MacDonald, and C. Wilkinson. 1996. Guidance and activation of murine macrophages by nanometric scale topography. *Exp. Cell Res.* 223, no. 2: 426–35.

Xia, T., M. Kovochich, J. Brant, M. Hotze, J. Sempf, T. Oberley, C. Sioutas, J. I. Yeh, M. R. Wiesner, and A. E. Nel. 2006. Comparison of the abilities of ambient and manufactured nanoparticles to induce cellular toxicity according to an oxidative stress paradigm. *Nano Letters* 6, no. 8: 1794–807.

Yamawaki, H. and N. Iwai. 2006. Mechanisms underlying nano-sized air-pollution-mediated progression of atherosclerosis—carbon black causes cytotoxic injury/inflammation and inhibits cell growth in vascular endothelial cells. *Circ. J.* 70, no. 1: 129–40.

Yim, E. K., R. M. Reano, S. W. Pang, A. F. Yee, C. S. Chen, and K. W. Leong. 2005. Nanopattern-induced changes in morphology and motility of smooth muscle cells. *Biomaterials* 26, no. 26: 5405–13.

8

Enhanced Cell Growth, Function, and Differentiation by TiO$_2$ Nanotube Surface Structuring

Karla S. Brammer
University of California, San Diego

Seunghan Oh
Wonkwang University

Christine J. Cobb
University of California, San Diego

Sungho Jin
University of California, San Diego

Advances in biomaterial surface structure and design have improved tissue engineering. We report specifically in this chapter on vertically aligned TiO$_2$ nanotube surface structuring for the optimization of titanium (Ti) implants utilizing nanotechnology. The TiO$_2$ nanotube surface structure formation, mechanism, biocharacteristics, and emerging role in tissue engineering and regenerative medicine are reviewed. The main focus will be on the unique 3-D tube-shaped nanostructure of TiO$_2$ and its effects on creating profound impacts on cell behavior. In particular, we discuss how the adhesion, proliferation, phenotypic functionality, and differentiation are enhanced on surfaces with TiO$_2$ nanotube surface structuring for advancing orthopedic and related applications. In fact, the presence of TiO$_2$ nanotube surface structuring on Ti for orthopedic applications had a critical effect that improved the proliferation and mineralization of osteoblasts *in vitro*, enhanced the bone bonding strength with rabbit tibia over conventional Ti implants *in vivo*, and induced human mesenchymal stem cell (MSC) differentiation into an osteogenic lineage because of the unique nanotopographical features and high-quality biocompatibility of the TiO$_2$ nanotube surface. The nanotopography of the TiO$_2$ nanotubular surface structure also has substantial influence on upregulating extracellular matrix (ECM) production in chondrocyte cultures for potential use in osteochondral bone/cartilage interface materials. This type of TiO$_2$ surface nano-configuration is advantageous in regulating many positive cell and tissue responses for various tissue engineering and regenerative medicine applications.

8.1 Introduction

Nanostructures have recently been of great interest due to their high surface-to-volume ratio and the higher degree of biological plasticity compared to microstructures. In terms of biomaterial development and implant technology, the cellular response can be affected by topographical circumstances. In the field of *in vitro* cell biology, there is a growing body of data that shows how cells respond positively to nanotopography (Brammer et al., 2008; Curtis et al., 2006; Dalby et al., 2001, 2007b, 2008, 2009; Gallagher et al., 2002; Oh et al., 2006; Park et al., 2007). It has been proven that cells sense and react to nanotopography, *in vitro* as well as *in vivo* by exhibiting changes in cell morphology, orientation, cytoskeletal organization, proliferation, signaling, and gene expression (Brammer et al., 2008; Curtis et al., 2006; Dalby et al., 2001, 2007b, 2008, 2009; Gallagher et al., 2002; Oh et al., 2006; Park et al., 2007). Researching the interactions between cells and nanotopography is a rapidly expanding field. By fabricating nanofeatures upon biomaterial surfaces, one provides interacting features that are on the same scale as cell features. Looking at what happens on different nanotextures can help to uncover signaling pathways that promote the desired cellular response for advanced tissue engineering therapies.

It is well known that Ti and its alloys have been used as implantable biomaterials, because they have high-quality mechanical properties, a native oxide layer that is resistant to corrosion, biocompatible, and bioactively react positively with native human tissue. In our recent studies reported here, vertically aligned TiO_2 nanostructures fabricated by electrochemical anodization have become apparent as primary candidates for the direct control of many types of cell behavior for progressing tissue engineering using nanotechnology.

8.2 The Mechanism of TiO_2 Nanotube Formation on a Ti Substrate

For this review, we describe TiO_2 nanotubes prepared by anodization in fluorine-ion containing electrolytes. In general, the mechanism of TiO_2 nanotube formation in fluorine-ion based electrolytes is said to occur as a result of three simultaneous processes: the field-assisted oxidation of Ti metal to form titanium dioxide, the field-assisted dissolution of Ti metal ions in the electrolyte, and the chemical dissolution of Ti and TiO_2 due to etching by fluoride ions, which is enhanced by the presence of H^+ ions (Prakasam et al., 2007). TiO_2 nanotubes are not formed on the pure Ti surface but on the thin TiO_2 oxide layer naturally present on the Ti surface. Therefore, the mechanism of TiO_2 nanotube formation is related to oxidation and dissolution kinetics.

Metallic Ti naturally contains a stable, passivation surface layer of TiO_2 that tends to inhibit further chemical reactions to occur on the Ti surface. When the passivation layer is damaged, the layer is generally restored quickly. This restoration reaction occurs when the TiO_2 layer is in contact with air or water. This reaction produces titanium oxide as well as hydrogen gas, according to the following reaction (Prakash et al., 2005):

$$Ti_{(s)} + 2H_2O_{(g)} \rightarrow TiO_{2(s)} + 2H_{2(g)} \tag{8.1}$$

When the Ti surface is in contact with the aqueous fluorine containing electrolyte solution, the TiO_2 layer forms rapidly. The detailed dissolution mechanism of TiO_2 with regard to the formation of TiO_2 nanotubes in fluorine-containing solutions has been proposed to be sufficiently described by the following reaction (Tao et al., 2008):

$$TiO_{2(s)} + 6F^-_{(soln)} + 4H^+_{(soln)} \rightarrow [TiF_6]^{2-}_{(soln)} + 2H_2O_{(soln)} \tag{8.2}$$

In this process, an intermediate layer (TiF_6^{2-}) is formed predominantly at the surface of Ti in the fluorine-containing solution. It is known that the TiO_2 nanotube pore formation is based on both the electrical field-assisted dissolution of the TiO_2 layer and the chemical dissolution by the fluorine-containing electrolyte. Both dissolution reactions occur at the same time and play a critical role in understanding the formation of TiO_2 nanotubes at the Ti surface. We have described this mechanism in detail in a previous work (Oh et al., 2009a). Briefly, when the Ti surface is first etched by the electrolyte solution, very small pits (sub-nanometer scale) are formed on the Ti surface and are rapidly restored to a TiO_2 layer. With continuous corrosion of the Ti surface by HF ions, the pits become nanoscale pores. As reaction time goes by, nanoscale pores become the main body of nanotubes, and the small pits which are still constantly formed at the latter stage of the processing become the interspaces between nanotubes. Another proposed mechanistic model further explains that prior to pit formation, there is an occurrence of microcracks in the TiO_2 layer, which further develop and guide the formation of the pits (Tao et al., 2008). The final fabricated structure is shown in Figure 8.1 with a schematic illustration of the electrochemical anodization apparatus, basic step-by-step procedure, and the TiO_2 nanotube arrays presented by scanning electron microscopy images (SEM) and a cross-sectional transmission electron microscopy (TEM) image.

Furthermore, based on the mechanism of nanotube formation, it is inherent that the nanotubular structure formation depends on both the intensity of applied voltage and the concentration of fluorine ions in solution. It is well known that by increasing the applied voltage, larger diameter nanotubes can be formed. We further discuss the effects of the diameter pore size by changing the voltage during anodization for optimizing the nanotube size for specific cell function and fate.

8.3 Tissue Engineering Applications

8.3.1 TiO₂ Nanotubes for Orthopedic Implant Materials

The most common and successful biomaterial being used for bone implants is Ti, which does not elicit an inflammatory response *in vivo*. The bone bonding generally occurs without the common connective

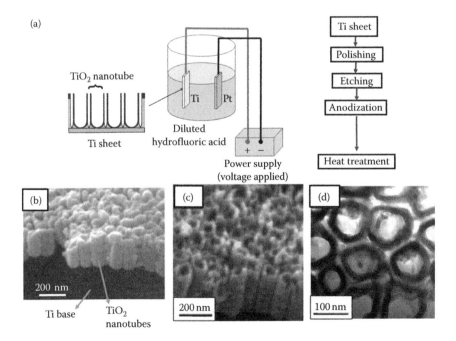

FIGURE 8.1 (**See color insert following page 10-24.**) TiO_2 nanotube surface structuring. (a) Schematic illustration of electrochemical anodization and experimental flowchart to form TiO_2 nanotube arrays. (b) SEM image showing vertically aligned TiO_2 nanotube arrays on a Ti sheet. (c) Higher magnification SEM image. (d) Cross-sectional TEM image.

tissue layer that forms from the body's immune response (foreign body reaction), between the implant metal and the underlying bone surface (Linder et al., 1988; Pillar et al., 1986; Satomi et al., 1988). Titanium surfaces seem to obtain their osseointegration (the direct structural and functional connection between living bone and implant) surface properties through mechanical interlocking. We have previously shown that heat-treated TiO_2 nanotube surfaces having a diameter and height of approximately 100 and 300 nm, respectively, elicit anchoring sites for osteoblast (bone-building cells) to adhere and grow directly into the nanotubes allowing significantly upregulated alkaline phosphatase (ALP) activity, accelerated proliferation, and increased mineralization (Oh et al., 2006). An important aspect of our nanotube system is that the nanotopography can feature a more defined, reproducible, natural, and reliable roughness than micro and macro-topography for enhanced bone cell function. It is also interesting to note that there are spaces in-between the nanotube walls (~10 nm) (Oh et al., 2005) which, even after the cell adhesion, can allow continued fluid flow of culture media and increased exchange spaces for gas, nutrients, and cell signaling molecules for an overall enhanced cell environment. In the following section, we shall further discuss nanostructure optimization by altering the size of the nanotube diameter and monitoring osteoblast behavior.

8.3.2 Nanotube Pore-Size Optimization and *In Vitro* Osteoblast Response

TiO_2 nanotube structures, already exhibiting a strongly osseointegrating implant material (Oh et al., 2006) offer encouraging implications for the development and optimization of novel orthopedics-related treatments with precise control toward desired cell and bone growth behavior. We further investigated the *in vitro* behavior of osteoblasts (bone building cells) cultured on various inner pore (30–100 nm) diameters of vertically aligned TiO_2 nanotubes and investigate the nanosize effect on osteoblast cell adhesion, morphology, and osteogenic functionality. A unique variation in cell behavior even within such a narrow range of nanotube dimensions was observed. Figure 8.2a shows the SEM micrographs of 30, 50, 70, and 100 nm TiO_2 nanotubes. The images show highly ordered, vertically aligned nanotubes with four different pore sizes between 30 and 100 nm, created by controlling potentials ranging from 5 to 20 V during the anodization fabrication processing. The nanotubes differ in diameter and height proportionally with a diameter to height ratio of 1:3. The nanotube surface on the anodized Ti substrate is robust and clear. For the purposes of our studies, the maximum size of TiO_2 nanotube diameter was limited to 100 nm in order to unify the experimental conditions and composition of electrolyte solution. For surface characterization, the nanotube pore size distribution, surface roughness, and surface contact angle for the different diameters are described in the chart in Figure 8.2b. The nanotopography significantly enhanced the roughness of the surface with Ra values ~13 nm and increased the hydrophilic surface characteristics showing contact angles less than 11°, while a flat Ti metal without a nanostructure is less rough with an Ra ~10 nm and more hydrophobic in nature with contact angle of ~54° (Ponsonnet et al., 2003).

When comparing the effect of different diameter of TiO_2 nanotubes, it was found that there were distinct size regimes for precisely controlling the cell behaviors of initial adhesion and growth versus elongation and increased ALP activity of osteoblasts. In terms of cell adhesion and morphology, adhesion was the greatest on the smallest 30 nm diameter nanotubes over all other larger sizes of nanotubes, but the nanotube surfaces with a lower density of cells started to show an increase in morphological elongation with increasing nanotube diameters as shown in Figure 8.2c. The trend of ALP activity seemed to correspond with the elongation trend where ALP activity increased with increasing diameters reaching a peak on the largest 100 nm diameter TiO_2 nanotube surfaces as displayed in Figure 8.2d. We observed that 100 nm TiO_2 nanotubes, having the most increased biochemical ALP activity of osteoblast cells, hold most promise for the greatest integration of material into the surrounding bone.

Furthermore, it has been suggested that the differences in cell responses can be explained by the presence of different curvature in the pores providing optimum compression and tension of cell

TiO$_2$ nanotube surface characteristics

(a)
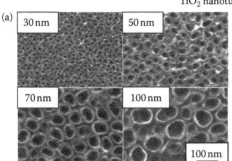

(b)

Sample	Estimated inner pore size (nm)	Roughness Ra (nm)	Contact angle (°)
Ti	NA	9.7	54 *
30 nm	27.02 ± 4.43	13.0	11
50 nm	46.37 ± 2.76	12.7	9
70 nm	69.55 ± 7.87	13.5	7
100 nm	99.61 ± 7.32	13.2	4

* Ponsonnet et al., 2003

(c)
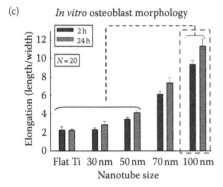

(d)
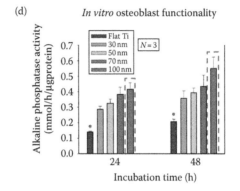

FIGURE 8.2 **(See color insert following page 10-24.)** (a) SEM micrographs of self-aligned TiO$_2$ nanotubes with different diameters. The images show highly ordered nanotubes with four different pore sizes between 30 and 100 nm. (b) Table with pore size distribution ± standard deviation, average roughness (Ra) from atomic force microscopy measurements, and surface contact angle measurements for Ti and 30–100 nm TiO$_2$ nanotube surfaces. (c) Quantification of osteoblast elongation on the different sized nanotube surfaces. (d) Bone-building functionality represented by ALP activity of osteoblasts on the different sized nanotube surfaces. (Reprinted from Brammer, K. S. et al., 2009. *Acta Biomaterialia* 5(8): 3215–3212. Copyright 2009 with permission from Elsevier.)

mechanoreceptors (Boyan et al., 1996; Ingber, 1993). It was also reported that the basement cell membrane specifically in contact with a nanostructured surface suffers tensile and relaxation mechanical forces that rearranges its components and/or open ion channels that trigger cell behavior (Martínez et al., 2009). This may help explain the slight difference in cellular responses by the different nanotube dimensions.

8.3.3 Osseointegration in Rabbit Tibia Enhanced by Nanotube Surface

In vivo osteoblasts adhere, proliferate, and mineralize regions of bone in direct contact with the orthopedic Ti implant. Instead of inserting materials purely for the mechanical support of the implants, the goal is to produce osteoinductive materials that integrate directly into the bone. To explore the *in vivo* animal response to the TiO$_2$ nanotube surface (100 nm diameter) versus conventional sandblasted Ti surfaces, five earloop rabbits were used in our studies. The details of the *in vivo* experimental procedures are given in a previous publication (Bjursten et al., 2010). Briefly, two planar surfaces on each rabbit tibia were prepared with a 5 mm diameter three-prong router during saline cooling. The Ti sandblasted disks or TiO$_2$ nanotubes were implanted according to a rotational scheme to ensure that any observed difference was due to the implant surfaces, rather than the implant positioning. Teflon caps were placed over the implant surfaces not in contact with the bone to prevent bone overgrowth. Figure 8.3 clearly indicates a direct growth of new bone onto the nanotube surface with no trapped

Ti sandblasted surface   vs.   TiO$_2$ nanotube surface

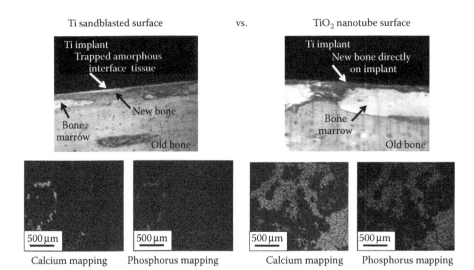

| Calcium mapping | Phosphorus mapping | Calcium mapping | Phosphorus mapping |

FIGURE 8.3 (See color insert following page 10-24.) Comparative osseointegration at bone implant surface. Cross-sectional microscopy of implant–new bone interface by histology and bone mineralization mapping on sandblasted Ti implant versus TiO$_2$ nanotube surface implant. (From Bjursten, L. M. et al., 2010. *J Biomed Mater Res Part A* 1:92(3): 1218–24. Copyright Wiley-VCH Verlag GmbH & Co. KGaA. Reproduced with permission.)

amorphous tissue layer at the implant-growing bone interface. In contrast, the sandblasted Ti implant (Figure 8.3) shows a new bone–implant interface with a trapped soft tissue layer, which contributes to the well-known bone-loosening problem and implant failure at the bone–implant interface. As well, mechanical pullout tests proved that the implant/bone bond with the nanotube surfaces was 9× stronger than the conventional sandblasted implant surfaces. Noticeably, nanotube surfaces exhibited greater bone formation and bone-implant contact compared with sandblasted surfaces. Comparative SEM energy-dispersive x-ray analysis (EDX) mapping after tensile testing exhibited strong signals for the component of bone, that is, the presence of calcium and phosphorus on the fractured interface of the TiO$_2$ nanotube surface, but not on the Ti sandblasted implant surface where only sporadic small regions showed calcium and phosphorus (Figure 8.3).

These data indicate that the interface bonding with TiO$_2$ nanotubes is so strong that a fracture actually occurs within the new growing bone, rather than at the implant–bone interface. Calcium and phosphorus, which are indicative of strong osseointegration, covered 41.7% of the nanotube implant surface area compared to 8.3% for the sandblasted surface.

8.3.4 Mesenchymal Stem Cell (MSC) Osteogenic Differentiation Dictated by Nanotube Size

8.3.4.1 Nanotopography in Stem Cell Research

Another approach to further advance the orthopedics technology is to introduce a combination of nanotechnology and stem cell treatment. MSCs are pluripotent adult stem cells available primarily from the bone marrow. For generation of osteoblasts, the MSCs need to be guided to selectively differentiate to osteoblasts, rather than differentiating into other types of cells such as myocytes, β-pancreatic islet cells, adipocytes, or neural cells.

In particular, nano-topography has recently been proven to have significant and favorable effects on stem cell commitment into mature lineages. In terms of bone cell (osteoblast) differentiation, Dalby et al. (2004, 2006, 2007a) have shown that random circular nanostructures promote and direct osteoblast differentiation of MSCs. This finding shows that the effect of nanoscale geometries alone can induce differentiation. These studies have demonstrated that different degrees of nanosymmetry or nanodisorder induces change in cell adhesion formation, which impacts on cytoskeletal tension, affects indirect mechanotransduction pathways, and imposes morphological changes on cells. The surface nanotopography directly induces pronounced changes of cell shape, and consequently gene expression, which can potentially mediate the differentiation of stem cells into various cell types.

Moreover, cell morphology/spreading dominates cell fate. McBeath et al. showed that the commitment of stem cell differentiation to specific lineages is dependent upon cell shape (Oh et al., 2009b). In single cell experiment with micropatterned surfaces, the critical role of cell spread/shape in regulating cell fate was determined. As well, a recent study showed MSCs in multicell islands differentiated into different lineages depending on the MSC location in population. Cells located at the edges of the island exhibit osteogenic characteristics, whereas cells located in the center are adipogenic (McBeath et al., 2004). These findings have been interpreted on the basis that cells at the edges of the micropatterns experience higher tension (higher stress) than cells at the center. The cellular tension/stress due to morphological shape control may provide the mechanical cues for controlling cell fate. Investigations with the manipulation of cell substrate rigidities have led to the same conclusion: MSCs on rigid surfaces (high tension) differentiated into osteogenic lineage, whereas MSCs on soft surfaces expressed neuron markers (Ruiz and Chen, 2008). All these recent evidences clearly demonstrated that the MSC fate is determined by their responses to the physical nature of the substrate.

By combining nanotechnology, cell biology, and bioengineering to guide stem cell osteogenesis *in vitro* and *in vivo* the goal of cell-based therapy for bone repair can be achieved. The realization of the full potential of MSCs in regenerative medicine requires selective differentiation. Our recent studies on nanotechnology osteogenic-related MSCs treatments have also shown the effects of nanotopography on specific differentiation by using only the geometric cues of the surface (Engler et al., 2007). On substrates made of TiO₂ nanotube surface structures, we induced selective osteoblast differentiation by creating stem cell elongation accompanied by increased cytoskeletal stress using large dimensions of nanotube diameters (~100 nm). It is hypothesized that different nanotube diameters control MSC fate by having different effects on the cell morphology and consequently cytoskeletal stresses which in turn modulates differentiation.

8.3.4.2 Mesenchymal Stem Cell (MSC) Elongation and Osteogenesis on TiO₂ Nanotubes

We have recently reported a novel discovery that the exposure of MSCs to substrates containing TiO₂ nanotubes with various diameters (Figure 8.2a) can induce differential fates. For TiO₂ nanotubes with a small diameter such as ~30 nm, the stem cell differentiation was suppressed while adhesion and growth was accelerated. Such cell enrichment and proliferation without differentiation is a beneficial application of stem cell technology to cell therapy. In contrast, when the MSCs were exposed to a larger diameter nanotube substrate such as ~100 nm, the cells were significantly stretched with ~10-fold elongation as observed by SEM analysis and by live cell imaging using fluorescein diacetate (FDA) staining shown in Figure 8.4a and b. We reported this type of morphological determination by altered nanotube dimension with osteoblast cells mentioned above (Brammer et al., 2009). The osteo-differentiation of these stretched MSCs was determined by PCR (Figure 8.4c) and immunostaining of the osteogenic markers ALP, osteopontin (OPN), and osteocalcin (OCN) (data not shown). Uniquely, MSCs on the largest 100 nm diameter TiO₂ nanotube surfaces had the highest upregulation of the osteogenic RNA transcription levels (Figure 8.4c) and were the only experimental samples that stained positively for OPN and OCN after 2 weeks of culture. The stem cell elongation and osteo-differentiation trends seem to correlate as shown in Figure 8.4a through c. The suggested mechanism is in agreement with the general notion that the morphological elongation induced increased cytoskeletal stress which in turn modulated differentiation into the specific osteoblast lineage.

The overall results indicated that the MSC adhesion was facilitated by small-diameter nanotubes, while their osteogenic differentiation was facilitated by large-diameter nanotubes. Thus, we have

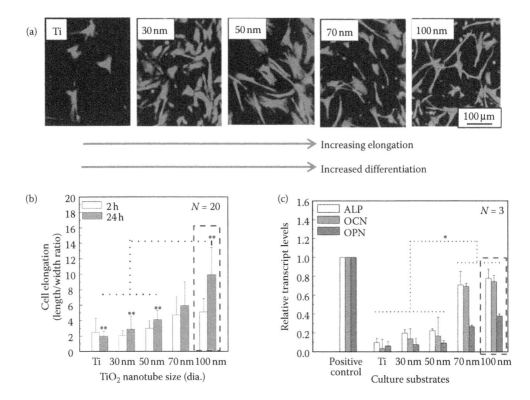

FIGURE 8.4 **(See color insert following page 10-24.)** *In vitro* MSC response to different sized nanotube surfaces. (a) Morphological observation of cells by FDA live staining. MSCs increase in elongation with increasing nanotube diameter. (b) Quantification of MSC elongation. (c) Comparative bar graph showing osteogenic differentiation on the different sized nanotube surfaces evaluated by PCR relative transcription levels for the primary osteogenic markers (ALP, OCN, and OPN). (Adapted from Oh, S. et al. 2009. *Proc Natl Acad Sci USA* 106(7): 2130–5.)

developed a concept of determining stem cell fate based solely on the geometric cues of the surface nanostructure and size of the nanotube diameter.

8.3.5 Nanotubes at the Osteochondral Interface for Cartilage Applications

Artificial cartilage prepared from cultured chondrocytes offers promise as a treatment for cartilage defects (Fedewa et al., 1998), but connecting this artificial soft tissue to bone in the attempts to restore the defected cartilage is difficult. One strategy we have employed is to develop a dually functional substrate that supports the growth and attachment of cartilage tissue on one extremity and encourages osseointegration on the other. This substrate should be an engineered interface between artificial cartilage and native bone (Zang et al., 2002). In our study, we hypothesize that nanotopographical cues, from porous nanotubular structured substrates made of TiO_2, already described above as a beneficial orthopedic biomaterial may also be a candidate for providing an alternative way to positively influence cartilage formation and the cellular behavior of cartilage chondrocytes.

We have recently observed interesting data regarding the chondrocyte cell response, morphological appearance, and ECM production based on our *in vitro* studies comparing nanotube versus flat substrata. The results of the study indicate that the nanotopography of the TiO_2 nanotubular surface structure has substantial influence on chondrocyte culture and this type of TiO_2 surface nanoconfiguration is advantageous over Ti surfaces without nanostructured topography in regulating ECM production and other positive chondrocyte responses *in vitro*. More specifically, the spherically round phenotypical chondrocyte shape and ECM production evaluated by glycosaminoglycan (GAG) secretion and PCR levels of aggrecan and collagen type-II was enhanced on TiO$_2$ nanotube surfaces.

Therefore, a Ti implant with all surfaces covered with the nanotubes can be potentially designed and utilized, for some specific types of articular cartilage injuries, to serve with the dual function of accelerated osseointegration to the existing articular bone surface at the bone-facing contact interface while the exposed nanotube surface can be applied for cartilage tissue regeneration by providing positive surface nanostructuring effects on chondrocyte ECM production.

8.4 Summary

The presence of vertically aligned TiO$_2$ nanotube surface structuring in biological tissue applications has critical and beneficial effects especially in the area of orthopedic implants. TiO$_2$ nanotubes improve the adhesion and mineralization of osteoblasts for accelerated bone healing and mechanical interlocking both *in vitro* and *in vivo*. MSC osteo-differentiation was determined by altering the size of the TiO$_2$ nanotube diameter for advanced therapies utilizing nanotechnology. Also, the enhanced cartilage chondrocyte response to the nanotopography indicated that TiO$_2$ nanotubes would be beneficial for osteo-chondral interface materials. The unique nano-topographical features and high-quality biocompatibility of the TiO$_2$ nanotube surface elicits many possibilities for tissue engineering applications using nanostructured constructs.

References

Bjursten LM, Rasmusson, L, Oh, S, Smith, GC, Brammer, and KS, Jin, S, 2010. Titanium dioxide nanotubes enhance bone bonding *in vivo*. *J Biomed Mater Res Part A* 1:92(3):1218–24.

Boyan BD, Humbert, TW, Dean, DD, and Schwartz, Z, 1996. Role of material surfaces in regulating bone and cartilage cell response. *Biomaterials* 17:137.

Brammer KS, Oh S, Gallagher JO, and Jin S, 2008. Enhanced cellular mobility guided by TiO$_2$ nanotube surfaces. *Nano Lett* 8:786.

Brammer KS, Oh S, Cobb CJ, Bjursten LM, van der Heyde H, and Jin S, 2009. Improved bone-forming functionality on diameter-controlled TiO$_2$ nanotube surface. *Acta Biomaterialia* 5(8):3215–23.

Curtis AS, Dalby M, and Gadegaard N, 2006. Cell signaling arising from nanotopography: Implications for nanomedical devices. *Nanomed* 1:67.

Dalby MJ, 2009. Nanostructured surfaces: Cell engineering and cell biology. *Nanomed* 4:247–8.

Dalby MJ, Andar A, Nag A, Affrossman S, Tare R, McFarlane S, and Oreffo RO, 2008. Genomic expression of mesenchymal stem cells to altered nanoscale topographies. *J R Soc Interface* 5:1055–65.

Dalby MJ, Gadegaard N, Curtis AS, and Oreffo RO, 2007a. Nanotopographical control of human osteoprogenitor differentiation. *Curr Stem Cell Res Ther* 2:129–38.

Dalby MJ, Gadegaard N, Herzyk P, et al. 2007b. Nanomechanotransduction and interphase nuclear organization influence on genomic control. *J Cell Biochem* 102:1234–44.

Dalby MJ, Riehle MO, Johnstone H, et al. 2001. In vitro reaction of endothelial cells to polymer demixed nanotopography. *Biomaterials* 23:2945.

Dalby MJ, McCloy D, Robertson M, et al. 2006. Osteoprogenitor response to semi-ordered and random nanotopographies. *Biomaterials* 27:2980–7.

Dalby MJ, Pasqui D, and Affrossman S, 2004. Cell response to nano-islands produced by polymer demixing: A brief review. *IEE Proc Nanobiotechnol* 151:53-61.

Engler AJ, Sweeney HL, Discher DE, and Schwarzbauer JE, 2007. Extracellular matrix elasticity directs stem cell differentiation. *J Musculoskelet Neuronal Interact* 7:335.

Fedewa MM, Oegema TR, Jr., Schwartz MH, MacLeod A, and Lewis JL, 1998. Chondrocytes in culture produce a mechanically functional tissue. *J Orthop Res* 16:227.

Gallagher JO, McGhee KF, Wilkinson CD, and Riehle MO, 2002. Interaction of animal cells with ordered nanotopography. *IEEE Trans Nanobioscience* 1:24.

Ingber DE, 1993. Cellular tensegrity: Defining new rules of biological design that govern the cytoskeleton. *J Cell Sci* 104:613.

Linder L, Carlsson A, Marsal L, Bjursten LM, and Branemark PI, 1988. Clinical aspects of osseointegration in joint replacement. A histological study of titanium implants. *J Bone Joint Surg Br* 70:550.

Martínez E, Engel E, Planell JA, and Samitier J, 2009. *Ann Anat* 191:126.

McBeath R, Pirone DM, Nelson CM, Bhadriraju K, and Chen CS, 2004. Cell shape, cytoskeletal tension, and RhoA regulate stem cell lineage commitment. *Dev Cell* 6:483–95.

Oh S, Brammer KS, Cobb CJ, Smith G, and Jin S, 2009a. TiO$_2$ nanotubes for enhanced cell and bone growth. In: Karlinsey R.L. (ed) *Recent Developments in Advanced Medical and Dental Materials Using Electrochemical Methodologies*. ISBN: 978-81-308-0335-7, Research Signpost, 199.

Oh S, Brammer KS, Li YS, Teng D, Engler AJ, Chien S, and Jin S, 2009b. Stem cell fate dictated solely by altered nanotube dimension. *Proc Natl Acad Sci USA* 106(7):2130–5. Epub 2009 Jan 28.

Oh S, Daraio C, Chen LH, Pisanic TR, Finones RR, and Jin S, 2006. Significantly accelerated osteoblast cell growth on aligned TiO$_2$ nanotubes. *J Biomed Mater Res A* 78:97.

Oh SH, Finones RR, Daraio C, Chen LH, and Jin S, 2005. Growth of nano-scale hydroxyapatite using chemically treated titanium oxide nanotubes. *Biomaterials* 26:4938.

Park J, Bauer S, von der Mark K, and Schmuki P, 2007. Nanosize and vitality: TiO$_2$ nanotube diameter directs cell fate. *Nano Lett* 7:1686.

Pillar RM LJ and Maniatopoulos C, 1986. Observation on the effect of movement on bone ingrowth into porous-surfaced implants. *Clin Orthop Rel Res* 208:108.

Ponsonnet L, Reybier K, Jaffrezic N, Comte V, Lagneau C, Liss M, and Martelet C, 2003. Relationship between surface properties (roughness, wettability) of titanium and titanium alloys and cell behaviour. *Materials Science and Engineering C* 23:551–560.

Prakasam HE, Shankar K, Paulose M, Varghese OK, and Grimes CA, 2007. A new benchmark for TiO$_2$ nanotube array growth by anodization. *J. Phys. Chem. C*, 111:7235–41.

Prakash S, Tuli GD, Basu SK, and Madan RD, 2005. *Advanced Inorganic Chemistry*, Vol. 2, S. Chand and Co Ltd.

Ruiz SA and Chen CS, 2008. Emergence of patterned stem cell differentiation within multicellular structures. *Stem Cells* 26:2921-7.

Satomi K, Akagawa Y, Nikai H, and Tsuru H, 1988. Bone-implant interface structures after nontapping and tapping insertion of screw-type titanium alloy endosseous implants. *J Prosthet Dent* 59:339.

Tao J, Zhao J, Tang C, Kang Y, and Li Y, 2008. Mechanism study of self-organized TiO$_2$ nanotube arrays by anodization. *New Journal of Chemistry* 32:2164-68.

Zhang K, Ma Y, and Francis LF, 2002. Porous polymer/bioactive glass composites for soft-to-hard tissue interfaces. *J Biomed Mater Res* 61:551.

9

Electrospun Pseudo Poly (Amino Acids) for Tissue Engineering Applications

Parth N. Shah
The University of Akron

Justin A. Smolen
The University of Akron

Anirban Sen Gupta
Case Western Reserve University

Yang H. Yun
The University of Akron

9.1 Introduction

An ideal tissue engineering scaffold should provide an architecture that promotes the exchange of nutrients and metabolites, provide structural integrity to the newly formed tissue, and possess the appropriate molecular composition for proper cellular function [1]. When examining the morphology of the extracellular matrix (ECM), collagen, elastin, and other proteins provide fibrous structures as well as a suitable environment for specific cellular interactions. While electrospun scaffolds have been shown to mimic the physical architecture of ECM, the choice of materials, which can be natural, synthetic, or a blend of both polymers, influences the biological properties of the resulting scaffold [2]. Unfortunately, natural polymers, such as collagen, generally lack the mechanical strength that is needed for proper tissue functions. Most synthetic polymers lack both the biological and mechanical characteristics needed for tissue engineering. Therefore an elastic biodegradable polymer with tunable degradation rate and with cellular recognition motifs is needed to properly engineer soft tissues.

9.2 Importance of Polyurethanes in Medical Devices

Segmented polyurethane elastomers are widely used biomaterials due to their favorable mechanical properties, such as high tensile and tear strength, fatigue and wear resistance, and elasticity [3,4]. These materials are a unique class of elastomeric block copolymers that generally exhibit a phase-segregated morphology due to the presence of rubbery soft segments and glassy or semicrystalline hard segments [5]. For these reasons, polyurethanes have been very attractive for biomedical applications, and many blood contacting devices, such as bypass grafts, catheters, and components of artificial hearts, have incorporated polyurethanes. Examples of commercial polyurethanes, their chemical compositions, and physical properties are provided in Table 9.1.

TABLE 9.1   Commercial Biomedical Polyurethanes

	Soft Segment	Hard Segment	Chain Extender	Applications	Tensile Strength	Ultimate Elongation
Polyester Polyurethanes						
Microthane (Surgitek Co.)[a]	DEG [67]	TDI [67]	AA [67]	Breast implant coating [67]	6900 psi [68]	590% [68]
BA-1011 Adhesive (Mila Chemical Corp.)[a]	PCL [68]	MDI [68]	BDO [68]	Medical adhesive [68]	NA	NA
Polyether Polyurethanes						
ChronoThane P (CardioTech International, Inc.)	PTMEG [69]	MDI [69]	BDO [69]	Substitute for Pellethane[b] [69]	5500 psi [69]	750% [69]
Tecoflex (Thermedics, Inc.)[a]	PTME [68]	HMDI [68]	BDO [68]	Vascular catheters [6], cardiac pacing leads [70], cardiac assist devices [71]	5300–8300 psi [72]	310–660% [72]
Tecophilic (Lubrizol Advanced Materials, Inc.)	PTMEG [73]	MDI [73]	BDO [73]	Wound dressing[b] [74]	700–2000 psi [75]	600–1000% [75]
Pellethane (Dow Chemical Co.)[a]	PTMEG [68]	MDI [68]	BDO [68]	Vascular catheters [6], cardiac pacing leads [70], blood bags [71]	5700 psi [70]	580% [70]
Biomer (Ethicon, Inc.)[a]	PTMEG [68]	MDI [68]	EDA [68]	Artificial heart [6], *in vivo* shunts [71]	7300 psi [76]	1200% [76]
Polycarbonate Polyurethanes						
ChronoFlex AR (CardioTech International, Inc.)	PCG [77]	HMDI [77]	BDO [77]	Coronary artery bypass graft [78], cardiac assist devices [71]	7500 psi [79]	500% [79]
Bionate (Polymer Technology Group, Inc.)	PHEC [77]	MDI [77]	BDO [77]	Cardiac assist devices [71]	6100 psi [77]	390% [77]

[a] Discontinued.
[b] Researched for use.

DEG–diethylene glycol, TDI–toluene diisocyanate, AA–adipic acid, PCL –polycaprolactone, MDI–methylene diisocyanate, BDO–butane diol, PTMEG–polytetramethylene ether glycol, HMDI–hexamethylene diisocyanate, EDA–ethylene diamine, PCG–polycarbonate glycol, PHEC–poly(1,6-hexyl 1,2-ethyl carbonate).

In the past, the majority of polyurethanes for biomedical implants have been primarily investigated for *in vivo* applications in which a key desired characteristic was the biostability of the material. Many of these polyurethanes have been discontinued due to their slow degradation via hydrolysis in which the degradation products are usually toxic, carcinogenic, and/or immunogenic [2]. Slow degradation can also compromise the structural integrity of the implant, such as cracking of the implant and causing premature failure.

To improve their overall biocompatibility, polyurethanes have been reformulated with alternative soft segments. These soft segments include, but are not limited to polycarbonates, hydrogenated polybutadienes, polydimethylsiloxanes, dimerized fatty acid derivatives, polycaprolactone (PCL), and polyethylene glycol (PEG) [6]. In addition, the choice of both the soft and hard segments must be made carefully since the degradation products must be relatively benign in order for biodegradable polyurethanes to be successful in tissue engineering applications where degradation of the polymer is highly desirable.

9.2.1 Biodegradable Polyurethanes

An apparent method of introducing biodegradable linkages in polyurethanes is through the incorporation of polyesters, such as polylactides and ε-PCL, and polyethers as the soft segments [7–11]. These biomaterials are commonly used for preparing many biodegradable devices. Since the majority of polyurethanes consist of a relatively large amount of soft segment linkages (50–75%), it is not surprising that the polymer properties are largely driven by the choice of the soft segments. However, the use of hydrolysable hard segments in combination with a variety of biodegradable soft segment chemistries provides additional control over the degradation and provides a distinct advantage over polyurethanes synthesized using only hydrolysable soft segments. Unfortunately, relatively few choices of hard segment diisocyanates are currently available for polyurethane synthesis [12], and the general practice is to incorporate hydrolysable hard segment chain extenders in the form of diols and diamines.

One of the strategies of synthesizing biodegradable polyurethanes is to use hard segment components, such as diisocyanates or use chain extenders based on amino acids [5,13]. These polymers are attractive biomaterials since amino acids are naturally occurring and their chemical structure offers functionalities that may be used for the attachment of drugs, crosslinking agents, or pendent groups that can be used for the modification of physico-mechanical properties of the polymer [6]. Due to these characteristics, poly (amino acids) have been investigated for biomedical applications, including controlled drug delivery devices [14–16], suture materials [17], and artificial skin substitutes [18]. Despite their apparent potential, the development of poly (amino acids) has been limited because of their insolubility in common organic solvents, high thermal transition temperatures, and difficulties associated with their processing [6]. In addition, these materials can induce an aggressive immune response depending upon their structure [19]. Since the problems associated with poly (amino acids) are associated with their chemical nature and hydrogen bonding occurring within the polymeric backbone, structural modification has been attempted by introducing nonamide linkages to replace the peptide linkages within the backbone [20]. Examples of these linkages include ester, imminocarbonate [21], carbonate [14], phosphate [22,23], or urethane bonds [13], and the resulting polymers are collectively known as "pseudo" poly (amino acids).

L-Tyrosine, a nonessential amino acid, has been used to synthesize a variety of "pseudo" poly (amino acids) by utilizing its functional groups to introduce a number of nonpeptide functionalities [24]. Primary reasons for the choice of L-tyrosine include the presence of a terminal hydroxyl group, which may be exploited for polymer synthesis, and the importance of L-tyrosine as a precursor of several neurotransmitters [25–29]. Polycarbonates, polyiminocarbonates, and polyarylates have been among the first L-tyrosine polymers to be successfully investigated for biomedical applications [20,21,24,30–32]. These materials demonstrate a considerable improvement in the physico-mechanical properties compared to amino acid based homopolymers; however, they are limited in their hydrolytic degradation and

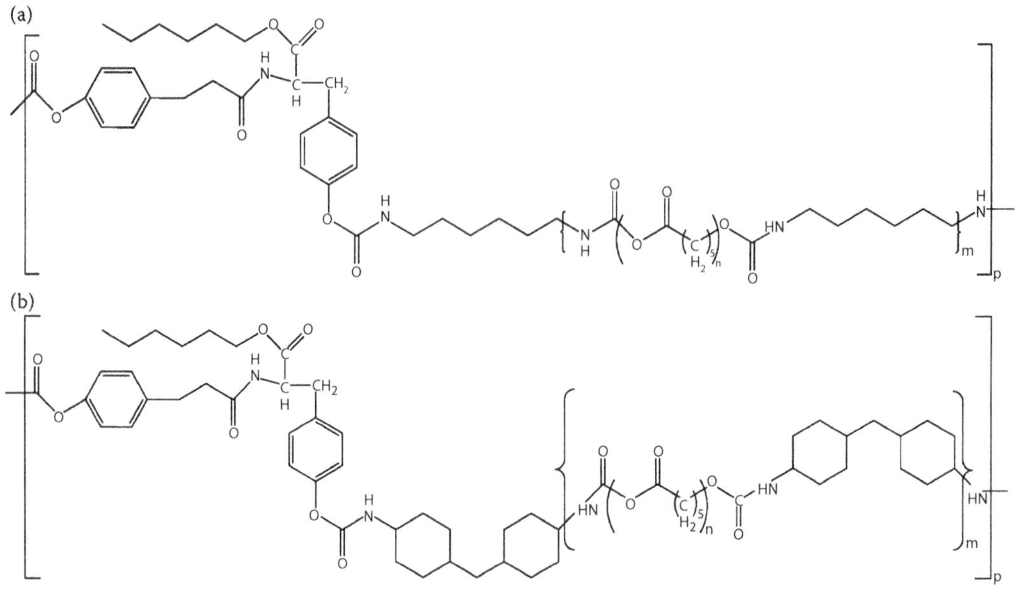

FIGURE 9.1 Chemical structures of L-tyrosine polyurethanes. (a) PCL-L-DTH and (b) PCL-C-DTH.

mechanical properties. Subsequently, L-tyrosine-based polyurethanes (LTUs) have been developed in an effort to obtain polymers with improved mechanical properties and degradation by both hydrolytic and enzymatic pathways [12,13,22,23,33–35].

Two LTUs (Figure 9.1) that have been extensively characterized for their physical properties are PCL-L-DTH and PCL-C-DTH (Table 9.2). These biodegradable polymers have similar tensile strength and elasticity to commercial polyurethanes that are designed to be biostable (Table 9.1). Thus, the introduction of both enzymatic and hydrolytic degradable components does not compromise their mechanical properties. The PCL-C-DTH electrospun scaffolds are generally stronger than PCL-L-DTH (ultimate

TABLE 9.2 Biomaterial Properties of LTUs

	PCL-L-DTH	PCL-C-DTH
Molecular Weight (Da)		
M_n	150,370	64,670
M_w	246,120	75,430
Thermal Properties (°C)		
Glass transition temperature of the soft segment	−37	−39
Melting temperature of the hard segment	173	—
Degradation temperature	~300	~300
Mechanical Properties		
Ultimate tensile strength (psi)	1022 ± 87	2698 ± 233
Modulus of elasticity (psi)	2608 ± 98	457 ± 41
Elongation at break (%)	643 ± 87	825 ± 29
Bulk Properties		
Water vapor permeability (mg/h*mm²*mm of Hg)	$9.11 \pm 1.32 \times 10^6$	7.73 ± 0.77
Swelling ratio	1.06 ± 0.01	1.21 ± 0.01
Degradation at 30 days (% mass loss)	7.8 ± 0.4	14.3 ± 1.2

tensile strength of 2698 vs. 1022 psi, respectively) and are more elastic (825 vs. 643%) but have a lower Young's modulus (457 vs. 2608 psi). These results show that the changing of the hard segment allows the alteration of both the mechanical and bulk properties of LTUs. However, by blending two LTUs with each other [12], or with other L-tyrosine-based polymers, biomaterials with tunable material properties and degradation rates can be fabricated [35].

9.2.2 Tuning Materials Properties of LTUs through Blending

For tissue engineering, scaffolds with tunable degradation properties are highly desirable since most biological mechanisms, such as cellular differentiation and wound healing, occur in stages. The two common methods for achieving the desired degradation rates are blending and copolymerization [36,37]. In general, blending two or more existing polymers is easier than the preparation of copolymers or co-block polymers [38]. Polymers that are blended generally possess better physical and mechanical properties in comparison to the individual polymers, and blending also potentially minimizes any undesired properties of the individual polymers. Depending on the compatibility and miscibility of the constituent polymers, the blend polymers exhibit a wide range of morphology that ranges from phase-mixed to phase-segregated structures [39]. By changing the composition of the polymers, the final properties of the blended material can be customized to the requirement for the desired applications.

Blends of PCL-L-DTH and PEG-L-DTH with three different compositions have been prepared by varying the mass ratios of these polymers (Table 9.3) [32]. The blended compositions, as determined by NMR and FTIR, closely match the theoretical compositions. The thermal characterization of the blended polymers confirms the presence of a two-phase morphology observed by scanning electron microscopy (SEM). Furthermore, the differential scanning calorimetry (DSC) also suggests the presence of amorphous hard segment domains with the presence of a short-range order, the absence of a long-range order, the lack of complete miscibility of the two LTU components, and the possibility of phase separation due to incompatibility between hydrophobic PCL and hydrophilic PEG soft segment.

Although the hard segments in both cases are similar and form a single phase, the presence of two different soft segments inhibits the ordering of hard segments into crystalline domains and alters the mechanical properties of the blends. While the mechanical properties of all blended polymers are intermediate to the parent LTUs, they—even for blends with higher PCL-L-DTH concentration—approximate the properties of PEG-L-DTH. These observations have been attributed to the amorphous nature of the hard segments, the absence of a long-range order, and the possible phase segregation between the parent LTUs. The incompatibility between PEG and PCL likely leads to the formation of a continuous PEG-L-DTH phase with PCL-L-DTH dispersed in it as discrete domains. Due to the immiscibility of the two phases, the micromechanical deformation of the individual polymers dominates over molecular deformation, causing the blend mechanical properties to be closer to those of PEG-L-DTH [40].

The blending of PCL-L-DTH and PEG-L-DTH also has distinct effects on the relative surface hydrophilicity, water absorption, and hydrolytic degradation characteristics. Phase separation leads to a heterogeneous surface for all of the blended polymers. The contact angle indicates that, initially, the blend surfaces are dominated by the hydrophobic PCL-L-DTH; however the hydrophilic PEG-L-DTH migrates to the surface in response to the applied water droplet [41]. As expected, the degree of phase separation

TABLE 9.3   Composition of PCL-L-DTH and PEG-L-DTH Blends

Blend Code	Percent Weight Ratio of PEG-L-DTH/PCL-L-DTH
PEG-L-DTH	100/0
Blend 1	67/33
Blend 2	50/50
Blend 3	33/67
PCL-L-DTH	0/100

within the blends increases with increasing PCL-L-DTH concentrations, causing the blended surfaces to become progressively more hydrophobic. The hydrophobic nature of the blended surface also influences the water absorption. While the data is not conclusive at the termination of the experiment at 17 h, due to onset of degradation, the water absorption increases with increasing PEG-L-DTH concentrations but does not approach the values of pure PEG-L-DTH due to the hydrophobicity of the blended surface.

During hydrolytic degradation studies, all of the blended films exhibit a rapid initial degradation followed by significantly slower degradation rates over a period of 30 days. These results could be caused by the rapid initial degradation of PEG-L-DTH followed by the slow degradation of hydrophobic and comparatively crystalline PCL-L-DTH. Furthermore, a higher mass loss is observed with increasing PEG-L-DTH content since the hydrophilic PEG component absorbs more water, leading to the degradation of hydrolytically labile urethane, amide, and ester linkages. Therefore, the soft segment characteristics are of particular importance in controlling the hydrolytic degradation of the blended LTUs.

9.3 Electrospinning of LTUs

While the development of biodegradable polyurethanes has lagged as compared to other biomaterials, electrospinning of these materials has received even lesser attention. Therefore, we have investigated the electrospinning of two biodegradable polyurethanes with an aim of developing tissue engineering scaffolds. To electrospin PCL-C-DTH and PCL-L-DTH, they have been initially dissolved in 1,1,1,3,3,3-hexafluoro-2-propanol (HFIP) at concentrations of 10%, 15%, 20%, and 25% (w/v). Each of the polymer solution mentioned above has been electrospun with a 10 gage stainless-steel tip, voltage of approximately 30 kV, a gap distance of 17 cm, and a flow rate of 0.035 mL/min. All of the resulting scaffolds show a porous structure comprised of randomly oriented nonwoven fibers with diameters ranging from hundreds of nanometers to a few microns (Table 9.4). Representative samples of scaffold morphologies are illustrated in Figure 9.2a–f. SEM images reveal that all PCL-L-DTH polymer concentrations lead to the formation of beaded nanofibers. The scaffolds with the most consistent fiber structure and a minimum amount of beads are observed upon increasing the polymer concentration to 20% (w/v). When the polymer concentration is increased to 25% (w/v), fibers form aggregates. In contrast, none of the electrospun PCL-C-DTH scaffolds show the presence of beads; rather, fibers show a smooth surface morphology.

Further study has been performed on electrospinning PCL-L-DTH using a cosolvent system consisting of 75% CHCl$_3$ and 25% HFIP, as opposed to 100% HFIP. The aim of this study is to reduce the amount of HFIP necessary to dissolve the PCL-L-DTH by adding another organic solvent. This cosolvent has been used to dissolve the PCL-L-DTH to a concentration of 20%. The additional changes in the parameters to accommodate successful electrospinning include reduction in the voltage to 20 kV, a flow rate of 1.5 mL/h, and the use of 21 gauge tip. As a result, a fibrous scaffold has been successfully electrospun. SEM images of the resultant fibers (Figure 9.3) show a random dispersion of fibers with beading.

Scaffolds obtained from electrospinning 15% PCL-L-DTH dissolved in HFIP (no cosolvent) exhibit a tight fiber diameter distribution with an average fiber diameter of 870 ± 12 nm. The fiber diameter

TABLE 9.4   Fiber Diameter of Electrospun LTUs

Polymer	Concentration (%)[a]	Average Fiber Diameter (nm)
PCL-L-DTH	15	870 ± 12
	20	890 ± 35
	25	930 ± 15
PCL-C-DTH	10	1201 ± 143
	15	2324 ± 83
	20	2596 ± 267

[a] By weight per volume. Data are presented as mean fiber diameter ± standard error.

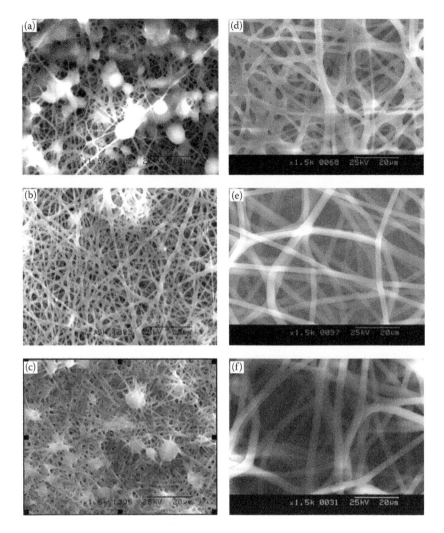

FIGURE 9.2 SEM micrographs of electrospun scaffolds obtained by using PCL-L-DTH (a) 15% (w/v) solution, (b) 20% (w/v) solution, and (c) 25% (w/v) and PCL-C-DTH (d) 10% (w/v) solution, (e) 15% (w/v) solution, and (f) 20% (w/v) solution.

increases with an increase in the polymer concentration. For PCL-C-DTH, the fiber diameters are in the micron range. In the case of the 10% PCL-C-DTH scaffolds, an average fiber diameter of 1201 ± 143 nm has been obtained by electrospinning. Similar to PCL-L-DTH scaffolds, increasing the polymer solution concentration results in scaffolds with larger diameters and wider fiber size distribution. Although both polyurethanes are influenced similarly by the polymer concentration, this effect is more pronounced for PCL-C-DTH.

In addition to the polymer itself, other parameters that influence the morphology and the fiber diameter of electrospun scaffolds include electrical force, gap distance, tip diameter, flow rate, and the solution parameters, such as concentration, viscosity, ionic strength, and conductivity. Of all of these parameters, the polymer concentration has been shown to be a determining factor in controlling the fiber morphology and size distribution by several researchers [42–45]. Our investigation performed by varying LTU concentrations keeping the other electrospinning parameters constant is in agreement with these findings by others. The increase in fiber diameters at higher polymer concentrations can be attributed to the viscoelastic forces associated with increasing viscosity, which resist the extension and

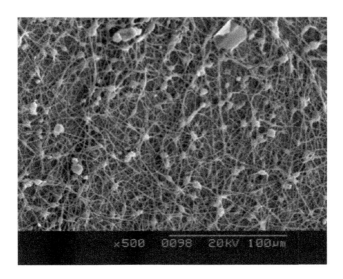

FIGURE 9.3   SEM of electrospun PCL-L-DTH scaffold in 75% $CHCl_3$ and 25% HFIP.

thinning of the jet thereby producing thicker fibers [46]. In addition to the effects of viscoelastic forces, the evaporation rates of the solution can also have an effect on the fiber diameters [47]. The higher viscosities of PCL-C-DTH solutions and the corresponding lower solvent evaporation rates may prevent a complete removal of the solvent by the time the fiber jet reaches the collection plate, thus facilitating fiber fusion and the formation of microfibers.

9.3.1 Evaluation of Physical Properties of Electrospun LTUs

Since the absorption of water influences both the mass transport and degradation characteristics of electrospun scaffolds, this parameter has been correlated to the polymer concentration. As evident from Table 9.5, the water absorption begins immediately upon incubation and continues to increase until equilibrium is reached (approximately 24 h of incubation), in which the swelling ratios for 15%, 20%, and 25% PCL-L-DTH scaffolds are 1.73 ± 0.13, 1.89 ± 0.08, and 2.14 ± 0.14, respectively. For PCL-C-DTH, equilibrium is also achieved at 24 h, and the swelling ratios for the 10, 15, and 20% scaffolds are 1.94 ± 0.01, 1.22 ± 0.04, and 1.34 ± 0.04, respectively. While an increase in the polymer concentration leads to an increase in the overall water absorption for PCL-L-DTH scaffolds, no such distinct trends are observed for PCL-C-DTH scaffolds. The maximum water absorption is observed for the 10% PCL-C-DTH scaffold. The water uptake process in polymeric scaffolds occurs primarily due to the presence of hydrophilic functional groups that are capable of forming hydrogen bonds with the water molecules [48]. The swelling ratios for the LTU scaffolds exhibit higher water content as compared to the solvent-cast

TABLE 9.5   Swelling Ratios of LTU Scaffolds

	PCL-L-DTH			PCL-C-DTH		
Time (h)	15%	20%	25%	10%	15%	20%
1	1.22 ± 0.03	1.26 ± 0.07	1.47 ± 0.04	1.19 ± 0.05	1.13 ± 0.02	1.19 ± 0.04
3	1.40 ± 0.05	1.68 ± 0.02	1.73 ± 0.11	1.46 ± 0.07	1.10 ± 0.02	1.24 ± 0.04
6	1.49 ± 0.03	1.60 ± 0.01	1.89 ± 0.20	1.89 ± 0.03	1.17 ± 0.06	1.31 ± 0.07
12	1.72 ± 0.10	1.87 ± 0.02	2.18 ± 0.20	1.95 ± 0.02	1.18 ± 0.06	1.33 ± 0.05
24	1.73 ± 0.13	1.89 ± 0.08	2.14 ± 0.14	1.94 ± 0.01	1.22 ± 0.04	1.37 ± 0.04

Data are presented as mean swelling ratio ± standard error at each time point.

LTU films, showing the importance of surface area for fluid transport processes within scaffolds. The porous structures are vital for the occurrence of nutrient and waste-exchange processes during tissue growth and remodeling. Furthermore, the swelling data also suggests the dependence of the water uptake process on the fiber diameter distribution, a factor that affects the scaffold's porosity.

To analyze the effects of *in vitro* hydrolytic degradation on the LTU scaffolds, mass-loss profiles for the electrospun scaffolds have been generated, and the morphology of the degraded scaffolds has been examined. Table 9.6 shows that the initial degradation rates for all PCL-L-DTH scaffolds are similar. Although the 25% scaffold seems to retain marginally more mass compared to the other scaffolds upon termination of the degradation studies at 28 days, these differences are not significant. Comparable results are also observed for the PCL-C-DTH scaffolds (Table 9.6), in which the 20% scaffold retains a slightly higher mass as compared to the 10 and 15% scaffolds following 28 days of *in vitro* hydrolytic degradation; however, these differences are not statistically different.

Although the mass loss of the scaffolds after degradation is similar, differences are observed when the surface morphology is evaluated for the degraded electrospun scaffolds. The structure and morphologies of degraded PCL-L-DTH scaffolds has been demonstrated in Figure 9.4a–c. In case of the 15% PCL-L-DTH scaffolds, the interconnected porous structure is completely degraded after 4 weeks of incubation in PBS, and the fiber-bonding points are fused together giving rise to a continuous molten structure with a few randomly interspersed fibers. A similar degradation pattern is also observed for the 20% scaffold; however, the bead formation is observed to occur to a lesser extent than in case of the 15% scaffold. In contrast, the fibrous structure of the 25% electrospun scaffold is still observed to be intact with the presence of a few beaded or molten structures, but the edges of the fibers appear to be frayed. Analysis of the post-degradation morphology for the PCL-C-DTH scaffolds (Figure 9.4d–f) suggests that the loss of fibrous structure is not as extensive as PCL-L-DTH. The 10% and 15% scaffolds mostly exhibit fusion of the individual fibers; however, some retention of the individual fiber structure is still observed. These results are in direct contrast to the PCL-L-DTH scaffolds, in which almost a complete loss of the fiber structure is observed. Furthermore, a decline in the scaffold pores and pore volume is also evident. The fusion of the individual fibers also seems to lead to thickening of the fiber structures. For 20% electrospun PCL-C-DTH scaffolds, the fiber structure and their diameters are extensively preserved. While some fusion of the fibers at the interconnected junctions is observed, the majority of the morphological features remain consistent with nondegraded scaffolds, except for the edges that appear frayed and the presence of spiky structures.

The *in vitro* degradation studies provide quantitative data on the resistance of PCL-L-DTH and PCL-C-DTH scaffolds against hydrolytic cleavage of the bonds present within the polymer backbone. These studies also provide an insight into the morphological and fiber structure changes as a function of the scaffold degradation process. Although the quantitative values for the mass loss are similar irrespective of the polymer utilized and its concentration, definitive differences in the morphology of the scaffolds as a function of these two parameters are observed postdegradation. The formation of fused fibrous structures at the fiber-overlap junctions and the congealing of the individual fibers possibly occurs due to a combination of mass loss (responsible for a reduction in the polymer intrinsic viscosity) and the

TABLE 9.6 Hydrolytic Degradation of LTU Scaffolds

Time (days)	PCL-L-DTH Scaffolds			PCL-C-DTH Scaffolds		
	15%	20%	25%	10%	15%	20%
1	98.3 ± 0.2	98.5 ± 0.3	96.7 ± 0.4	96.9 ± 0.7	96.4 ± 0.2	96.8 ± 0.4
7	93.6 ± 0.7	92.6 ± 1.0	92.5 ± 0.2	91.5 ± 0.3	91.5 ± 0.7	92.1 ± 0.4
14	86.9 ± 0.4	88.6 ± 0.1	88.7 ± 0.3	83.8 ± 0.4	88.5 ± 0.3	87.5 ± 0.3
21	84.8 ± 0.4	84.7 ± 0.3	87.7 ± 0.3	81.2 ± 0.3	83.4 ± 0.7	86.5 ± 0.5
28	82.9 ± 0.4	83.1 ± 0.1	85.3 ± 0.3	81.1 ± 0.4	82.2 ± 0.3	83.9 ± 0.2

Data are presented as mean ± standard error and indicates percent mass remaining at each time point.

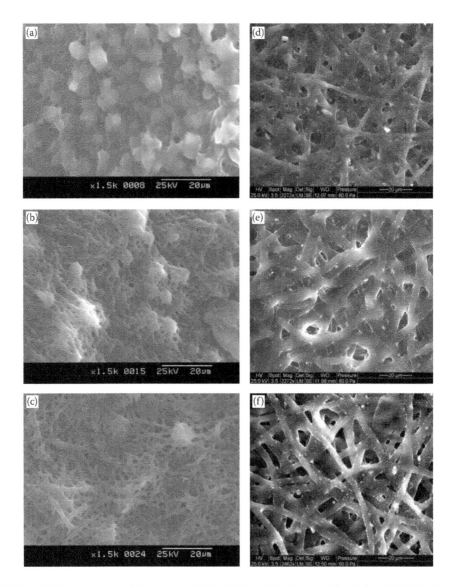

FIGURE 9.4 SEM micrographs of electrospun PCL-L-DTH scaffolds degraded for 28 days (a) 15% (w/v) solution, (b) 20% (w/v) solution, and (c) 25% (w/v) solution and PCL-C-DTH scaffolds degraded for 28 days (d) 10% (w/v) solution, (e) 15% (w/v) solution, and (f) 20% (w/v) solution.

glass transition of the LTUs (T_g's of PCL-L-DTH and PCL-C-DTH are −37°C and −39°C) being lower than the physiological temperature. Furthermore, a comparison of 10% w/v solvent cast films and electrospun scaffolds for PCL-L-DTH shows 10–12% mass loss over a period of 30 days, versus 18–20% for the electrospun scaffolds. These differences are further magnified in the case of PCL-C-DTH (2–5% mass loss for the films compared to 18–20% for the scaffolds). The higher mass loss of the scaffolds likely occurs due to a combination of several factors. In the case of PCL-L-DTH, the presence of a linear diisocyanate within the polymeric backbone permits the packing of the soft segment chains, thereby generating a partially phase-segregated semicrystalline structure for dense films. However, these soft segment chains may align together, and the semicrystalline nature of the material may be lost during electrospinning. Another factor that aids in a faster hydrolytic degradation is the presence of a highly porous structure, which is absent in the case of dense films. The presence of a porous structure facilitates the entry of water and causes an increase in the degradation rate, and the mechanism of hydrolytic degradation is primarily by a surface-erosion mechanism since both PCL-L-DTH and PCL-C-DTH are moderately hydrophobic [32,35]. Unfortunately, these *in vitro* tests do not measure the effect of enzymatic degradation that will occur once these materials are implanted.

9.3.2 Cytotoxicity of LTUs

Apart from the investigation of the physico-chemical and mechanical properties, the biocompatibility of a material is an important consideration for tissue engineering applications [49]. Cytotoxicity studies have been performed with PCL-L-DTH and PCL-C-DTH films and with their degradation products to determine the possibility of any detrimental effects. Primary dermal human fibroblasts exposed to 20 mg/mL PCL-L-DTH and PLGA control films for 24 h (Figures 9.5 and 9.6, respectively) exhibit cells with a spindle-shaped morphology, which is typical of human fibroblasts, and an excellent cell viability according to the LIVE/DEAD® Cell Viability Assay (Invitrogen). Table 9.7 summarizes the data obtained from PCL-L-DTH and PCL-C-DTH cytotoxicity studies and provides a comparison between the viability of human fibroblasts after exposure to various treatments. The cell viability is 97% or greater for all treatments with no significant differences among the treatment groups.

A further investigation into the possible cytotoxic effects of LTUs has been performed by exposure of primary dermal human fibroblasts to PCL-L-DTH and PCL-C-DTH degradation products. Degradation products obtained at two different time points (days 21 and 42) have been utilized at two different dosages (500 and 800 μg/mL) and the resulting data has been compared to the cell viabilities obtained using PLGA degradation products at similar dosages (Table 9.7). High fibroblast viabilities are seen following incubation with 500 μg/mL of LTU degradation products, which suggests the absence of cytotoxicity for the degradation products at this dosage. Upon increasing the dosage to 800 μg/mL degradation products, the cell viabilities are found to decline slightly as compared to similar treatments at 500 μg/mL and compared to PLGA controls. Specifically, the viability values are approximately 93–94%. At these dosages, microscopy of fibroblasts shows most cells are normal in their morphology. However, a population of cells has an enlarged nucleus along with disturbed cellular membranes even though their spindle shaped morphology is preserved and homeostasis is maintained as indicted by the LIVE/DEAD Cell Viability Assay. Fibroblasts exposed to 800 μg/mL PLGA degradation products have a rounded

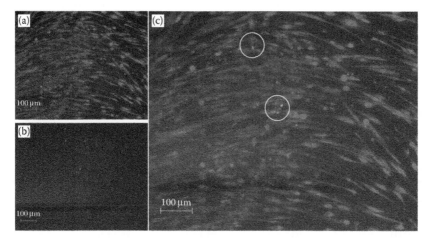

FIGURE 9.5 **(See color insert following page 10-24.)** LIVE/DEAD cell assay analysis of cells exposed to 20 mg/mL PCL-L-DTH polyurethane film (a) dead cells, (b) live cells, and (c) combined image. Circles in yellow highlight representative dead cell nuclei.

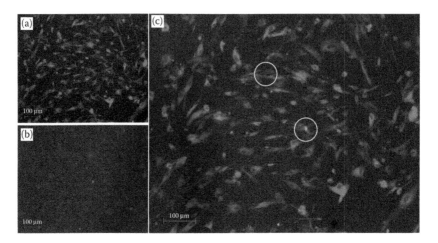

FIGURE 9.6   (See color insert following page 10-24.) LIVE/DEAD cell assay analysis of cells exposed to 20 mg/mL PLGA film (a) dead cells, (b) live cells, and (c) combined image. Circles in yellow highlight representative dead cell nuclei.

morphology, and they too have the ability to maintain homeostasis. As with numerous cyclic and aromatic diisocyanates, 4,4′-Methylenebis (cyclohexyl isocyanate) used for the synthesis of PCL-C-DTH is cyclic and may be cytotoxic at higher concentrations [6,50,51]. However, the translation of cytotoxic effects of polyurethane degradation products to *in vivo* conditions is ambiguous [6,50,52] since the threshold concentrations may never be exceeded *in vivo*.

9.3.3 Cellular Adhesion onto Electrospun LTUs

Cell adhesion and proliferation on biomaterial surfaces is an important marker of biocompatibility and positive cell–biomaterial interactions are crucial to the success of biodegradable scaffolds for tissue engineering. Cell interaction with biomaterial surfaces has been found to be a function of several parameters, of which surface chemistry, surface wettability, surface charge, and topography [53–59] are perhaps the most important. Rajaraman et al. have found that the process of cell adhesion and proliferation consists of a series of events occurring in a sequential order: initial cell attachment, filopodial growth, cytoplasmic webbing, flattening of the cell mass, and the ruffling of the peripheral cytoplasm [60]. While the surface chemistry appears to have a direct influence on the attachment of cells onto the surface, the cellular adhesion occurs by interaction with the proteins adsorbed on the substrate surface instead of specific interactions. The nature of the surface, including the chemistry and wettability, influences the composition and the confirmation of the adsorbed protein layer, which in turn influences the subsequent cellular adhesion and spread [61,62]. In the case of the moderately hydrophobic PCL-L-DTH and PCL-C-DTH surfaces, a high degree of protein adsorption is likely to occur, which in turn favors cell attachment and spreading.

TABLE 9.7   Cell Viability Comparison of LTU and Their Degradation Products

Polymer	Films (%)	500 µg Degradation Products (%)		800 µg Degradation Products (%)	
		at 21 Days	at 42 Days	at 21 Days	at 42 Days
PCL-L-DTH	97.0 ± 0.6	98.3 ± 0.4	98.4 ± 0.6	98.2 ± 0.2	97.9 ± 0.1
PCL-C-DTH	97.1 ± 1.0	98.8 ± 0.2	98.9 ± 0.1	94.0 ± 0.3	93.4 ± 0.1
PLGA	97.4 ± 0.4	97.5 ± 0.4	—	99.4 ± 0.2	—

Data are presented as mean cell viability percentage ± standard error.

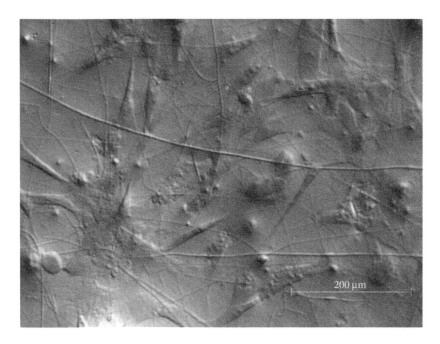

200 μm

FIGURE 9.7   (See color insert following page 10-24.) Attachment of human dermal fibroblasts to PCL-L-DTH fiber.

The adhesion of human dermal fibroblasts to electrospun PCL-L-DTH fibers has been tested on molded polydimethylsiloxane (PDMS) stubs. PDMS is a frequently used biomaterial for cell adhesion studies due to its tendency to inhibit cellular attachment [63]. In this study, human dermal fibroblasts have been seeded onto PCL-L-DTH fiber-covered PDMS stubs at a density of 25,000 cells/cm^2 and incubated over a 48-h period. Afterwards, the samples are washed, fixed in formaldehyde, and treated with nuclear fast red. Microscope images of the cells (Figure 9.7) reveal that the fibroblasts have taken on their typical spindle-shaped morphology and have aligned along the electrospun fibers. In order to visualize the attachment of human dermal fibroblasts to the electrospun PCL-L-DTH fibers, immunofluorescence staining for vinculin has also been performed using the same setup. In this case, the fibroblasts are fixed in formaldehyde, washed with newborn calf serum (NCS) to prevent nonspecific antibody binding, incubated with mouse anti-vinculin primary antibody, washed again with NCS, and incubated with tetramethyl rhodamine iso-thiocyanate (TRITC) conjugated rabbit anti-mouse secondary antibody. Visualization of the fluorescence-labeled vinculin was performed with a fluorescent microscope (Figure 9.8). In order to visualize the fibroblasts, samples are also treated with Alexa Fluor® 488 phalloidin stain for actin and Hoechst for nuclear stain. Separate fluorescence channels are used to visualize the actin (green), nucleus (blue), and vinculin attachment (red). The fluorescence channels are overlain on differential interference contrast (DIC) images of the scaffold, showing the relative positions of the fibroblasts with the electrospun PCL-L-DTH fibers.

Since the surface of the PDMS stub is nonadhesive with respect to cells, Figure 9.7 demonstrates that the PCL-L-DTH fibers are able to support nonspecific adhesion of human dermal fibroblasts. Overall, the results reveal a large number of fibroblasts interacting with the PCL-L-DTH fibers, and the immunofluorescence staining shown in Figure 9.8 demonstrate direct attachment between the fibroblasts and the fibers via vinculin, which is stained in red. Vinculin appears at the edge of the fibroblast, is aligned with the fibers (Figure 9.8b), and shows clear indication of focal adhesion. As expected, the vinculin and actin stains are not colocalized and confirms that the fibroblasts are attaching directly to the PCL-L-DTH fibers.

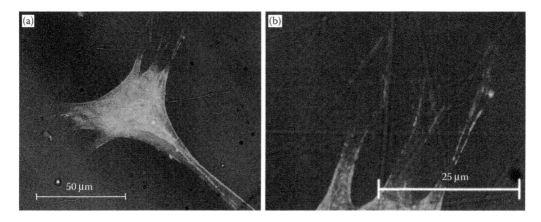

FIGURE 9.8 **(See color insert following page 10-24.)** Vinculin immunofluorescence staining of human dermal fibroblast attachment to PCL-L-DTH fibers. Green color represents staining of actin using Alexa Fluor 488 phalloidin, blue represents Hoechst nuclear staining, and red represents anti-vinculin antibody conjugated with TRITC. (a) Image of a single cell and (b) close up of focal adhesion sites.

9.4 Conclusions

Generating a synthetic tissue engineering scaffold is a challenging undertaking that necessitates the design of a three-dimensional network that not only provides the appropriate architectural qualities, such as the geometrical shape and scale of pores and fibers, but also requires the necessary mechanical, biological, and chemical properties. A promising foundation has been set for creating an effective tissue engineering scaffold that is able to support cellular attachment, via focal adhesion, by electrospinning biodegradable L-tyrosine polyurethanes. These biomaterials have shown to be capable of being fabricated into scaffolds with ECM-like architecture that have mechanical properties similar to non-biodegradable commercial polyurethanes, support cellular attachment, and degrade hydrolytically into byproducts with minimal cellular toxicity. While these results are encouraging, further study is needed. The mechanical properties of these electrospun polyurethane scaffolds, including tensile strength, modulus of elasticity, and maximum strain, should be investigated with respect to the scaffold degradation to determine how well they would function under the mechanical stresses of the body. Further study is also needed into cell adhesion and proliferation with more than one cell types and under dynamic deformation. While these scaffolds have shown to perform well in cellular viability and cytotoxicity studies, immunological studies are needed to determine the degree to which these polyurethanes incite an inflammatory response. Finally, the electrospinning process provides an effective means of integrating drugs, such as antibiotics, proteins, and genes, into the scaffold to be released over a period of time [64–66]. The ability to incorporate drugs and genes into these biodegradable polyurethanes could provide control over the environment of the tissue engineering scaffold and enhance cell proliferation and tissue regeneration.

References

1. Van Blitterswijk, C. 2008. *Tissue Engineering.* Ed. J. Bronzino. 1st ed., Academic Press Series in Biomedical Engineering. New York: Elsevier.
2. Lannutti, J., D. H. Reneker, T. Ma, et al. 2007. Electrospinning for tissue engineering scaffolds. *Materials Science and Engineering C* 27:504–509.
3. Lamba, N. M. K., K. A. Woodhouse, and S. L. Cooper. 1998. *Polyurethanes in Biomedical Applications.* Boca Raton: CRC Press.

4. Yoda, R. J. 1998. Elastomers for biomedical applications. *Journal of Biomaterials Science,* Polymer Edition 9:561–626.

5. Skarja, G. A. and K. A. Woodhouse. 2000. Structure-property relationships of degradable polyurethane elastomers containing an amino acid chain extender. *J. of Appl. Polym. Sci.* 75:1522–1534.

6. Coury, A. J., R. J. Levy, B. D. Ratner, et al. 2004. Degradation of materials in the biological environment. In *Biomaterials Science: An Introduction to Materials in Medicine,* Eds. B. D. Ratner, A. S. Hoffman, F. J. Schoen and J. E. Lemons. San Diego: Elsevier Academic Press.

7. Hatakeyama, H., Y. Izuta, K. Kobashigawa, et al. 1998. Synthesis and physical properties of polyurethanes from saccharide-based polycaprolactones. *Macromolecular Symposia* 130:127–138.

8. Gogolewski, S. and A. J. Pennings. 1983. An artificial skin based on biodegradable mixtures of polylactides and polyurethanes for full-thickness skin wound covering. *J. Macromol Rapid Commun* 4:675–680.

9. Bruin, P., J. Smedinga, A. J. Pennings, et al. 1990. Biodegradable lysine diisocyanate-based poly(glycolide-co-epsilon (Porson)-caprolactone)-urethane network in artificial skin. *Biomaterials* 11:291–295.

10. Storey, R. F., J. S. Wiggins, and A. D. Puckett. 1994. Hydrolyzable poly(ester-urethane) networks from L-lysine diisocyanate and D,L-lactide/epsis-caprolactone homo- and copolyester triols. *Journal of Polymer Science Part A: Polymer Chemistry* 32:2345–2363.

11. Kylma, J. and J. V. Seppala. 1997. Synthesis and characterization of a biodegradable thermoplastic poly(ester–urethane) elastomer. *Macromolecules* 30:2876–2882.

12. Gogolewski, S. 1989. Selected topics in biomedical polyurethanes. A review. *Colloid Polymer Science* 267:757–785.

13. Gupta, A. S. 2003. Synthesis and characterization of L-tyrosine based novel biodegradable polyphosphates and polyurethanes for biomedical applications. Dissertation, The University of Akron.

14. Pulapura, S. and J. Kohn. 1992. Tyrosine-derived polycarbonates: Backbone-modified ldquopseudordquo-poly(amino acids) designed for biomedical applications. *Biopolymers* 32:411–417.

15. Anderson, J. M. 1985. *Macromolecules as drugs and as carriers for biologically active materials.* Eds. D. A. Tirell, L. G. Donaruma and A. B. Turek. New York: The New York Academy of Sciences.

16. Gonsalves, K. E. and P. M. Mungara. 1996. Synthesis and properties of degradable polyamides and related polymers. *Trends in Polymer Science* 4:25–31.

17. Miyamae, T., S. Mori, and Y. Takeda. 1968. Poly-L-glutamic acid surgical sutures. United States of America. U. S. Patent number 3,371,069.

18. Spira, M., J. Fissette, C. W. Hall, et al. 1969. Evaluation of synthetic fabrics as artificial skin grafts to experimental burn wounds. *Journal of Biomedical Materials Research* 3:213–234.

19. Williams, D. F., ed. 1985. *Biocompatibility of Tissue Analogs.* Boca Raton, FL: CRC Press.

20. Kohn, J. and R. Langer. 1984. A new approach to the development of bioerodible polymers for controlled release applications employing naturally occurring amino acids. In *Polymeric Materials, Science and Engineering.* Washington DC: American Chemical Society.

21. Li, C. and J. Kohn. 1989. Synthesis of thermotropic liquid crystalline side-chain polymers via chemical modification of polymeric carboxylic acids. *Macromolecules* 22:2036–2039.

22. Gupta, A. S. and S. T. Lopina. 2004. Synthesis and characterization of image-tyrosine based novel polyphosphates for potential biomaterial applications. *Polymer* 45:4653–4662.

23. Gupta, A. S. and S. T. Lopina. 2005. Properties of L-tyrosine based polyphosphates pertinent to biomedical applications. *Polymer* 46:2133–2140.

24. Kohn, J. and R. Langer. 1985. Non-peptide poly(amino acids) for biodegradable drug delivery systems. Paper read at Proceedings of the 12th International Symposium on Controlled Release of Bioactive Materials, at Lincolnshire, IL.

25. Bogdanzki, M. and A. Bogdanzki. 1984. *The Practice of Peptide Synthesis.* Berlin: Springer-Verlag.

26. Hao, S., Y. Avraham, O. Bonne, et al. 2001. Separation-induced body weight loss, impairment in alternation behavior, and autonomic tone: Effects of tyrosine. *Pharmacology, Biochemistry and Behavior* 68:273–281.

27. Neri, D. F., D. Wiegmann, R. R. Stanny, et al. 1995. The effects of tyrosine on cognitive performance during extended wakefulnless. *Aviation, Space, and Environmental Medicine* 66:313–319.

28. Reinstein, D. K., H. Lehnert, and R. J. Wurtman. 1985. Dietary tyrosine suppresses the rise in plasma corticosterone following acute stress in rats. *Life Sciences* 37:2157–2163.

29. Deijen, J. B. and J. F. Orlebeke. 1994. Effect of tyrosine on cognitive function and blood pressure under stress. *Brain Research Bulletin* 33:319–323.

30. Kohn, J. and R. Langer. 1987. Polymerization reactions involving the side chains of alpha-L-amino acids. *Journal of the American Chemical Society* 109:817–820.

31. Kohn, J. and R. Langer. 1986. Poly(iminocarbonates) as potential biomaterials. *Biomaterials* 7:176–182.

32. Sarkar, D., J.-C. Yang, A. S. Gupta, et al. 2009. Synthesis and characterization of L-tyrosine based polyurethanes for biomaterial applications. *Journal of Biomedical Materials Research* 90A:263–271.

33. Sarkar, D. 2007. Development and characterization of L-tyrosine based polyurethanes for tissue engineering applications, The University of Akron.

34. Sarkar, D. and S. T. Lopina. 2008. Structure-property relationship of L-tyrosine-based polyurethanes for biomaterial applications. *Journal of Applied Polymer Science* 108:2345–2355.

35. Shah, P. N., R. L. Manthe, S. T. Lopina, et al. 2009. Electrospinning of L-tyrosine polyurethanes for potential biomedical applications. *Polymer* 50:2281–2289.

36. Buchanan, C. M., S. C. Gedon, A. W. White, et al. 1992. Cellulose acetate butyrate and poly(hydroxybutyrate-co-valerate) copolymer blends. *Macromolecules* 25:7373–7381.

37. Shimamura, E., K. Kashuya, C. Kobayashi, et al. 1994. Physical properties and biodegradability of microbial of poly(3-hydroxybutyrate-co-3-hydroxyhexanoate). *Macromolecules* 27:878–880.

38. Paul, D. R. and S. Newman. 1978. *Polymer Blends.* New York: Academic Press.

39. Park, T. G., S. Cohen, and R. Langer. 1992. Poly(L-lactic acid)/pluronic blends: characterization of phase separation behavior, degradation, and morphology and use as protein releasing matrices. *Macromolecules* 25:116–122.

40. Simon, G. P. 2003. *Polymer Characterization Techniques and Their Application to Blends.* New York: Oxford University Press.

41. Sarkar, D. 2007. Development and characterization of L-tyrosine based polyurethanes for tissue engineering applications, PhD dissertation, Chemical Engineering, The University of Akron, Akron, OH.

42. Luu, Y. K., K. Kim, B. S. Hsiao, et al. 2003. Development of a nanostructured DNA delivery scaffold via electrospinning of PLGA and PLA-PEG block copolymers. *Journal of Controlled Release* 89:341–353.

43. Ding, B., H. K. Kim, S. C. Lee, et al. 2002. Preparation and characterization of a nanoscale poly(vinyl alcohol) fiber aggregate produced by an electrospinning method. *Journal of Polymer Science Part B: Polymer Physics* 40:1261–1268.

44. Lee, K. H., H. Y. Kim, M. S. Khil, et al. 2003. Characterization of nano-structured poly(var epsilon-caprolactone) nonwoven mats via electrospinning. *Polymer* 44:1287–1294.

45. Deitzel, L. M., J. Kleinmeyer, D. Harris, et al. 2001. The effect of processing variables on the morphology of electrospun nanofibers and textiles. *Polymer* 42:261–272.

46. Gu, S. Y. and J. Ren. 2005. Process optimization and empirical modeling for electrospun poly(D,L-lactide) fibers using response surface methodology. *Macromolecular Materials and Engineering* 290:1097–1105.

47. Tripatanasuwan, S., Z. Zhong, and D. H. Reneker. 2007. Effect of evaporation and solidification of the charged jet in electrospinning of poly(ethylene oxide) aqueous solution. *Polymer* 48:5742–5746.

48. Diez-Pena, E., I. Quijada-Garrido, and J. M. Barrales-Rienda. 2002. Hydrogen-bonding effects on the dynamic swelling of P(N-iPAAm-co-MAA) copolymers. A case of autocatalytic swelling kinetics. *Macromolecules* 35:8882-8888.

49. Pachence, J. M. and J. Kohn. 1997. Biodegradable polymers for tissue engineering. In *Principles of Tissue Engineering*, Eds. R. Lanza, R. Robert and W. Chick. New York: Academic Press.

50. Szycher, M., A. M. Reed, and A. Siciliano. 1991. In vivo testing of a biostable polyurethane. *Journal of Biomaterials Applications* 6:110–130.

51. Blais, P. 1990. Letter to the editor. *Journal of Applied Biomaterials* 1:197.

52. Chen, M., P. O. Zamora, P. Som, et al. 2003. Cell attachment and biocompatibility of polytetrafluoroethylene (PTFE) treated with glow-discharge plasma of mixed ammonia and oxygen. *Journal of Biomaterials Science, Polymer Edition* 14 (9):917–935.

53. El Sayegh, T. Y., R. M. Pilliar, and C. A. McCulloch. 2002. Attachment, spreading, and matrix formation by human gingival fibroblasts on porous-structured titanium alloy and calcium polyphosphate substrates. *Journal of Biomedical Materials Research* 61:482–492.

54. Zhu, B., Q. Lu, J. Yin, et al. 2004. Effects of laser-modified polystyrene substrate on CHO cell growth and alignment. *Journal of Biomedical Materials Research Part B: Applied Biomaterials* 70:43–48.

55. Ikada, Y. 1994. Surface modification of polymers for medical applications. *Biomaterials* 15:725–736.

56. Van Wachem, P. B., A. H. Hogt, T. Beugeling, et al. 1987. Adhesion of cultured human endothelial cells onto methacrylate polymers with varying surface wettability and charge. *Biomaterials* 8:323–328.

57. Wang, Y. W., Q. Wu, and G. Q. Chen. 2003. Reduced mouse fibroblast cell growth by increased hydrophilicity of microbial polyhydroxyalkanoates via hyaluronan coating. *Biomaterials* 24:4621–4629.

58. Lee, J. H., G. Khang, J. W. Lee, et al. 1998. Interaction of different types of cells on polymer surfaces with wettability gradient. *Journal of Colloid and Interface Science* 205:323–330.

59. Van Kooten, T. G., H. T. Spijker, and H. J. Busscher. 2004. Plasma-treated polystyrene surfaces: model surfaces for studying cell–biomaterial interactions. *Biomaterials* 25:1735–1747.

60. Rajaraman, R., D. E. Rounds, S. P. S. Yen, et al. 1974. A scanning electron microscope study of cell adhesion and spreading in vitro. *Experimental Cell Research* 88:327–339.

61. Wei, J., M. Yoshinari, S. Takemoto, et al. 2007. Adhesion of mouse fibroblasts on hexamethyldisiloxane surfaces with wide range of wettability. *Journal of Biomedical Materials Research Part B: Applied Biomaterials* 81B:66–75.

62. Carbonetto, S. T., M. M. Gruver, and D. C. Turner. 1982. Nerve fiber growth on defined hydrogel substrates. *Science* 216:897–899.

63. Silva, M. N. D., R. Desai, and D. J. Odde. 2004. Micro-patterning of animal cells on PDMS substrates in the presence of serum without use of adhesion inhibitors. *Biomedical Microdevices* 6:219–222.

64. Sill, T. J. and H. A. Recum. 2008. Electrospinning: Applications in drug delivery and tissue engineering. *Biomaterials* 29:1989–2006.

65. Kim, K., Y. K. Luu, C. Chang, et al. 2004. Incorporation and controlled release of a hydrophilic antibiotic using poly(lactide-co-glycolide)-based electrospun nanofibrous scaffolds. *Journal of Controlled Release* 98:47–56.

66. Verreck, G., I. Chun, J. Rosenblatt, et al. 2003. Incorporation of drugs in an amorphous state into electrospun nanofibers composed of a water-insoluble, nonbiodegradable polymer. *Journal of Controlled Release* 92:349–360.

67. Amin, P., J. Wille, K. Shah, et al. 1993. Analysis of the extractive and hydrolytic behavior of microthane poly(ester-urethane) foam by high pressure liquid chromatography. *Journal of Biomedical Materials Research* 27:655–666.

68. Szycher, M., A. Reed, and R. Case. 1993. *Biocompatible Polyurethanes: Medical and Pharmaceutical Applications*, Lancaster, PA: Technomic.

69. ChronoThane™ P Thermoplastic Polyurethane Elastomers. 2008. Wilmington, MA: AdvanSource Biomaterials Corp.

70. Stokes, K., R. McVenes, and J. M. Anderson. 1995. Polyurethane elastomer biostability. *Journal of Biomaterials Applications* 9:321–354.

71. Zdrahala, R. J. and I. J. Zdrahala. 1999. Biomedical applications of polyurethanes: A review of past promises, present realities, and a vibrant future. *Journal of Biomaterials Applications* 14:67–90.

72. Tecoflex® Clear: Technical data sheet. 2007. Wilmington, MA: Lubrizol Advanced Materials, Inc.

73. Lin, W.-C., C.-H. Tseng, and M.-C. Yang. 2005. In-vitro hemocompatibility evaluation of a thermoplastic polyurethane membrane with surface-immobilized water-soluble chitosan and heparin. *Macromolecular Bioscience* 5:1013–1021.

74. Williams, T. R. 2007. Fabrication and characterization of electrospun tecophilic scaffolds for gene delivery, Dissertation, Biomedical Engineering, University of Akron, Akron, OH.

75. Tecophilic® solution grade TPUs: Technical data sheet. 2007. Wilmington, MA: Lubrizol Advanced Materials, Inc.

76. Orang, F., C. J. G. Plummer, and H.-H. Kausch. 1996. Effects of processing conditions and *in vitro* ageing on physical properties of Biomer®. *Biomaterials* 17:485–490.

77. Khan, I., N. Smith, E. Jones, et al. 2005. Analysis and evaluation of a biomedical polycarbonate urethane tested in an in vitro study and an ovine anthroplasty model. Part I: Materials selection and evaluation. *Biomaterials* 26:621–631.

78. Szycher, M. 2002. CardioPass™ coronary artery bypass graft: A progress report. Wilmington, MA: CardioTech International Inc.

79. Fact Sheet: Chronoflex® AR: Biodurable medical grade polyurethane. 2008. Wilmington, MA: AdvanSource Biomaterials Corp.

10

Nanotechnologies for Peripheral Nerve Regeneration

Chandra M. Valmikinathan
Stevens Institute of Technology

Harinder K. Bawa
Stevens Institute of Technology

Radoslaw Junka
Stevens Institute of Technology

Xiaojun Yu
Stevens Institute of Technology

10.1 Introduction

All biological entities in the human anatomy originate at the nanoscale.[1] Further understanding of the biology, materials engineering, and basic chemistry has led to a better understanding of biological systems or native tissues and what it takes to create, repair, or even regenerate whole functional tissues. It has also been recently evident that nanoscale features on the grafts greatly aid cellular signaling processes and play a major role in the regeneration processes. Based on these findings over the years, it is very obvious that in order to repair and regenerate lost or damaged tissues, nanotechnology and its applications play a key role.

There are several applications originating from the harmony of nanotechnology to biological systems, especially for the regeneration in the nervous system.[1] First and foremost of the applications is the fabrication of scaffolds that aid in better cell surface interactions, therefore enhancing the formation of axon guiding cues that aid in regeneration along large gaps, in the peripheral and central nervous system. The other major applications being studied for these systems lies in the fabrication of neural electrodes for seamless integration of host and brain tissue, matrices for growth factor and gene therapy, imaging tools for the brain and central nervous system (CNS) and most importantly systems that aid in better understanding of the regeneration processes, broadly described as systems for neurobiology.

Current limitations related to the fabrication of uniform features at the nanoscale in *three* dimensions (3D) originate from to most applications being in the *two* dimensional (2D) platforms.[2] In such applications, surface moieties, topographies, growth factors, extracellular matrix (ECM) proteins are presented at the surface of the substrates.[3] The interaction of primary cells and cell lines are evaluated before transferring the technologies to the 3D spaces. However, there are several limitations associated with 2D systems as compared to 3D systems. It has been illustrated before that in the case of 2D systems; the boundaries for protein concentrations, growth factors, and the density of the molecules that are available for influencing the effect are very steep.[4,5] The native tissue is a 3D matrix that allows uniform and complete distribution of factors in 3D spaces, which is not available in the case of 2D systems.[6]

Owing to the complexity of the peripheral and the central nervous systems, it is important to design 3D systems with optimal properties such as mechanical integrity, porosity, and orientation of the matrix.[7] The electrical conductivity also plays a major role in the regeneration and functional performance of the graft post regeneration. As described by Schmidt et al.,[7] an ideal guidance channel should also be nonimmunogenic, noncytotoxic, and biodegradable. The porosity, pore size, and pore interconnectivity control cell migration into the scaffolds,[8] with a supply from the host's own population of either glial cells or stem cells.[9,10]

Before proceeding to the studies performed using nanoscale features on the process of regeneration, it is vital to understand the biology of the nervous system, the components that form the nervous system, and the short and long-term effects of damaged tissues in the nervous system.

10.1.1 Physiology of the Nervous System

The nervous system is composed of the central nervous system (CNS) and peripheral nervous system (PNS). The CNS, which includes the brain and spinal cord, interprets and coordinates all incoming signals providing sensory information as well as controlling outgoing motor commands to the PNS. The PNS consists of all neural tissue outside the CNS, which includes the cranial nerves arising from the brain, the spinal nerves that arise from the spinal cord, and all sensory nerve cells, also known as dorsal root ganglia. These peripheral nerves are responsible for innervating muscle tissue and transmitting sensory and excitatory stimuli to (afferent) and from (efferent) the spinal column.

The nervous system is mainly comprised of neurons and neuroglia, two cell types essential for nerve cell communication and regulation of the neural environment. Neurons are the core structural and functional elements of nervous system that process and transmit information; they consist of a cell body (soma), a dendritic tree (arbor), and an axon. A dendritic tree, more commonly referred to as dendrites, is the cellular extension that has numerous branches close to the cell body (rarely longer than 1–2 mm). Dendrites are specialized for receiving and processing synaptic inputs and then transmitting electrical signals to the neural soma. An axon, on the other hand, typically extends from the soma to targets that can be up to a meter or further. They conduct electrical impulses away from the cell body to dendrites of other nerve cells. Neurons communicate across a synapse, a gap between the axon of the transmitting cell and the dendrites of the receiving cell, through electrochemical signals to and from the brain at speeds that can reach up to 200 mph.

Neuroglia, or glial cells, are more abundant than neurons (account for 90% of total cell numbers in the brain) and have diverse functions that are necessary for the proper function of the complex nervous system. These include Schwann cells in the PNS and astrocytes and oligodendrocytes in the CNS. Glial cells regulate the myelin coating of axons in both the CNS and PNS, an essential element in increasing the speeds at which electrical impulses propagate along an axon. Schwann cells form myelin around a single peripheral nerve axon and line up along the axon with distinct gaps, called the nodes of Ranvier, between adjacent cells. On the other hand, one oligodendrocyte can extend itself and myelinate several central nerve axons. Astrocytes, the major glial cells in the CNS, serve to structurally support neurons as well as maintain water balance, ion homeostasis, and regulate neurotransmitters amongst other key functions. Neuronal structure and the intricate networks formed with glial cells in both the CNS and PNS prove to be crucial when it comes to nerve injury and regeneration.

Both the brain and the spinal cord are composed of gray matter (neuronal cell bodies) and white matter (myelinated axons). More in depth, gray matter contains the cell bodies of excitatory neurons, glial cells, and blood vessels, whereas white matter consists of axons and glial cells. In the brain, the outer layer consists of gray matter and the deep inner parts consist of white matter. The center of the spinal cord is composed of a butterfly-shaped region of gray matter which is then surrounded by white matter. This helps to protect and insulate the spinal cord in addition to the protection provided by the vertebrae and protective membranes. Axons project from the white matter of the spinal column in bundles, called fascicles, travel through the PNS–CNS transition zone, and enter the PNS. In general, sensory nerves enter the spinal column as dorsal roots and motor nerves exit the spinal column as ventral roots. The transition zone, also named the Obersteiner–Redlich zone, is a clearly defined region where the glial cells of the CNS are distinctly separated from those of the PNS.

Peripheral nerve axons, both motor and sensory, are organized and bundled together by connective tissues to form an anatomically defined trunk. Individual axons and their Schwann cell myelin sheaths are surrounded by a connective tissue containing small diameter collagen fibers termed as the endoneurium. These nerve fibers are then surrounded by the perineurium, connective tissue formed from many layers of flattened cells and collagen, to form fascicles. Finally, the epineurium, composed of loose fibrocollagenous tissue, binds several nerve fascicles into a nerve trunk. Peripheral nerves are also well vascularized by the capillaries that are incorporated within the connective tissue and by blood vessels that penetrate the nerve from surrounding veins and arteries.

10.1.2 Neuronal Injury, Degeneration, and Regeneration

In either the CNS or PNS, if an axon of a neuron is focally destroyed (i.e., cut, crushed, or frozen), the part of the axon that is disconnected from the cell body, in other words the "distal" portion of the axon, begins to fragment and degenerate. This event is called anterograde or Wallerian degeneration, as Waller first described these changes in transected nerve segments of frog glossopharyngeal and hypoglossal nerves.[11] The axonal cytoskeleton of the distal portion begins to degenerate as a result of calcium-dependent protease activity and separation from the metabolically active nerve cell bodies.[12] The proximal portion of the axon may degenerate a short distance, referred to as retrograde degeneration, but generally survives in the short term.

In the PNS, after the cytoskeleton and membrane degradation, Schwann cells surrounding the distal end of the axon shed their myelin lipids. Schwann cells in the proximal and distal nerve portions of the transected nerve cell begin to proliferate together with the influx of macrophages, the two cell types phagocytose myelin and the degenerated axon fragments of the distal nerve segment.[13] In the CNS, however, the influx of phagocytotic cells entering the injury site is far less. Therefore myelin and axonal debris can take months to clear in the CNS while it takes only a few weeks in the PNS. Although Wallerian degeneration is seen in both the PNS and CNS, each responds differently to traumatic injuries in terms of degeneration and the eventual nerve regeneration.

10.1.3 Peripheral Nervous System Injury and Regeneration

Peripheral nerve injuries occur frequently and are a major source of disabilities as they can range from being traumatic, nontraumatic, to surgical in nature. The ability of a peripheral nerve to regenerate following injury largely depends on the severity of the injury. Sir Sydney Sunderland defined five degrees of peripheral nerve injury ranging from mild to severe.[14] Neuropraxia, a first-degree injury, is the mildest form of nerve injury involving the partial or complete conduction failure of a nerve without any evident structural changes. A nerve can recover its full functionality from neuropraxia without any intervention within a few days. Axonotmesis, a second-degree injury, is the interruption of axons within a nerve without any damage to its supporting structures. Such a lesion is usually caused by the crushing, pinching, or stretching of a nerve and is subject to Wallerian degeneration immediately after the insult. Third, fourth, and fifth-degree injuries are collectively known as neurotmesis as they all involve damage to the support structures. While partial regeneration is possible in the mildest form or neurotmesis (third degree), surgical intervention to reconnect the distal and proximal nerve stumps is imperative for regaining nerve function.[15-17] The degree of injury greatly affects the regeneration ability of the nerve.

Along with the clearance of debris at the site of injury, Schwann cells and macrophages produce cytokines, which leads to enhance axon growth.[18] Mast cells around the injury site release histamine and heparin, both of which dramatically increase the endoneurial vessel size and vascular permeability and facilitate the entry of yet more macrophages. Afterwards, these mast cells degranulate and further contribute to the degradation of myelin debris.[19] Additionally, mast cell numbers significantly increase at the injury site and contribute to nerve regeneration by releasing the nerve growth factor (NGF) and vascular endothelial growth factor (VEGF).[20-22] Regeneration begins at the proximal end and continues toward the distal end. Schwann cells produce a growth-promoting environment by proliferating and aligning into conduits within the basal lamina, known as the Bands of Büngner, which provides a substrate for the axons to grow.[23] These cells also produce a specialized ECM and various neurotrophic factors (i.e., NGF, brain-derived neurotrophic factor (BDNF), and ciliary neurotrophic factor (CNTF)) that are essential for the survival of neurons and neuronal migration.[24,25] The various factors that play a role in regeneration are discussed later in the text. Axons must continue to extend until they reach their distal end in order to gain functionality. As axon regeneration occurs at a rate of 2–5 mm/day, significant injuries can take several months to heal.[26]

In peripheral nerve injuries that are mild (degrees 1–3), Schwann cells proliferate and successfully fill the gap between the proximal and distal nerve ends and promote nerve regeneration. In more severe injuries (degrees 4–5), however, Schwann cells form a dense mass at the injury site through which regenerating axons are unable to navigate. In such cases, surgical intervention is required either to ligate the severed nerve ends or to provide an artificial conduit that bridges the gap between the distal and proximal nerve ends.[27]

10.2 Critical Parameters for Peripheral Nerve Regeneration

Peripheral nerve injuries can be broadly classified into two categories, large gaps (greater than 4 mm) and small gaps (less than 4 mm).[28,29] There are several treatment options that currently exist, with some of them showing great promise in the clinic trails. For the regeneration of peripheral nerve injuries, the gold standard is an autograft, in which the injured nerve gap is filled with a patient's own nerve.[29] However, the autograft is adopted only when coaptation (approximation and suture of the 2 ends) of the nerve is not possible owing to the length of the gap created by the injury.[30] Specifically, in the case of large nerve defects, an autograft is usually extracted from the sural nerve, located near the ankle, and is placed at the site of injury. However, in cases of trauma or tumor, where large nerve sections and several nerve sections are required, an autograft was not sufficient to repair all the injuries.

In most cases, the scaffold is a guidance approach that allows for guiding severed axons across the gap. This is the most vital component in the regeneration of nerve injuries. A few decades ago, several guidance strategies were attempted to repair large nerve defects.[31] One of the earliest approaches to guide axons across nerve injuries was the application of tube-like structures usually made of autologous tissues, a fat sheath,[32] tendons,[33] veins,[34,35] or sub-mucosa[36] in most cases. However, inherent to these techniques was the fact that these nerve grafts did not mimic the native nerve microstructure of the actual nerve. Also, optimal growth factors and ECM proteins that are needed for guiding the axons across the ends were not sufficient.[37]

In order to alleviate drawbacks associated with the autografts, several researchers have adopted allograft-based techniques to repair and regenerate large nerve defects.[38] However, the allografts possess the risk of disease transmission, unfavorable immune response, and more importantly lack of donors. In order to mitigate drawbacks associated with these techniques, several tissue engineering strategies were adopted to study the regeneration process in the nervous system.

Tissue engineering is composed of three major components: the scaffolds, proteins (in the form of growth factors and surface tethered ECM proteins), and most importantly the cells, which are composed of the glial support cells and the main neurons in the case of nerve tissue engineering. These critical parameters for peripheral nerve regeneration are summarized in Figure 10.1 and are discussed below in detail.

10.2.1 Optimal Physical Properties of Scaffolds

The conventional approach in the fabrication of functional tissue engineered grafts is creation of biodegradable grafts with optimal physical properties, that support and promote axonal growth from the proximal end to the distal ends, and cause functional recovery. Porosity plays a major role in the regeneration process. First, it allows the migration of cells, specifically the glial cells, and more importantly the neural processes or axon growth across the scaffold. Second, porosity allows medium or blood vessel influx into the scaffold. The blood circulation is a vital source of nutrients for the survival of the nerves as well as a major source of debris clearance when the scar tissues, polymer graft, and sutures are cleared from the site of injury.[39] However, the porosity, degradability, and mechanical properties are all interrelated and changes in one of the parameters alternatively affect the other.

Mechanical properties play a vital role in the success of the peripheral nerve regeneration process. Ideally, the engineered grafts should match a native acellular nerve graft, which has to be a factor of consideration, during scaffold design and material selection. An acellular nerve graft has tensile stress of about 0.2–0.5 MPa and a modulus of 1–5 MPa.[40]

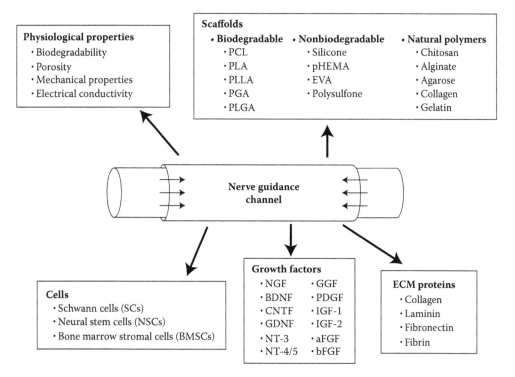

FIGURE 10.1 Critical parameters for nerve regeneration: scaffolds, physiological properties, cells, growth factors, and extracellular matrix proteins.

10.2.2 Materials for Scaffold Fabrication

Many biodegradable and biocompatible materials have been developed and tested for applications in the regeneration of the peripheral nerve injuries. There have been several natural materials as well as synthetic materials that have been applied for filling the nerve guidance channel (NGC) as well as fabrication of the whole graft by various techniques. Some of the most common natural materials that have been used for nerve tissue engineering include collagen (described above),[41,42] chitosan,[43,44] alginate,[45] dextran,[46] gelatin,[47] fibrin,[48] and fibronectin.[49] These materials possess several properties that make them attractive for use as nerve grafts, especially in filling guidance channels. They form a hydrogel-like matrix, which mimics the soft-tissue architecture of the nerve, and a large amount of critical growth factors such as NGF, neurophin-3 (NT-3), or BDNF can be encapsulated into the systems. There are also some nonbiodegradable systems that have been used extensively for nerve tissue engineering. Agarose is one of the most common nonbiodegradable hydrogel that has been evaluated for PNS and CNS regeneration.[50] Another versatile platform, which is biocompatible but nonbiodegradable is poly(hydroxyethyl methacrylate) (PHEMA). PHEMA has shown great promise as a substitute for regeneration.[51]

However, inherent to the hydrogel-based system is the fact that it is mechanically very weak and therefore in most cases needs a housing system like the silicone tube. Therefore, several synthetic materials have been developed that have ideal mechanical properties, degradation rates as well as do not need an external system, like silicone to form the NGCs. Some of the most common materials used for the fabrication of nerve grafts include polycaprolactone (PCL),[52] poly lactide (PLLA),[53] polyglycolide (PGA), and their copolymers.[54] These materials have a stable degradation period *in vivo* and produce by-products that can be easily cleared by system. Also, by changing the ratio of the polymers (PGA and PLLA) the degradation rates can be precisely controlled. There are several other materials that have been used for the fabrication of scaffolds for tissue engineering, including electro-conductive materials such as polypyrrole (ppy).[55,56] Several review articles[7,57,58] have dwelled on the materials aspect of nerve tissue engineering, and would give a more detailed perspective on the materials used.

10.2.3 Protein Factors for Regeneration

10.2.3.1 Extracellular Matrix Proteins

During the development and repair of the nervous system, glial cells, especially Schwann cells, play a key role.[59] They have been regarded as a potential guide towards the regeneration process, and have been attributed to the success of autografts as compared to other NGCs.[60] They provide vital molecules for the regeneration process, either as diffusible cues (growth factors) or as substrate bound proteins (ECM proteins), such as collagen, fibronectin, and laminin.[61] They are also a major source of signaling molecules that enhance the migration of Schwann cells into the injury site, macrophages for debris clearance, and more importantly axons towards the proximal end.

Collagen: Collagen is the most prominent protein in the PNS and the CNS. Collagen exists in the form of nanofibers that are oriented in the scaffolds and aid in the guidance of the cells and axons across the nerve. They also have several motifs that allow for cell surface interactions and also house several growth factors that are produced by the cells.[62]

Laminin: The second most prominent ECM protein in the nervous system is laminin. They are usually present in the basement membrane of cells and play vital roles in cell migration, adhesion, proliferation, differentiation, and neurite outgrowth in the nervous system during development and regeneration.[63,64] There is considerable evidence that laminin is a vital component in the embryonic development stages as well during the process of regeneration. Laminin at optimal concentrations promotes axonal and glial cell attachment, migration, differentiation, survival, and overall development. However, at larger concentrations, it tends to affect the normal development processes and aid in the formation of glial scars that might retard neurite growth.[65]

Other surface bound proteins that are vital to the regeneration processes are, fibronectin, which is over-expressed immediately postinjury and plays a major role in the regeneration and wound healing process; NCAM and N-cadherin, have significant impact in the signaling processes.[66]

10.2.3.2 Neurotrophic Factors

Neurotrophic factors, also known as growth factors, are soluble agents found in the extracellular fluid surrounding most cells and account for differentiation, proliferation, gene expression, proper networking, as well as survival of neurons.[67,68] There are several neurotrophic factors whose effects have been extensively studied in neural tissue regeneration; NGF, BDNF, CNTF, glial cell line-derived growth factor (GDNF), NT-3, neurophin-4/5 (NT-4/5), acidic and basic fibroblast growth factor (aFGF, bFGF) are all important neurotrophic factors.[69,70] Local delivery of growth factors through use of nanoparticles, scaffolds, or gels is highly desirable in order to compete with the inhibitory agents present after trauma to the nervous system. The following part gives a more detailed insight into the critical growth factors that affect the nerve regeneration process.

NGF: Amongst all the neurotrophic factors, NGF is possibly the best-characterized growth factor as it has shown importance in peripheral nerve regeneration. NGF is a dimeric (27 kDa) neurotrophic factor that is produced in the target organs of the sympathetic and sensory nerves.[71] Normally, sympathetic and sensory nerves contain a low concentration of NGF as compared to their target organs.[24] However, following axotomy, Schwann cells in the distal stump start producing NGF, which has been shown to stimulate and promote the survival of sensory ganglia and nerves.[72,73] Two distinct receptors for NGF exist, including a high affinity trkA receptor and a low affinity p75 receptor.[74] Activation of NGF receptors initiates a cascade of signaling events and leads to neuronal differentiation.[75] Although NGF has shown success in the growth and development of sensory neurons, its effects are limited with respect to motor neuron regeneration.[76–80] Nonetheless, the delivery of NGF to neuronal injuries has been studied extensively.[81,82]

BDNF: BDNF is another neurotrophic factor that promotes the axonal growth of sensory neurons.[83] Additionally, BDNF supports survival and axonal growth of motor neurons.[84,85] Although research investigating the effects of BDNF on nerve regeneration has led to some inconclusive results in the PNS, it has been noted that BDNF must be delivered locally at high concentrations to have an effect on nerve regeneration.[78,86]

NT-3 and NT-4/5: Similar to BDNF, NT-3 promotes motor neurons survival and outgrowth, as well as sensory nerve axonal growth.[86,87] It has shown promising results *in vivo* with respect to the regeneration of peripheral nerves.[88,89] NT-4/5 can promote the survival of motor neurons[86,90] and sensory neurons.[91] This factor aids in growth of sensory axons from dorsal root ganglia into the spinal cord,[92,93] and also promotes axonal outgrowth in motor neurons[86,91] and the regeneration of peripheral nerves.[94]

CNTF: Similar to the other growth factors, CNTF accounts for survival and outgrowth of motor neurons.[95–97] Its increased mRNA levels near the spinal cord injury indicate that CNTF might be involved in a healing response mechanism. It has also shown promise in the regeneration of peripheral nerves[98] and spinal cord. However, some literature indicates that the introduction of CNTF into spinal cord injuries leads to glial scarring, which inhibits the regeneration process in spinal cord injuries.[99]

GDNF: GDNF supports sensory,[100,101] autonomic,[102] and motor[103] neurons' survival, it has been shown as most effective survival and tropic factor for motor neurons.[86,104,105] It can also increase peripheral nerve regeneration.[106–108] Its effects on sensory neural growth are greater than those of NGF and NT-3.[93,94]

aFGF and bFGF: aFGF and bFGF have been shown to increase the regeneration of peripheral nerve.[109,110] Like several other neurotrophic factors, these fibroblast growth factors significantly increase angiogenesis levels which in turn helps heal injury to a nerve.[111] bFGF has also been linked to increased sensory neural outgrowth. However, FGF has limited effectiveness at regenerating axons over a prolonged period of time.[112]

In summary, neurotrophic factors encourage a variety of neural responses that include the survival of motor and sensory nerves in the PNS amongst others. Due to different methods of delivering growth factors, *in vivo* responses are not always consistent. As a result, the development of highly controllable delivery devices is required and currently part of ongoing research.

10.3 Nanotechnology Approaches to Peripheral Nerve Regeneration

The scaffold architecture at the macro, micro, and nanoscale provides the necessary cues to a successful system, which can then be implanted to repair or regenerate lost tissues. Several fabrication techniques have been used to create highly complex 3D networks for nerve tissue engineering applications. At the macroscale, the scaffolds have to provide ideal pore architectures and porosities, meanwhile at the microscale allow easy cell penetration, pore interconnectivity, and even allow media influx into the 3D spaces. More importantly, it has been understood that the native nerve is composed of oriented collagen fibrils that are 66 nm in diameter,[113] which enhances the surface area for easier cell migration, attachment, and other cell surface interactions. The potential of nanotechnology-based approaches stems from the similarity at the length scales as well as the ability to functionalize substrates at the cellular microenvironment. Despite several promising approaches and results at the microscale, several researchers have shown that scaffolds containing nanoscale features promote better nerve regeneration by enhancing the cell material contact, allowing more cells to attach per unit surface area and also show enhanced functionalization with growth factors and ECM proteins.

10.3.1 Nanoscale Topographies for Peripheral Nerve Regeneration

Nanoscale topographies on the surface have been shown to enhance the activity of support cells (glial cells) as well provide a suitable path for oriented or guided neuron outgrowth.[2,114] There have been several approaches to the creation of scaffolds with nanoscale topographies for peripheral nerve regeneration (Table 10.1). Some of the most common approaches are electrospinning, micro and nanopatterning, photolithography, e-beam lithography, and self-assembly based approaches.

One of the very first methods to create nanoscale features for peripheral nerve regeneration includes chemical and physical etching. Etching using suitable reagents were used to create patterns on 2D substrates, with feature sizes ranging from 2 to 800 nm,[115] based on exposure time and the concentration of the etchant. Some of the most common etchants used are hydrofluoric acid[116] and sodium hydroxide. However, most of the systems created using this technique were applicable only to 2D platforms and have not yet been totally successful in creating patterns in 3D. Also, owing to the nature of the technique, it is very difficult to create dense patterns on the surfaces and most patterns tend to be either nano or microscale grooves, with high order of repeatability in terms of pitch and feature sizes.

Fan et al., showed the fabrication of nanotopography or surface roughness in the range of 2–800 nm. A Fluoric acid-based etchant was used to create the nanotopographies on the surface of silicon chips.[117] The depth and feature size were controlled by the duration of exposure to the etchant. They also reported that a feature in the range of 25 nm produces two orders of magnitude increase in neuronal differentiation, as compared to feature sizes that are much larger. It was also noted that as the size of the patterns increased (100–200 nm) and even at the microscale (2–5 μm) the response of the neuronal cells reduced indicating the effectiveness of the nanotopography to influence neuronal cell performance.

Another extension of the above mentioned technique is the application of electrochemical moieties to create specific nanoscale patterns on 2D substrates. Most of the substrates prepared by this technique are microscale or nanoscale pores on silicon or ceramic substrates. Moxon et al.,[118] showed the ability to create microporous substrates using the above technique on silicon and studied PC12 cell adhesion and advantages of similar features on surfaces. However, this technique is limited to 2D substrates and not yet explored for 3D applications.

TABLE 10.1 Nanoscale Fabrication for Neural Tissue Engineering

Fabrication Method	Feature Sizes	Advantages	Disadvantages
Phase separation	Pore sizes ≥1 nm	Good for creating porous scaffolds. Porosity is easily controlled. Simple, no special equipment necessary	Organized patterning not possible
Polymer demixing	Vertical: ≥13 nm	Simple, fast, and inexpensive	Only sample features can be created (e.g., islands, pits, ribbons)
Chemical etching	Dependent on etchant used, time, and many other factors	Simple, fast, and no special equipment needed	Specific feature geometries not possible
Nanoporous membranes as scaffolds	≥1 nm	Relatively easy fabrication, inexpensive, and allows for precise control over pore size and distribution	Material strength can be insufficient to withstands physiological loads
Photolithography (near-UV)	≥0.5 nm	Can create precise geometries and patterns	Expensive equipment, feature size is the largest of reviewed methods
Electron beam lithography	For positive results: ≥3–5 nm for a single feature. ≥30–40 nm for arrays of features	Precise geometries and computer-controlled patterns can be created. No mask is needed	Expensive equipment, time consuming, small surface area coverage. Increasing area, lowers resolution. Negative resists have even lower resolution
Nanofiber scaffolds electrospinning	Allows for 3D scaffolds to be created that are ≥3 nm	Can create aligned fibrous meshes. Ability to be used with biological polymers such as collagen	Can only create fibers
Self-assembly	Tailored by molecule design	Molecules undergo spontaneous self-assembly into higher order structures	Requires engineering of molecules that will self-assemble

10.3.1.1 Micro and Nanopatterning Using Poly(Dimethylsiloxane) (PDMS) Stamps

Over the last decade, several other techniques have evolved to create microscale and nanoscale patterns on 3D substrates. One of the earliest techniques was the micropatterning-based approach to create channels or protein containing patterns on 3D surfaces. In such applications, first a master mold is prepared that has the pattern which can be transferred or imprinted to surfaces, either in 2D or 3D.[119] Photolithography-based techniques, common to semiconductor applications, are used to create the master. Common materials used for the fabrication of the master are poly(dimethylsiloxane) (PDMS).[120,121] This material is photo-cross-linkable and upon exposure to light, at specific wavelengths, through specific patterns, it creates patterns, otherwise called stamps. Based on current technology, distinct and clear patterns can be formed with feature size ranging from 50 nm to 20 μm in width.

Miller et al., created microscale patterns on PLLA-based scaffolds prepared by phase separation. Using the adsorption-based technique, they showed the localization of laminin into the microgrooves and studied dorsal root ganglion (DRG) neurite outgrowth in the patterns. They also studied Schwann cell attachment and alignment into the grooves with and without laminin. The authors reported that in the presence of oriented Schwann cells and laminin, an enhanced neurite outgrowth was observed, as compared to microgrooves without Schwann cells or laminin. They observed oriented neurites in the same direction as the microgrooves, even in the case of shallow micropatterns. Similar results were also reported by Thompson et al.,[122] where bovine serum albumin (BSA) was coupled to laminin and cross-linked to microgrooves that were 20 μm wide. They reported that 94% of the Schwann cells oriented along the microgrooves after 24 h after seeding.

10.3.1.2 Electron Beam Lithography

Recent developments in science have led to the use of electron beam lithography-based techniques to create nanopatterns on surfaces. E-beam lithography creates nanoscale features using a high energy focused electron beam by patterning on to photo-resist-like materials, which undergo physical and chemical changes upon exposure to an electron beam. The cross-linking, or changes in physical and chemical attributes is marked by molecular resistance to movement through interlocking of molecules that happens when they come into contact with the e-beam, leads to pattern formation. Unlike other traditional light-based techniques, this technique does not need a mask to create the pattern. However, a programmable unit is needed to control the beam location on the substrate.

E-beam lithography allows the creation of patterns that are 3–5 nm in size, at a very high density. However, this technique is not very applicable in cases bulk 3D substrates owing to the limitations of penetration depth of the electron beam. Krsko et al.,[123] showed the fabrication of nanoscale patterns on a silicon substrate coated with polyethylene glycol (PEG). The PEG is cross-linked as the electron beam is restored on the surface, and the un-cross-linked PEG can be released from the surface by washing in water. The density and the mechanical properties of the gels can be controlled based on the dosage and time of exposure.[124] Krsko et al., reported that the stiffer the gels were, the greater the attachment and interaction with the cells. They also used an amine terminated PEG and showed the creation of functional surfaces by crosslinking laminin to the nanoscale patterns.[125] DRG neurite attachment and neurite extension were studied on the substrate and with increasing pattern density neurite outgrowth reduced. It was observed that growth cones migrated into the scaffolds, especially at regions where no hydrogels were present.

10.3.1.3 Peptide-Based Nanofibers Produced by Self-Assembly

Peptide and protein-based scaffolds have recently been explored to generate 3D scaffolds for peripheral nerve regeneration. The building blocks are usually small peptides, which self assemble to form 3D hydrogel-like constructs. Usually the peptides chosen have a hydrophilic backbone and hydrophobic heads. Specific peptides sequences can be selected to create hydrogels based on given cells or organ of interest. Specifically, for PNS applications, a peptide sequence composed of isoleucine–lysine–valine–alanine–valine (IKVAV) has shown the ability to promote axonal elongation.

Silva et al., showed the fabrication of one such hydrogel system, wherein the head groups were composed of IKVAV peptide sequence. They showed that self-assembly takes place when the peptides are introduced into a cell suspension at 37°C owing to ionic or Van der Waals interaction between the peptides.[126] The peptides self-assemble to form a hydrogel-like 3D structure composed of nanofibers that are few microns in length and a have diameter of 5–8 nm. These hydrogels showed enhanced differentiation and neurite outgrowth as compared to control laminin coated controls. They also showed faster rates of differentiation as compared to the control scaffolds.

10.3.1.4 Electrospun Nanofibrous Scaffolds for Peripheral Nerve Regeneration

Over the last decade, electrospinning has been regarded as one of the most suitable approaches to fabricate scaffolds for tissue engineering applications. The nanofibers produced through electrospinning mimic native ECM, and have enhanced surface area to promote cell attachment, proliferation, and migration.[127] Electrospinning is a technique wherein nanofibers are produced by the application of high voltage to a flowing viscous solution of any polymer. Owing to the flexibility of the system, scaffolds can be created with varying diameter, orientations, and thickness of the graft by varying the viscosity of the solution used, flow-rate of the process, and even the voltage used. The other important feature of electrospinning is the fact that almost all polymers either water soluble or organic solvent soluble can be electrospun. In addition, the electrospinning setup can be modified to collect various fiber morphologies ranging from braided scaffolds, aligned nanofibers, random nanofibers, and even porous nanofibers. It is also versatile enough to spin fibers that contain biological compounds such as drugs,[128] growth factors,[129] ECM proteins,[130] and even cells.[131]

Gupta et al.,[132] fabricated aligned and random electrospun PCL/gelatin scaffolds for peripheral nerve tissue engineering applications. The nanofibers hence produced were 240 nm in diameter and had a porosity of about 90%, which closely matches the porosity of native nerve tissues. They also observed that on blending gelatin with PCL, they had enhanced mechanical properties as compared to pure PCL-based scaffolds. They studied Schwann cell attachment and proliferation on the scaffolds and reported an enhanced cell attachment and proliferation on gelatin-containing scaffolds as compared to pure PCL-based scaffolds. From the scanning electron micrographs, it was evident that the Schwann cells oriented along the direction of the nanofibers, in the case of aligned scaffolds and no significant orientation was observed in the case of random nanofibers.

Koh et al.,[133] experimented with the electrospinning of laminin functionalized PLLA nanofibers. They studied three different methods to include laminin in the nanofibers such as electrospinning a blend of the polymer with laminin, adsorption of laminin on the nanofiber template, and covalent binding of laminin using basic carbodiimide chemistry. The nanofibers fabricated were in the range of 100–500 nm and the authors suggested that no significant difference in the fiber diameter was observed when laminin was electrospun with PLLA as a blend. On the evaluation of laminin-loaded content in the nanofibers using the three treatments, the author reports that the blended scaffold had a significantly higher loading efficiency as compared to the other two techniques. They also observed that inclusion of laminin into the nanofibers enhanced PC12 cells attachment, proliferation, and differentiation. An increased neurite outgrowth was observed in the case of laminin-blended PLLA scaffolds as compared to other scaffold types, perhaps due to the increased laminin loading in such fibers. However, no significant difference in cell proliferation was observed between all other scaffold types, incorporated with laminin or even control PLLA scaffolds without laminin.

Bini et al.,[134] showed the fabrication of braided scaffolds produced by electrospinning aligned PLGA based nanofibers. The nanofiber system was tested with C 17.2 cells and showed good attachment and proliferation of the cells. However, the authors observed that post differentiation, the cells oriented in random directions and did not follow the orientation of the nanofibers.

Bellamkonda et al.,[135] showed the fabrication of scaffolds composed of aligned nanofibers inside a polysolfone nerve guidance channel. They fabricated aligned electrospun nanofibers from polyacrylonitrile methacrylate (PAN-MA) that were 400–600 nm in diameter. They also fabricated randomly oriented PAN-MA nanofibers as controls. These scaffolds were first tested *in vitro* using primary DRG cells. From their data, it was evident that the neurites as well as the Schwann cells that migrated from the DRGs, elongated in the direction of orientation. In the case of random nanofiber no significant direction was observed. In the case of aligned nanofibrous scaffolds, a longer neurite length was observed as compared to scaffolds with random nanofibers. They also reported the application of the same type of scaffold *in vivo*. It was observable that the scaffolds that had the aligned nanofibers showed improved regeneration at the proximal and distal ends. Meanwhile the scaffolds that had the random nanofibers showed regeneration only closer to the proximal ends and minimal regeneration at the distal end.

Chew et al.,[136] showed the importance of alignment on glial cell attachment, proliferation, and maturation. Electrospun PCL fibers, with either aligned or random orientation were fabricated and evaluated for Schwann cell attachment, proliferation, and gene expression. Even though the fibers they produced had a diameter around 1 μm, the effect of fiber orientation on Schwann cell maturation was apparent. From their data, it is evident that on aligned and random fiber scaffolds the expression of vital factors such as NGF, GDNF, and MAP were higher as compared to thin film-based scaffolds.

From the previous examples, it is understandable that electrospinning can yield scaffolds that have a substrate that mimics native ECM in terms of alignment, architecture, and even in terms of porosity and mechanical properties. However, it is extremely challenging to create 3D scaffolds from electrospun nanofibers with optimal mechanical properties. In order to mitigate this drawback and also enhance surface areas available for cell attachment, spiral shaped scaffolds were developed by coating aligned or random nanofibers onto PLGA microsphere-based sintered scaffolds.[39] The sintered scaffolds provide necessary mechanical stability (tensile properties) to prevent collapse of the scaffold, meanwhile the spiral shape enhances surface area. The open scaffold architecture allows media influx into and waste removal from the scaffold.

There are several other references indicating the applicability of the electrospinning process to neural tissue engineering applications, especially for functionalization, growth factor release, DNA release, which have been discussed in the appropriate sections in the text below.

10.4 Nanotechnology Platforms for Controlled Release of Growth Factors and DNAs for Peripheral Nerve Regeneration

10.4.1 Nanotechnology for Delivery of Growth Factors

Various techniques of growth factor delivery from scaffolds have been developed for peripheral nerve regeneration. The approachs used are based on compatibility among many variables such as material used, drug delivered, and application. Degradation/diffusion-based delivery technique utilizes the materials' physical properties, pore size, crosslinking density, and scaffold degradation time, to diffuse the drug. On the other hand, other techniques rely on covalent and noncovalent interactions between the growth factor and the scaffolds. The duration of the release in covalently bonded growth factor depends on the degradation of the scaffold.[58] Nanoscale techniques allow greater interaction between the target cell's ECM, improved transport properties, and *in vivo* pharmacokinetics.[137,138]

10.4.1.1 Nanoparticles

Nanoparticles have advantages with respect to diffusion, solubility, biodistribution, and immunogenicity.[139] Nanoparticles can be tuned to target specific tissues, as well as limit their concentration in tissues nearby. Nanoparticles are thought to be able to solve the transport and pharmacokinetics of growth factor delivery because of their advantageous size that allows them to penetrate deep into the tissues.[146] Polyesters, polyphosphazenes, poly(alkyl cyano-acrylate), polyanhydrides, block copolymers, alkyl vinyl ethers, and hemiesters of copolymers of maleic anhydride have been used to manufacture nanoparticles.[140] Growth factors are incorporated into nanoparticles via covalent and noncovalent means.[147]

Nkasah et al., had studied the delivery of CNTF through nanospherical PLGA particles. The particles were 314.9 ± 24.9 nm in diameter. The release was sustained over 14 days, after which neural stem cells exhibited astrocytes as well as heightened expression in oligodendrocytic and neuronal markers.[141] significantly, cells treated with CNTF released by nanospheres promoted differentiation found in the control CNTF of equivalent concentration, proving its potency after encapsulation.

Another example of nanoparticulate delivery system of growth factors is quantum dots. Growth factors are able to successfully bind to these semiconductor nanoparticles (2–10 nm).[142] Another advantage of quantum dots is their photostability, which allows better resolutions during imaging.[143] This allows the quantum dots to be used in qualitative as well as quantitative data collection. Successful attachment and transport of NGF to quantum dots made it a considerable alternative for growth factor transport.[147,144]

Naka and coworkers had studied the delivery of neurotrophin-coated nanoscale magnetic beads, 250 nm in diameter, to promote the survival and differentiation.[145] The beads coated with NGF or BDNF exhibited similar effects on neurite outgrowths of neurons as found in soluble NGF or soluble BDNF. Upon an increase of the volume of NGF-coated bead solution, the number of outgrowths increased. Beads coated with both NGF and BDNF induced outgrowths in PC12h cells, something not found with the use of BDNF alone. With a use of a magnet, NGF-coated beads were concentrated in a desired area, promoting neurite outgrowths in neurons nearby.

10.4.1.2 Nanofibers

Owing to the versatility of the electrospinning process, there have been several references where drugs, growth factors, and other proteins were incorporated into the nanofiber matrix. Chew et al., successfully incorporated bNGF into the copolymer of e-caprolactone and ethyl ethylene phosphate (PCLEEP) system through electrospinning.[146] The nanofibers hence produced were about 0.5–5 μm in diameter and had a loading efficiency of about 5–10%. They also showed NGF release in a sustained fashion over a 3-month period, further proving that this approach was suitable for growth factor delivery to the nerves. The released NGF was shown to be bioactive over the entire study period as evaluated by the neurite differentiation assay; however, the percentage differentiation was significantly lower at 40 days and beyond as compared to earlier time points.

Valmikinathan et al., also used electrospinning and a combination of PCL and BSA to deliver NGF.[147] The addition of BSA reduced the degradation period as well as loading efficiency, previously reduced by the hydrophobic nature of PCL. A sustained release of NGF was obtained for at least 28 days. The diameters of the fibers were in the range of 548.89 ± 214.37 nm. The encapsulation efficiency of the NGF in PCL scaffolds was 26.3 ± 1.4%. This indicated a reduced loading of NGF in PCL nanofibers as well as an initial burst release. The PCL nanofibers alone did not sustain release for 28 days while the PCL-BSA nanofibers exhibited an encapsulation efficiency of 88.6 ± 4.7% and more stable release over a period of time.

Wang et al., sought to improve upon bioactivity of the NGF by using the coaxial electrospinning method. The fibers were composed of BSA/NGF core covered with P(LLA-CL) shell on the outside. The 8-week study showed that PC12 cells achieved differentiation into neurons and that NGF remained bioactive for the duration of study qualifying the method of sustained delivery.[148] The average size of the fibers ranged from 500 nm to 840 nm. The encapsulation efficiency of BSA in PLLACL was at 78.5 ± 4.6% for 5% BSA and 80.2 ± 5.1% for 10% BSA. The release was sustained for 108 h, where 70% of the total amount was released. Coaxially electrospun nanofibers exhibited an increased encapsulation efficiency of 93.2 ± 5.4% for 5% BSA and 89.7 ± 5.9% for 10% BSA.

10.4.2 DNA Delivery

DNA delivery is an indirect technique used to deliver neurotrophins into the injury site. The DNA structure is more stable than that of protein, because proteins' bioactivity is sensitive to its delicate 3D confirmation. Two popular methods used for this type of delivery are plasmid-based transfection,[149] and viral transduction.[150]

10.4.2.1 Virus-Based Transfection

Virions are biologically occurring transfection agents that survive solely through transfection of host cells and exist either as an infectious virion particle or as a provirus integrated in the host genome. Viral-mediated transfection occurs in general through the attachment or adsorption of the virion to the host membrane, penetration of the plasma membrane, un-coating, and delivery of genetic material into the host genome.[151] Commonly, adenovirus[152] and retroviruses are employed; however, other classes of viruses have been used as well.[163] Virus-based transfection entails splicing a gene of interest into a viral genome usually of an attenuated virus to reduce immunogenic complications. Virions have the advantage of high transfection efficiency when compared to other systems as well as permanent effects as opposed to other forms of transfection bar artificial chromosome construction. This concept has been applied to a neuronal system by Liu et al., to deliver the GDNF gene to sciatic nerves in diabetic rats afflicted with demyelination and inhibited GDNF/Akt signaling cascade. Post-transfection showed increased signaling, normal levels of GDNF production, and halted demyelination.[168]

As can be seen with patients infected with common cold, rhinovirus, virions, and molecules composing the capsid and envelope are immunogenic and antigenic. This was seen with the first adenoviral-mediated gene therapy trial death, Jesse Gelsinger.[153] Also, the lack of specificity in the location of insertion of the provirus has been shown to cause genetic defects and even cancer.[154]

10.4.2.2 Liposomes

Another way of delivering DNA to a target site is through lipoplexes, plasmid DNA (pDNA), and cationic lipid complexes. These complexes are used in transient transfection.[155] Nonetheless, they have weak stability *in vivo*, consequently reducing the efficacy of such delivery.[156–158] Delivery of pDNA through polymer matrices is limited by the questionable effectiveness *in vitro* and the difficulty for supplying a large amount of DNA required *in vivo*.[159]

Shea and colleagues had devised PLG/lipoplex system for a sustained release of pDNA for NGF.[160] The lipoplex release was maintained for 50 days while transfecting about 48% of NIH3T3 cells. The lipofected PC12 cells produced bioactive NGF while transfected HEK293T cells exhibited outgrowth by dorsal root ganglia. Similarly, Okano and coworkers transfected the BDNF gene into NIH3T3 by lipofection into cochlea cells.[161] The cells exhibited increased production in BDNF.

10.4.2.3 Self-Assembled Complexes

In gene therapy, the integration of ligands is essential for specific cell targeting.[162–165] Ligands recognize specific cell receptors in a cell and bind to them. Ligand integration improves efficiency of the delivery by eliminating possibility of DNA reaching undesired cells. However, these conjugation reactions present a risk to bioactivity proteins or peptides. Zeng et al., used charge interactions between poly-ethylenimine (PEI), plasmid DNA, and positively charged targeting peptides to achieve ternary complexes. These complexes are used to deliver genes into cells expressing the NGF receptor, TrkA. The complexes enhanced the expression of luciferase reporter gene by 1000-fold *in vitro*. *In vivo*, the transfection of dorsal root ganglia, where TrkA-expressing neurons are located, was improved 59-fold. Finally, the complexes did not present any signs of toxicity in neuronal cells.[166]

10.5 Nanotechnology for Generating Protein Gradients for Peripheral Nerve Regeneration

During the development of the nervous system, axonal growth is directed by several extrinsic cues that include haptotactic and chemotactic signaling molecules to which the growth cone responds.[167–169] Growth cones, located at the nerve fiber terminus, are highly motile structures that are believed to guide axonal growth toward its target by sampling the environment for either positive or negative signals using filopodial and lamellar protrusions.[170,171] Similarly, axons during nerve regeneration are guided by the growth cone's interpretation of its environment, believed to be a concentration gradient-dependent procedure,[172] where the relative steepness of the gradient is more important than the mean concentration of the guidance molecule.[173,174] In detail, it has been suggested that growth cones navigate over long distances depending on two conditions: (a) cell surface receptors are not saturated by the concentration of the given molecule and (b) the concentration gradient is adequately steep for growth cone detection.[175,176] Generic tissue engineered scaffolds, which contain growth factors and ECM proteins, which promote nerve regrowth and regeneration cues are normally distributed at uniform concentrations throughout. However, in native state, the critical promontory and inhibitory molecules are usually presented in a spatially and temporally controlled manner.[177–179]

Controlled spatially and temporally, the two kinds of molecules that play an important role in nerve regeneration include haptotactic proteins, which are substrate-bound or cell-surface bound ECM proteins that include laminin and collagen amongst others, and diffusible chemotactic proteins, such as NGF, BDNF, and CNTF.[180] It is critical for neural development and regeneration, that the proteins be present at the appropriate concentrations, time, and location. As a result, neural regeneration poses unique challenges when designing scaffolds to promote neurite outgrowth across a nerve gap in both the

CNS and PNS. Typically, biomaterial scaffolds are used for the spatial control of proteins between the severed ends of the nerve. Equally imperative is to control the amount of protein delivered over a period of time since it can take several months for regeneration to occur.

There are many requirements that need to be met when designing such scaffolds, including generating a biocompatible environment that allows cell infiltration and restoration of lost neuronal connections. In addition, the scaffolds should be able to deliver appropriate cues for promoting nerve regeneration in a controlled and localized manner. Tissue engineered scaffolds using neurostimulatory molecules can be of two types: isotropic scaffolds in which biomolecules are distributed uniformly throughout the scaffold or anisotropic scaffolds in which biomolecules are incorporated in a gradient. Isotropic scaffolds do not provide the necessary guidance cues to regenerating axons, due to the absence of a protein concentration gradient. As a result, there are several techniques that have been employed to prepare scaffolds of the latter type as protein gradients have shown great promise in the field of nerve regeneration.

10.5.1 Lipid Microtubules

There are several lipid-based systems that have been developed to release biomolecules including liposomes and cochleates.[181,182] These systems, however, often involve the use of organic solvents, such as dichloromethane, which can easily denature proteins, a characteristic highly not desirable in drug delivery.[183] Alternatively, lipid microtubules, also known as microcylinders, are lipid-based structures that have the ability to release proteins without the above-mentioned problems. Lipid microtubules were initially described by Yager and Schoen as cylinders formed by the polymerization of lipids upon heating and further treatment with ultraviolet light.[184] Microtubules are hollow, open-ended tubules with a diameter of approximately 500 nm and varying length. They spontaneously form while passing through a phase transition temperature during a controlled cooling process in which the chiral interactions between the lipid molecules cause the bilayers to twist into a tubular structure.[185,186] Molecules are released via the two ends of each microtubule, due to highly structured and ordered packing of the lipid molecules. As a result, the length of the microtubules controls the time period in which the desired molecule needs to be released.[187]

There are several studies in which lipid microtubules were loaded with neurotrophic factors and then embedded in within hydrogel scaffolds. Such systems are capable of creating a two-step slow release system that aids axonal regeneration in the PNS: first the diffusion of the neurotrophic factor from the microtubules into the scaffold and then the release of the neurotrophic factor into the nerve gap. Neurotrophic factors can be loaded into these lipid microtubules at different concentrations and then can be loaded into a scaffold at varying concentrations to create a gradient. Specifically, NGF was loaded into microtubules that were embedded in an agarose hydrogel. The slow release system allowed the NGF to last longer in the nerve gap and two months postimplantation a nerve cable formed in which the number of myelinated axons was considerably increased.[188] The lipid microtubule-hydrogel delivery system can be fabricated for use in a wide variety of release applications, which can be fine-tuned by adjusting several parameters including the average microtubule length, concentration of microtubules used, loading concentration of release agent, and the porosity of the hydrogel used to embed the microtubules.

10.5.2 Covalent Immobilization of Biomolecules

A different approach to controlled protein release involves the covalent immobilization of proteins on the scaffold. In this manner, the desired protein will not be lost by diffusion. Time period in which the release takes place will be comparable to the lifetime of the scaffold. However, when designing such substrate-bound gradient systems, considerable attention must be given to ensure that the process of immobilization does not affect the viability of the target biomolecules. Equally important is to make certain that the target protein does not need to be internalized by the cell in order to produce the desired effect. A variety of techniques have been developed to covalently bond molecules to scaffolds: photochemical immobilization and chemical immobilization.

Valmikinathan et al. described a technique in which protein gradients were fabricated onto electrospun nanofibers using an external magnetic field.[189] Specifically, a gradient of laminin was created on nanofibrous scaffolds, with a diamater of 500–700 nm, using an external magnetic field. They used ferritin, which has a magnetically inducible core and surface-active amino and carboxylic acid groups. The laminin was cross-linked to ferritin, which was in turn deposited on electrospun nanofibers under the influence of the magnetic field. Schwann cell attachment was increased with increasing concentrations of laminin along the length of the scaffold.

Summary

Given the complexity of the nervous system, the repair and regeneration of large gaps in the peripheral nerves is very challenging. The applications of nanotechnology-based platforms for evaluation, control, and understanding of the PNS has significantly improved the quality and performance of 2D and 3D systems for PNS regeneration over the last decade. However, further studies precisely for control nanoscale features and structures at three dimensions are still necessary and vital to allow the development of clinical useful platforms for the successful regeneration of PNS.

Acknowledgments

The authors would like to acknowledge the National Institute of Health (R03 NS058595) for providing funding support.

References

1. Silva GA, 2004. Introduction to nanotechnology and its applications in medicine. *Surg Neurol*, 61(3), 216–220.
2. Chang WC, Kilot M, Sretavan DW, 2008. Microtechnology and nanotechnology in nerve repair. *Neurol Res*, 30(1), 1053–1062.
3. Adams DN, Kao EY, Hypolite CL, Distefano MD, Hu WS, Letourneau PC, 2005. Growth cones turn and migrate up an immobilized gradient of the laminin IKVAV peptide. *J Neurobiol*, 62, 134–147.
4. Halfter W, 1996. The behavior of optic axons on substrate gradients of retinal basal lamina proteins and merosin. *J Neurosci*, 16, 4389–4401.
5. McKenna MP, Raper JA, 1998. Growth cone behavior on gradients of substratum bound laminin. *Dev Biol*, 130, 232–236.
6. Clark P, Britland S, Connolly P, 1993. Growth cone guidance and neuron morphology on micropatterned laminin surfaces. *J Cell Sci*, 105(1), 203–212.
7. Schmidt CE, Leach JB, 2003. Neural tissue engineering: Strategies for repair and regeneration. *Ann Rev Biomed Eng*, 5, 293–347.
8. Aebischer P, Guenard V, Brace S, 1989. Peripheral nerve regeneration through blind-ended semipermeable guidance channels: Effect of molecular weight cutoff. *J Neurosci*, 9, 3590–3595.
9. Bryan DJ, Wang KK, Chakalis-Haley DP, 1996. Effect of Schwann cells in the enhancement of peripheral nerve regeneration. *J Reconstr Microsurg*, 12, 439–446.
10. Choi BH, Zhu SJ, Jung JH, et al., 2005. Transplantation of cultured bone marrow stromal cells to improve peripheral nerve regeneration. *Int J Oral Maxillofac Surg*, 34, 537–542.
11. Waller A, 1850. Experiments on the section of the glossopharyngeal and hypoglossal nerves of the frog, and observations of the alterations produced thereby in the structure of their primitive fibers. *Philos Trans R Soc London*, 140, 423–429.
12. George EB, Glass JD, Griffin JW. 1995. Axotomy-induced axonal degeneration is mediated by calcium influx through ion-specific channels. *J Neurosci*, 15(10), 6445–6452.

13. Stoll G, Griffin JW, Trapp BD, et al., 1989. Wallerian degeneration in the peripheral nervous system: Participation of both Schwann cells and macrophages in myelin degradation. *J Neurocytol*, 18, 671–683.

14. Sunderland S, 1965. The connective tissues of peripheral nerves. *Brain*, 88, 841–854.

15. Sunderland S, 1970. Anatomical features of nerve trunks in relation to nerve injury and nerve repair. *Clin Neurosurg*, 17, 38–62.

16. Sunderland S, 1990. The anatomy and physiology of nerve injury. *Muscle & Nerve*, 13, 771–784.

17. Møller AR, 2006. *Neural Plasticity and Disorders of the Nervous System*. Cambridge University Press, Cambridge, pp. 51–53.

18. Chaudhry V, Glass JD, Griffin JW, 1992. Wallerian degeneration in peripheral nerve disease. *Neurol Clin*, 10, 613–627.

19. Esposito B, De Santis A, Baccari GC, et al., 2002. Mast cells in Wallerian degeneration: Morphological and ultrastructural changes. *J Comp Neurol*, 445(3), 199–210.

20. Zochodne DW, Cheng C, 2000. Neurotrophins and other growth factors in the regenerative milieu of proximal nerve stump tips. *J Anat*, 196(Pt 2), 279–283.

21. Norrby K, 2002. Mast cells and angiogenesis. *Apmis*, 110(5), 355–371.

22. Rosenstein JM, Krum JM, 2004. New roles for VEGF in nervous tissue–beyond blood vessels. *Exp Neurol*, 187(2), 246–253.

23. Bunge RP, 1993. Expanding roles for the Schwann cell: Ensheathment, myelination, trophism and regeneration. *Curr Opin Neurobiol*, 3(5), 805–809.

24. Heumann R, Korsching S, Thoenen H, et al., 1987. Changes of nerve growth factor synthesis in nonneuronal cell in response to sciatic nerve transaction. *J Cell Biol*, 104, 1623–1631.

25. Martini R, 1994. Expression and functional roles of neural cell surface molecules and extra-cellular matrix components during development and regeneration of peripheral nerves. *J Neurocytol*, 23(1), 1–28.

26. Jacobsen S, Guth L, 1965. An electrophysiological study of the early stages of peripheral nerve regeneration. *Exp Neurol*, 11, 48–60.

27. Ngo TT, Waggoner PJ, Smith GM, et al., 2003. Poly(L-lactide) microfilaments enhance peripheral nerve regeneration across extended nerve lesions. *J Neurosci Res*, 72(2), 227–238.

28. Aebischer P, Salessiotis AN, Winn SR, 1989. Basic fibroblast growth factor released from synthetic guidance channels facilitates peripheral nerve regeneration across long nerve gaps. *J Neurosci Res*, 23, 282–289.

29. Yu X, Bellamkonda RV, 2003. Tissue-engineered scaffolds are effective alternatives to autografts for bridging peripheral nerve gaps. *Tissue Eng*, 9(3), 421–430.

30. Bellamkonda RV, 2006. Peripheral nerve regeneration: An opinion on channels, scaffolds and anisotropy. *Biomaterials*, 27(19), 3515–3518.

31. Fawcett JW, 1990. Peripheral nerve regeneration. *Ann Rev Neurosci*, 13, 43–60.

32. Kirk EG, 1915. Fascial tubulization in the repair of nerve defects. *JAMA*, 65, 486–492.

33. Brandt J, Dahlin LB, Lundborg G, 1999. Autologous tendons used as grafts for bridging peripheral nerve defects. *J Hand Surg [Br]*, 24, 284–290.

34. Chiu DT, Janecka I, Krizek TJ, Wolff M, Lovelace RE, 1982. Autogenous vein graft as a conduit for nerve regeneration. *Surgery*, 91, 226–233.

35. Chiu DT, Lovelace RE, Krizek TJ, et al., 1988. Comparative electrophysiological evaluation of nerve grafts and autogenous vein grafts as nerve conduits: An experimental study. *J Reconstr Microsurg*, 4, 303–309.

36. Hadlock TA, Sundback CA, Hunter DA, Vacanti JP, 2001. A new artificial nerve graft containing rolled Schwann cell monolayers. *Microsurgery*, 21(3), 96–101.

37. Evans GR, 2001. Peripheral nerve injury: A review and approach to tissue engineered constructs. *Anat Rec*, 263, 396–404.

38. Mackinnon SE, Hudson AR, Bain JR, 1987. A peripheral nerve allograft—An assessment of regeneration in the immunosuppressed host. *Plastic Reconstr Surg*, 79(3), 445–451.

39. Valmikinathan CM, Tian J, Wang J, Yu X, 2008. Novel nanofibrous spiral scaffolds for neural tissue engineering. *J Neural Eng* 5, 422–432.

40. Borschel GR, Kia KF, Dennis RG, 2003. Mechanical properties of acellular nerve grafts. *J Surg Res*, 114, 133–139.

41. Yao CC, Yao P, Wu H, Zha ZG, 2007. Absorbable collagen sponge combined with recombinant human basic fibroblast growth factor promotes nerve regeneration in rat sciatic nerve. *J Mater Sci: Mater Med*, 18, 1969–1972.

42. Mahoney MJ, Krewson C, Miller J, Saltzman WM, 2006. Impact of cell type and density on nerve growth factor distribution and bioactivity in 3-dimensional collagen gel cultures. *Tissue Eng*, 12(7), 1915–1927.

43. Crompton KE, Goud JD, Bellamkonda RV, Gengenbach TR, Finkelstein DI, Horne MK, Forsythe JS, 2007. Polylysine-functionalised thermoresponsive chitosan hydrogel for neural tissue engineering. *Biomaterials*, 28(3), 441–449.

44. Freier T, Koh HS, Kazazian K, Shoichet MS, 2005. Controlling cell adhesion and degradation of chitosan films by N-acetylation. *Biomaterials*, 26(29), 5872–5878.

45. Prang P, Muller R, Weidner N, et al., 2006. The promotion of oriented axonal regrowth in the injured spinal cord by alginate-based anisotropic capillary hydrogels. *Biomaterials*, 27(19), 3560–3569.

46. Levesque SG, Shoichet MS, 2006. Synthesis of cell-adhesive dextran hydrogels and macroporous scaffolds. *Biomaterials*, 27(30), 5277–5285.

47. Gamez E, Goto Y, Nagata K, Iwaki T, Sasaki T, Matsuda T, 2004. Photofabricated gelatin-based nerve conduits: Nerve tissue regeneration potentials. *Cell Transpl*, 13(5), 549–564.

48. Sakiyama SE, Schense JC, Hubbell JA, 1999. Incorporation of heparin-binding peptides into fibrin gels enhances neurite extension: An example of designer matrices in tissue engineering. *Faseb J*, 13(15), 2214–2224.

49. Ahmed Z, Underwood S, Brown RA, 2003. Nerve guide material made from fibronectin: Assessment of *in vitro* properties. *Tissue Eng*, 9(2), 219–231.

50. Balgude AP, Yu X, Szymanski A, Bellamkonda RV, 2001. Agarose gel stiffness determines rate of DRG neurite extension in 3D cultures. *Biomaterials*, 22(10), 1077–1084.

51. Carone TW, Hasenwinkel JM, 2006. Mechanical and morphological characterization of homogeneous and bilayered poly(2-hydroxyethyl methacrylate) scaffolds for use in CNS nerve regeneration. *J Biomed Mater Res B Appl Biomater*, 78(2), 274–282.

52. Clavijo-Alvarez JA, Nguyen VT, Santiago LY, Doctor JS, Lee WP, Marra KG, 2007. Comparison of biodegradable conduits within aged rat sciatic nerve defects. *Plast Reconstr Surg*, 119(6), 1839–1851.

53. Athanasiou KA, Niederauer GG, Agrawal CM, 1996. Sterilization, toxicity, biocompatibility and clinical applications of polylactic acid/polyglycolic acid copolymers. *Biomaterials*, 17(2), 93–102.

54. Gunatillake PA, Adhikari R, 2003. Biodegradable synthetic polymers for tissue engineering. *Eur Cell Mater*, 5, 1–16.

55. Wang X, Gu X, Yuan C, Chen G, et al., 2004. Evaluation of biocompatibility of polypyrrole *in vitro* and *in vivo*. *J Biomed Mater Res A*, 68(3), 411–422.

56. Richardson RT, Thompson B, O'Leary S, et al., 2007. The effect of polypyrrole with incorporated neurotrophin-3 on the promotion of neurite outgrowth from auditory neurons. *Biomaterials*, 28(3), 513–523.

57. Willerth SM, Sakiyama-Elbert SE, 2007. Approaches to neural tissue engineering using scaffolds for drug delivery. *Adv Drug Deliv* 59, 325–338.

58. Valentini RF, Aebischer P, 1997. Strategies for the engineering of the peripheral nervous system, *Principles of Tissue Engineering*, RG Landes Company, ed. Lanza et al., Chapter 42, 671–685.

59. Bunge RP, 2003. Expanding roles for the Schwann cell: Ensheathment, myelination, trophism and regeneration. *Curr Opin Neurobiol*, 3, 805–809.

60. Keilhoff G, Pratsch F, Wolf G, Fansa H, 2005. Bridging extra large defects of peripheral nerves: Possibilities and limitations of alternative biological grafts from acellular muscle and Schwann cells. *Tissue Eng*, 11, 1004–1014.

61. Ansselin AD, Fink T, Davey DF, 1997. Peripheral nerve regeneration through nerve guides seeded with adult Schwann cells. *Neuropathol Appl Neurobiol*, 23, 387–398.

62. Choi BH, Zhu SJ, Kim SH, Kim BY, Huh JH, Lee SH, Jung JH, 2005. Nerve repair using a vein graft filled with collagen gel. *J Reconstr Microsurg*, 21, 267–272.

63. Letourneau PC, Condic ML, Snow DM, 1994. Interactions of developing neurons with the extracellular matrix. *J Neurosci*, 14, 915–928.

64. Reichardt LF, Tomaselli KJ, 1991. Extracellular matrix molecules and their receptors: Functions in neural development. *Annu Rev Neurosci*, 14, 531–570.

65. Rivas RJ, Burmeister DW, Goldberg DJ, 1992. Rapid effects of laminin on the growth cone. *Neuron*, 8, 107–115.

66. Edgar D, 1985. Nerve growth factors and molecules of the extracellular matrix in neuronal development. *J Cell Sci Suppl*, 3, 107–113.

67. Babensee JE, McIntire LV, Mikos AG, 2000. Growth factor delivery for tissue engineering. *Pharm Res*, 17, 497–504.

68. Lanza RP, Langer R, Chick WL, 1997. *Principles of Tissue Engineering*, Austin, TX: Academic Press.

69. Davies AM, 1994. The role of neurotrophins in the developing nervous system. *J Neurobiol*, 25, 1334–1348.

70. Henderson CE, 1996. Role of neurotrophic factors in neuronal development. *Curr Opin Neurobiol*, 6, 64–70.

71. Barde YA, 1989. Trophic factors and neuronal survival. *Neuron*, 2(6), 1525–1534.

72. Levi-Montalcini R, 1987. The nerve growth factor 35 years later. *Science*, 237(4819), 1154–1162.

73. Theonen H, Barde YA, Davies AM, Johnson JE, 1987. Neurotrophic factors and neuronal death. *Ciba Found Symp*, 126, 82–95.

74. Raivich G, Kreutzberg GW, 1993. Peripheral nerve regeneration: Role of growth factors and their receptors. *Int J Dev Neurosci*, 11(3), 311–324.

75. Schanen-King C, Nel A, Williams LK, Landreth G, 1991. Nerve growth factor stimulates the tyrosine phosphorylation of MAP2 kinase in PC12 cells. *Neurons*, 6, 915–922.

76. Tuszynski MH, Gabriel K, Meyer S, et al., 1996. Nerve growth factor delivery by gene transfer induces differential outgrowth of sensory, motor, and noradrenergic neuritis after adult spinal cord injury. *Exp Neurol*, 137, 157–173.

77. Oudega M, Hagg T, 1996. Nerve growth factor promotes regeneration of sensory axons into adult rat spinal cord. *Exp Neurol*, 140, 218–229.

78. Matheson CR, Carnahan J, Zhang TJ, et al., 1997. Glial cell line-derived neurotrophic factor (GNDF) is a neurotrophic factor for sensory neurons: Comparison with the effects of the neurotrophins. *J Neurobiol*, 32, 22–32.

79. Dawbarn D, Allen SJ, 2003. Neurotrophins and neurodegeneration. *Neuropathol Appl Neurobiol*, 29, 211–230.

80. Huang EJ, Reichardt LF, 2001. Neurotrophins: Roles in neuronal development and function. *Annu Rev Neurosci*, 24, 677–736.

81. Lundborg G, 2000. A 25-year perspective of peripheral nerve surgery: Evolving neuroscientific concepts and clinical significance. *J Hand Surg [Am]*, 25, 391–414.

82. Yin Q, Kemp GJ, Frostick Sp, 1998. Neurotrophins, neurons and peripheral nerve regeneration. *J Hand Surg [Br]*, 23, 433–437.

83. Oudega M, Hagg T, 1999. Neurotrophins promote regeneration of sensory axons in the adult rat spinal cord. *Brain Res*, 818, 431–438.

84. Braun S, Croizat B, Poindron P, et al., 1996. Neurotrophins increase motoneurons' ability to innervate skeletal muscle fibers in rat spinal cord-human muscle cocultures. *J Neurol Sci*, 136, 17–23.

85. Henderson CE, Camu W, Poulsen K, et al., 1993. Neurotrophins promote motor neuron survival and are present in embryonic limb bud. *Nature*, 363, 266–270.

86. Jones LL, Oudega M, Tuszynski MH, et al., 2001. Neurotrophic factors, cellular bridges and gene therapy for spinal cord injury. *J Physiol*, 533, 83–89.

87. Dijkhuizen PA, Hermens WT, Verhaagen J, et al., 1997. Adenoviral vector-directed expression of neurotrophin-3 in rat dorsal ganglion explants results in a robust neurite outgrowth response. *J Neurobiol*, 33, 172–184.

88. Bloch J, Fine EG, Zurn AD, Aebischer P, et al., 2001. Nerve growth factor and nurotrophin-3-releasing guidance channels promote regeneration of transected rat dorsal root. *Exp Neurol*, 172, 425–432.

89. Sterne GD, Brown RA, Terenghi G, et al., 1997. Neurtrophin-3 delivered locally viz fibronectin mats enhances peripheral nerve regeneration. *Eur J Neurosci*, 9, 1388–1396.

90. Schmalbruch H, Rosenthal A, 1995. Neurotrophin-4/5 postpones the death of injured spinal motoneurons in newborn rats. *Brain Res*, 700, 254–260.

91. Stucky C, Shin JB, Lewin GR, 2002. Neurotrophin-4: A survival factor for adult sensory neurons. *Curr Biol*, 12, 1401–1404.

92. Ramer MS, Priestley JV, McMahon SB, 2000. Functional regeneration of sensory axons into the adult spinal cord. *Nature*, 403, 312–316.

93. Priestley JV, Ramer MS, Brown RA, et al., 2002. Stimulating regeneration in the damaged spinal cord. *J Physiol Paris*, 96, 123–133.

94. Yin Q, Kemp GJ, Frostick SP, et al., 2001. Neurotrophin-4 delivered by fibrin glue promotes peripheral nerve regeneration. *Muscle Nerve*, 24, 345–351.

95. Sendtner M, Kreutzberg GW, Thoenen H, 1990. Ciliary neurotrophic factor prevents the degradation of motor neurons afteraxonomy. *Nature*, 345, 440–441.

96. Gravel C, Gotz R, Sendtner M, et al., 1997. Adenoviral gene transfer of ciliary neurotrophic factor and brain-derived neurotrophic factor leads to long-term survival of axotomized motor neurons. *Nat Med* 3, 765–770.

97. Oyesiku NM, Wigston DJ, 1996. Ciliary neurotrophic factor stimulates neurite outgrowth from spinal cord neurons. *J Comp Neurol*, 364(1), 68–77.

98. Newman JP, Verity AN, Terris DJ, et al., 1996. Ciliary neurotrophic factors enhances peripheral nerve regeneration. *Arch Otolaryngol Head Neck Surg*, 122, 399–403.

99. Ishii K, Bergman BS, et al., 2006. Neutralisation of ciliary neurotrophic factor reduces astrocyte production from transplanted neural stem cells and promotes regeneration of corticospinal tract fibers in spinal cord injury. *J Neurosci Res*, 84, 1669–1681.

100. Matheson CR, Carnahan J, Zhang TJ, et al., 1997. Glial cell line-derived neurotrophic factor (GDNF) is a neurotrophic factor for sensory neurons: Comparison with the effects of the neurotrophins. *J Neurobiol*, 32, 22–32.

101. Levison SW, Ducceschi MH, Wood TL, et al., 1996. Acute exposure to CNTF *in vivo* induces multiple components of reactive gliosis. *Exp Neurol*, 141, 256–268.

102. Blesch A, Tuszynski MH, 2001. GNDF gene delivery to injured adult CNS motor neurons promotes axonal growth, expression of the tropic neuropeptide CGRP, and cellular protection. *J Comp Neurol*, 436, 399–410.

103. Henderson CE, Philips HS, Davies AM, Lemeulle C, et al., 1994. GNDF: A potent survival factor for motoneurons present in peripheral nerve and muscle. *Science*, 266, 1062–1064.

104. Li L, Houenou LJ, et al., 1995. Rescue of adult mouse motoneurons from injury-induced cell death by glial cell line-derived neurotrophic factor. *Proc Natl Acad Sci USA*, 92, 9771–9775.

105. Oppenheim RW, Lo AC, et al., 1995. Developing motor neurons rescued from programmed and axonomy-induced cell death facial motor neurons. *Nature*, 373, 341–344.

106. Fine EG, Decosterd I, Aebischer P, et al., 2002. GNDF and NGF released by synthetic guidance channels support sciatic nerve regenerationacross a long gap. *Eur J Neurosci*, 15, 589–601.
107. Barras FM, Zurn AD, et al., 2002. Glial cell line-derived neurotrophic factor released by synthetic guidance channels promotes facial nerve regeneration in the rat. *J Neuroci Res*, 70, 746–755.
108. Piquilloud G, Papaloizos MY, et al., 2007. Variations in glial cell line-derived neurotrophic release from biodegradable nerve conduits modify the rate of functional motor recovery after rat primary nerve repairs. *Eur J Neurosci*, 26, 1109–1117.
109. Cordeiro PG, Seckel BR, Wagner J, et al., 1989. Acidic fibroblast growth factor enhances peripheral nerve regeneration *in vivo*. *Plast Reconstr Surg*, 83, 1013–1019.
110. Danielsen N, Pettmann B, Varon S, et al., 1988. Fibroblast growth factor effects on peripheral nerve regeneration in a silicone chamber model. *J Neurosci Res*, 20, 320–330.
111. Friesel RE, Maciag T, 1995. Molecular mechanisms of angiogenesis: Fibroblast growth factor signal transduction. *FASEB J*, 9, 919–925.
112. Trigg DJ, Toriumi DM, et al., 1998. Peripheral nerve regeneration: Comparison of laminin and acidic fibroblast growth factor. *Am J Otolat*, 19(1), 29–32.
113. Desai TA, Norman JJ, 2006. Methods of fabrication of nanoscale topography for tissue engineering scaffolds. *Annals of Niomed Eng*, 34(1), 89–101.
114. Johannson F, Carlberg P, Danielsen N, Kanje M, 2006. Axonal outgrowth on nanoimprinbted patterns. *Biomaterials*, 27, 1251–1258.
115. Akin T, Najafi K, Smoke RH, Bradley RM, 1994. A micromachined silicon sieve electrode for nerve regeneration applications. *IEEE Trans Biomed Eng*, 41(4), 305–313.
116. Thapa A, Webster TJ, Haberstroh KM, 2003. Polymers with nano-dimensional surface features enhance bladder smooth muscle cell adhesion. *J Biomed Mater Res A*, 15, 67(4), 1374–1383.
117. Fan YW, Cui FZ, Lee LS, et al., 2002. Culture of neural cells on silicon wafers with nanoscale surface topography. *J Neurosci Methods*, 120, 17–23.
118. Moxon KA, Hallman S, Aslani A, Kalkhoran NM, Lelkes PI, 2007. Bioactive properties of nano-structured porous silicon for enhancing electrode to neuron interfaces. *J Biomater Sci Polym Ed*, 18(10), 1263–1281.
119. Buzanska L, Ruiz A, Coecke S, et al., 2009. Patterned growth and differentiation of human cord blood-derived neural stem cells on bio-functionalized surfaces. *Acta Neurobiol Exp (Wars)*, 69(1), 24–36.
120. Ostuni E, Whitesides GM, Ingber DE, Chen CS, 2009. Using self-assembled monolayers to pattern ECM proteins and cells on substrates. *Methods in Molecular Biology*, 522, 183–194.
121. Chen CS, Mrksich M, Huang S, Whitesides GM, Ingber DE, 1997. Geometric control of cell life and death. *Science*, 276(5317), 1425–1428.
122. Thompson DM, Buettner HM, 2006. Neurite outgrowth is directed by Schwann cell alignment in the absence of other guidance cues. *Annals of Biomedical Engg*, 34, 161–174.
123. Krsko P, McCann TE, Thach TT, Laabs TL, Geller HM, Libera MR, 2009. Length-scale mediated adhesion and directed growth of neural cells by surface-patterned poly(ethylene glycol) hydrogels. *Biomaterials*, 30(5), 721–729.
124. Krsko P, Sukhishvili S, Mansfield M, Libera M, 2003. Electron-beam surface-patterned poly(ethylene glycol) microhydrogels. *Langmuir*, 19(14), 5618–5625.
125. Hong Y, Krsko P, Libera M, 2004. Protein surface patterning using nanoscale PEG hydrogels. *Langmuir*, 20, 25, 7, 11123–11126.
126. Silva GA, Czeisler C, Niece KL, Beniash E, Stupp SI, 2004. Selective differentiation of neural progenitor cells by high-density epitope nanofibers. *Science*, 303, 1352–1355.
127. Venugopal J, Prabhakaran MP, Deepika G, Ramakrishna S, 2008. Nanotechnology for nano-medicine and delivery of drugs. *Curr Pharmaceut Des*, 14(22), 2184–2200.
128. Huang HH, He CL, Wang HS, Mo XM, 2009. Preparation of core-shell biodegradable microfibers for long-term drug delivery. *J Biomed Mater Res Part A*, 90A(4), 1243–1251.

129. Ashammakhi N, Ndreu A, Piras AM, Reis RL, 2007. Biodegradable nanomats produced by electrospinning: Expanding multifunctionality and potential for tissue engineering. *J Nanosci Nanotechnol*, 7(3), 862–882.

130. Neal RA, McClugage SG, Link MC, Botchwey EA, 2009. Laminin nanofiber meshes that mimic morphological properties and bioactivity of basement membranes. *Tissue Eng Part C: Methods*, 15(1), 11–21.

131. Jayasinghe SN, Irvine S, McEwan JR, 2007. Cell electrospinning highly concentrated cellular suspensions containing primary living organisms into cell-bearing threads and scaffolds. *Nanomedicine*, 2(4), 555–567.

132. Gupta D, Venugopal J, Ramakrishna S, et al., 2009. Aligned and random nanofibrous substrate for the *in vitro* culture of Schwann cells for neural tissue engineering. *Acta Biomater* 5(7), 2560–2569.

133. Koh HS, Yong T, Chan CK, Ramakrishna S, 2008. Enhancement of neurite outgrowth using nanostructured scaffolds coupled with laminin. *Biomaterials*, 9(26), 3574–3582.

134. Bini TB, Gao S, Wang S, Ramakrishna S, 2006. Poly(L-lactide-*co*-glycolide) biodegradable microfibers and electrospun nanofibers for nerve tissue engineering: An *in vitro* study. *J Mater Sci*, 41, 6453–6459.

135. Kim YT, Haftel VK, Kumar S, Bellamkonda RV, 2008. The role of aligned polymer fiber-based constructs in the bridging of long peripheral nerve gaps. *Biomaterials*, 29(21), 3117–3127.

136. Chew SY, Mi R, Hoke A, Leong KW, 2007. Aligned protein-polymer composite fibers enhance nerve regeneration: A potential tissue-engineering platform. *Adv Funct Mater*, 17(8), 1288–1296.

137. Seidlits SK, Lee Y, Schmidt CE, 2008. Nanostructured scaffolds for neural applications. *Nanomedicine*, 3, 183–199.

138. Panyam J, Lebhastetwar V, 2003. Biodegradable nanoparticles for drug and gene delivery to cells and tissue. *Adv Drug Deliv Rev*, 55, 329–347.

139. Zhang S, Uludag H, 2009. Nanoparticulate systems for growth factor delivery. *Pharm Res*, 26, 1561–1580.

140. Chinellini F, Piras AM, Chiellini E, et al., 2008. Micro/nanostructured polymeric systems for biomedical and pharmaceutical applications. *Nanomedicine*, 3, 367–393.

141. Nkansah MK, Tzeng SY, Lavik EB, et al., 2008. Poly(lactic-*co*-glycolic acid) nanospheres and microspheres for short- and long-term delivery of bioactive ciliary neurotrophic factor. *Biotechnol. Bioeng*, 100, 1010–1019.

142. Chung BG, Khademhosseini A, et al., 2007. Micro- and nanoscale technologies for tissue engineering and drug discovery applications. *Exp Opin Drug Discov*, 2, 1–16.

143. Gao X, Petros JA, et al., 2005. *In vivo* molecular and cellular imaging with quantum dots. *Curr Opin Biotechnol*, 16(1), 63–72.

144. Echarte MM, Pietrasanta LI, et al., 2007. Quantitative single particle tracking of NGF-receptor complexes: Transport is bidirectional but biased by longer retrograde run lengths. *FEBS Lett*, 581, 2905–2913.

145. Naka Y, Shimizu N, 2004. Neurite outgrowths of neurons using neurotrophin-coated nanoscale magnetic beads. *J Biosci Bioeng*, 98(5), 348–352.

146. Chew SY, Wen J, Leong KW, et al., 2005. Sustained release of proteins from electrospun biodegradable fibers. *Biomacromol*, 6, 2017–2024.

147. Valmikinathan CM, Defroda S, Yu X, 2009. Polycaprolactone and bovine serum albumin based nanofibers for controlled release of nerve growth factor. *Biomacromol*, 10(5), 1084–1089.

148. Yan S, Lianjiang T, Xiumei M, et al., 2009. Poly(L-lactide-*co*-epsilon-caprolactone) electrospun nanofibers for encapsulating and sustained releasing proteins. *Polymer*, 50(17), 4212–4219.

149. Moller JC, Shooter EM, et al., 1998. Subcellular localization of epitopetagged neurotrophins in neuroendocrine cells. *J Neurosci Res*, 51(4), 463–472.

150. Hendriks WT, Ruitenberg MJ, Verhaagen J, et al., 2004. Viral vector-mediated gene transfer of neurotrophins to promote regeneration of the injured spinal cord. *Prog Brain Res*, 146, 451–476.

151. Barretm JT, 1998. *Microbiology and Immunology Concepts*. Philadelphia, PA: Lippincott-Raven, 111–112.
152. Sharma A, Suresh K, et al., 2009. Adenovirus receptors and their implications in gene delivery. *Virus Research*, 143(2), 184–194.
153. Hollon T, 2000. Researchers and regulators refect on first gene therapy death. *Nat Med*, 6, 715–745.
154. Rezazadeh A, Kloecher G, et al., 2008. The role of human Papilloma virus in lung cancer: A review of the evidence. *Am J Med Sci*, 338(1), 64–67.
155. Audouy S, Hoekstra D, 2001. Cationic lipid-mediated transfection *in vitro* and in vivo. *Mol Membr Biol*, 18(2), 129–143.
156. Nchinda G, Uberla K, Zschornig O, 2002. Characterization of cationic lipid DNA transfection complexes differing in susceptability to serum inhibition. *BMC Biotechnol*, 2(1):12.
157. Yang JP, Huang L, 1998. Time-dependent maturation of cationic liposome–DNA complex for serum resistance. *Gene Ther*, 5(3), 380–387.
158. Li S, Tseng WC, Huang L, et al., 1999. Dynamic changes in the characteristics of cationic lipidic vectors after exposure to mouse serum: implications for intravenous lipofection. *Gene Ther*, 6(4), 585–594.
159. Shea LD, Smiley E, Mooney DJ, et al., 1999. DNA delivery from polymer matrices for tissue engineering. *Nat Biotechnol*, 17(6), 551–554.
160. Whittlesey KJ, Shea LD, 2006. Nerve growth factor expression by PLG-mediated lipofection. *Biomaterials*, 27, 2477–2486.
161. Okano T, Ito J, et al. 2006. Cell–gene delivery of brain-derived neurotrophic factor to the mouse inner ear. *Mol Ther*, 14(6), 866–871.
162. Wu GY, Wu CH, 1987. Receptor-mediated *in vitro* gene transformation by a soluble DNA carrier system. *J Biol Chem*, 262, 4429–4432.
163. Wu GY, Wu CH, 1988. Evidence for targeted gene delivery to Hep G2 hepatoma cells in vitro. *Biochem*, 27, 887–892.
164. Wagner E, Birnstiel ML, et al., 1990. Transferrin–polycation conjugates as carriers for DNA uptake into cells. *Proc Natl Acad Sci USA*, 87, 3410–3414.
165. Fajac I, Monsigny M, et al., 2002. Targeting of cell receptors and gene transfer efficiency: A balancing act. *Gene Ther*, 9, 740–742.
166. Zeng J, Wang S, et al., 2007. Self-assembled ternary complexes of plasmid DNA, low molecular weight polyethylenimine and targeting peptide for nonviral gene delivery into neurons. *Biomaterials*, 28, 1443–1451.
167. Dickson BJ, 2002. Molecular mechanisms of axon guidance. *Science*, 298(5600), 1959–1964.
168. Goodman CS, 1996. Mechanisms and molecules that control growth cone guidance. *Ann Rev Neurosci*, 19, 341–371.
169. Tessier-Lavigne M, Goodman CS, 1996. The molecular biology of axon guidance. *Science*, 274, 1123–1133.
170. Mueller BK, 1999. Growth cone guidance: first steps towards a deeper understanding. *Ann Rev Neurosci*, 22, 351–388.
171. Gallo G, Letourneau PC, 2004. Regulation of growth cone actin filaments by guidance cues. *J Neurobiol*, 58(1), 92–102.
172. Zheng JQ, Wan JJ, Poo MM, 1996. Essential role of filopodial in chemotropic turning of nerve growth cone induced by a glutamate gradient. *J Neurosci*, 16(3), 1140–1149.
173. Rosoff WJ, Urbach JS, Goodhill GJ, et al., 2004. A new chemotaxis assay shows the extreme sensitivity of axons to molecular gradients. *Nat Neurosci*, 7(6), 678–682.
174. Guan KL, Rao Y, 2003. Signaling mechanisms mediating neuronal responses to guidance cues. *Nat Rev Neurosci*, 4, 941–956.
175. Zigmond SH, 1981. Consequences of chemotactic peptide receptor modulation for leukocyte orientation. *J Cell Biol*, 88, 644–647.

176. Goodhill GJ, 1997. Diffusion of axon guidance. *Eur J Neurosci*, 9, 1414–1421.

177. Song H, Poo M, 2001. The cell biology of neuronal navigation. *Nat Cell Biol*, 3, E81–E88.

178. Bonhoeffer F, Huf J, 1982. *In vitro* experiments on axon guidance demonstrating an anterior-posterior gradient on the tectum. *EMBO J*, 1, 427–431.

179. Bonner J, O'Connor TP. 2001, The permissive cue laminin is essential for growth cone turning *in vivo*. *J Neurosci*, 21, 9782–9791.

180. Edgar D, 1985. Nerve growth factors and molecules of the extracellular matrix in neuronal development. *J Cell Sci Suppl*, 3, 107–113.

181. Gregoriadis G, 1995. Engineering liposomes for drug delivery: Progress and problems. *Trends Biotechnol*, 13(12), 527–537.

182. Santangelo R, Paderu P, Delmas G, Chen ZW, Mannino R, Zarif L, Perlin DS, 2000. Efficacy of oral cochleates-amphotericin B in a mouse model of systemic candidiasis. *Antimicrob Agents Chemother*, 44(9), 2356–2360.

183. Raghuvanshi RS, Goyal S, Singh O, Panda AK, 1998. Stabilization of dichloromethane-induced protein denaturation during microencapsulation. *Pharmaceut Dev Technol*, 3(2), 269–276.

184. Yager P, Schoen PE, 1983. Formation of tubules by a polymerizable surfactant. *Mol Crys Liquid Crys*, 106(3–4), 371–381.

185. Schnur JM, 1993. Lipid tubules: A paradigm for molecularly engineered structures. *Science*, 262(5140), 1669–1676.

186. Spector MS, Selinger JV, Schnur JM, 1997. Thermodynamics of phospholipid tubules in alcohol/water solutions. *J Am Chem Soc*, 119(36), 8533–8539.

187. Meilander NJ, Yu X, Ziats NP, Bellamkonda RV, 2001. Lipid-based microtubular drug delivery vehicles. *J Control Release*, 71(1), 141–152.

188. Yu X, Bellamkonda RV, 2003. Tissue-engineered scaffolds are effective alternatives to autografts for bridging peripheral nerve gaps. *Tissue Eng*, 9(3), 421–430.

189. Valmikinathan CM, Wang J, Smiriglio S, Golwala NG, Yu X, 2009. Magnetically induced protein gradients on electrospun nanofibers. *Combin Chem High Throughput Screen*, 12(6), 1–8.

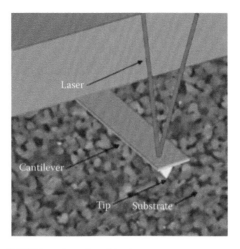

FIGURE 1.1 Representation of AFM imaging of a gold substrate.

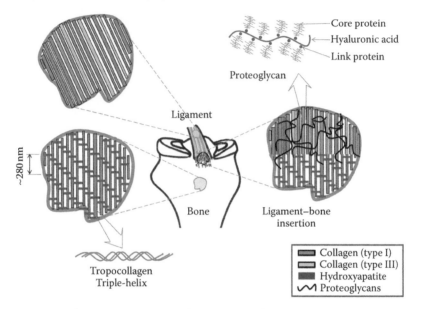

FIGURE 2.1 Overview of the nanoscale structural organization of bone, ligament/tendon, and direct ligament/tendon-to-bone insertion site.

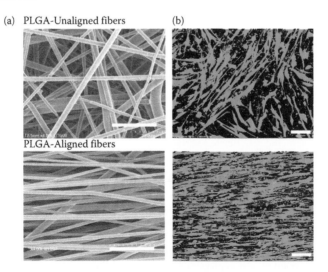

FIGURE 2.2 (a) Aligned and unaligned nanofiber scaffolds evaluated with scanning electron microscopy (SEM) (4000×, bar = 10 µm); (b) Human rotator cuff tendon fibroblasts cultured on aligned and unaligned PLGA (85:15) nanofiber scaffolds (day 14, 20×, bar = 100 µm).

Ligament	Tissue	Cell type	Major matrix composition
	Ligament/tendon	Fibrolasts	Collagen types I, III
	Non-mineralized fibrocartilage	Ovoid chondrocytes	Collagen types I, II proteoglycans
	Mineralized fibrocartilage	Hypertrophic chondrocytes	Collagen type X
	Bone	Osteoblast, osteocytes, osteoclasts	Collagen type I

FIGURE 2.3 Structure and composition of direct insertion site (ACL-to-bone interface, FTIR-I).

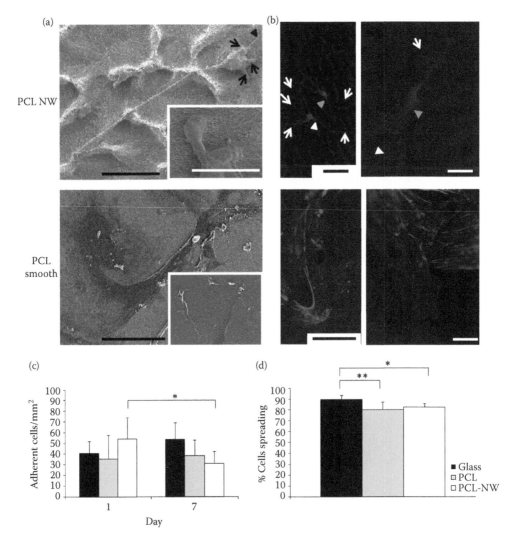

FIGURE 3.3 Human umbilical vein endothelial cells cultured for 7 days. (a) SEM image of cells on smooth and nanowire PCL. Cells cultured on nanowire PCL sprout and extend multiple long, narrow processes with round tips, whereas cells cultured on smooth PCL are flat and well spread, forming lamellipodia for motility. Black arrows point to examples of sprouting. Black arrowhead points to filopodia associated with new sprouting process. (b) Cells cultured on nanowire and smooth PCL stained for actin by rhodamine phalloidin and nucleus by DAPI. White arrows point to examples of branched processes. Gray arrow heads point to concentrated actin at growth sprout, white arrowheads point to actin aggregates. (c) Number of adherent live cells after 1 and 7 days in culture. (d) Percent of spreading (nonrounded) cells after 24 h in culture. Black scale bars = 50 μm, white scale bars = 20 μm. $*p < 0.05$, $**p < 0.01$.

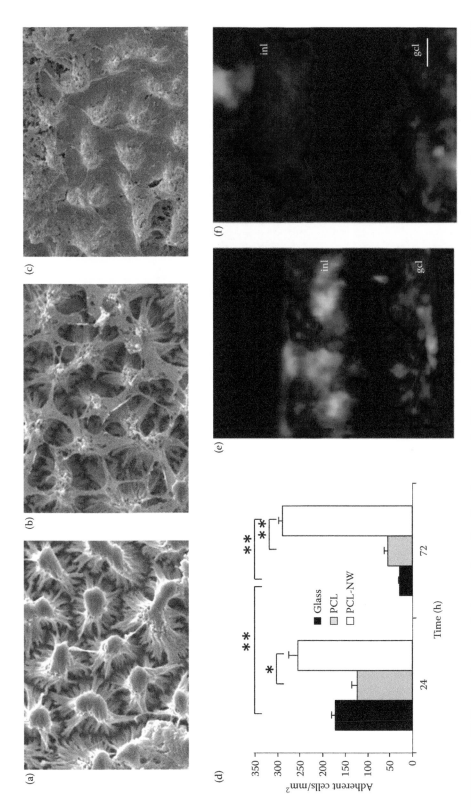

FIGURE 3.4 SEM images of mouse retinal progenitor cells cultured on nanowire PCL at (a) day 1, (b) day 3, and (c) day 7. (d) Number of adherent cells after 24 and 72 h in culture on glass, smooth PCL, and nanowire PCL. (e) Integration of RPCs cultured on nanowire PCL into Rho −/− retinal explants, with high migration into the inner nuclear and ganglion cell layers. (f) RPCs cultured on smooth PCL with little integration of RPCs into Rho −/− retinal explants. Note that the ONL is absent from the 8- to 10-week Rho −/− retina due to degeneration. Black scale bar = 2 μm. White scale bar = 100 μm. (With kind permission from Springer Science+Business Media: Redenti, S. et al. 2008. *Journal of Ocular Biology, Dieases, and Informatics* 1(1):19–29. Copyright 2008.)

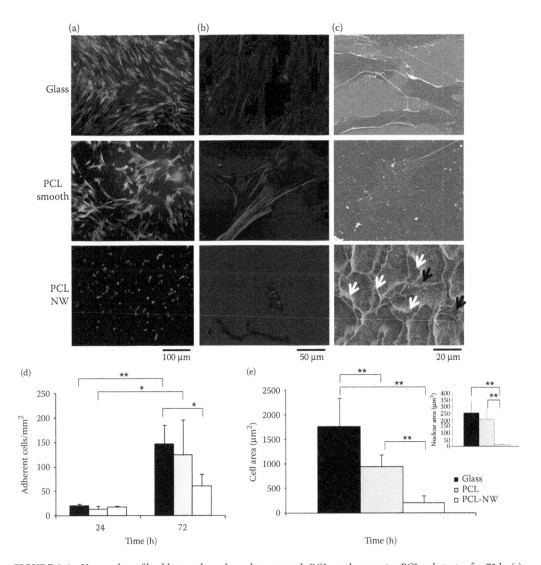

FIGURE 3.6 Human lung fibroblasts cultured on glass, smooth PCL, and nanowire PCL substrates for 72 h. (a) Live cells stained by 5-chloromethylfluorescein diacetate. (b) Actin stained by rhodamine phalloidin and nucleus stained by DAPI. (c) SEM image of cell morphology. Cells cultured on glass elongated, while cells on smooth PCL appeared triangular and motile. Cells cultured on nanowire PCL were either conformed to the top of the nanowire cluster (white arrows) or were spread between clusters (black arrows). (d) Number of adherent live cells after 24 and 72 h in culture. (e) Cell area after 72 h in culture. Inset shows nuclear area. $*p < 0.05$, $**p < 0.01$. (Reprinted from Tao, S. L. and T. A. Desai. 2007. *Nano Lett* 7 (6):1463–1468. With permission. © 2007 American Chemical Society.)

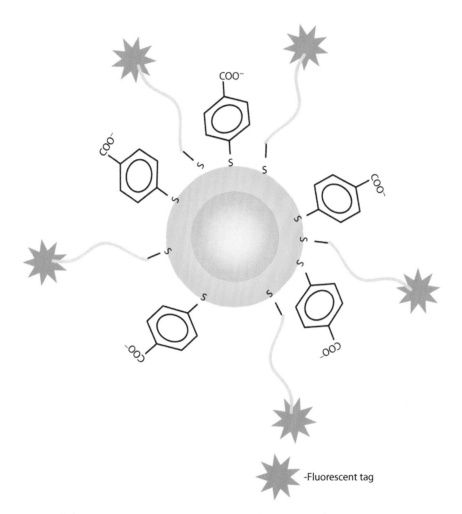

FIGURE 5.6 Multifunctional pH sensor using a mixed monolayer system of 4-MBA and Cys-PEG-Fl.

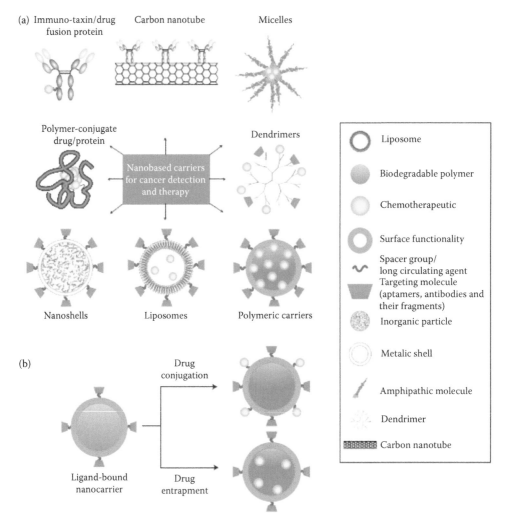

FIGURE 6.1 Examples of nanoparticles/nanocarriers for targeting cancer. (a) A whole range of delivery agents are possible but the main components typically include a nanoparticle/nanocarrier, a targeting moiety conjugated to the nanoparticle/nanocarrier, and a cargo (such as the desired chemotherapeutic drugs). (b) Schematic diagram of the drug conjugation and entrapment processes. The chemotherapeutics could be bound to the nanoparticle/nanocarrier, as in the use of polymer–drug conjugates, dendrimers and some particulate carriers, or they could be entrapped inside the nanoparticle/nanocarrier. (Reprinted by permission from Macmillan Publishers LTD: Peer, D. et al., 2007. *Nat. Nanotechnol.* 2:751–760. Copyright 2007.)

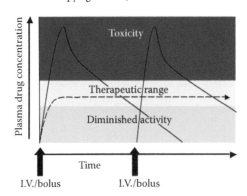

FIGURE 6.2 Concept of controlled drug delivery. Plasma concentration versus time curve for intravenous drug administration showing first-order kinetics (——). Plasma concentration versus time curve for sustained release profile of zero-order kinetics (-----).

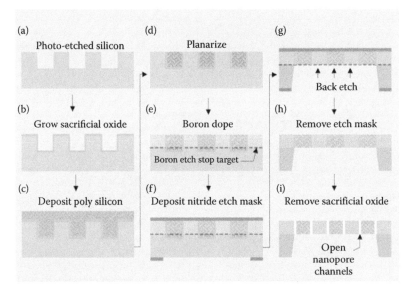

FIGURE 6.5 Schematic of key steps in the silicon nanopore membrane fabrication process. (From Martin, F. et al., 2005. *J. Control. Release* 102:123–133. With permission.)

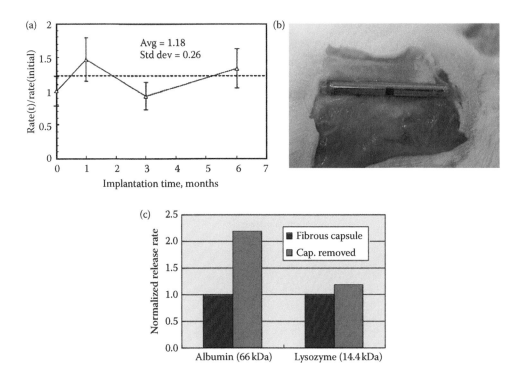

FIGURE 6.9 (a) Ratio of pre- and postimplantation glucose diffusion rates from the NanoGATE device. (b) *Ex vivo* analysis of implanted devices after the sacrifice of a rat. Note the lack of tissue attachment to both the Ti shell, Si device, and polymethyl methacrylate plugs in device. (c) Postimplantation diffusion testing (with and without tissue capsule). The normalized release rates were obtained by dividing the biomolecular release rates from the implant before and after the tissue capsule was removed from the implant surface after explantation. (With kind permission from Springer Science+Business Media: Walczak, R. et al., 2005. *Nanobiotechnology* 1(1): 35–42. Copyright 2005.)

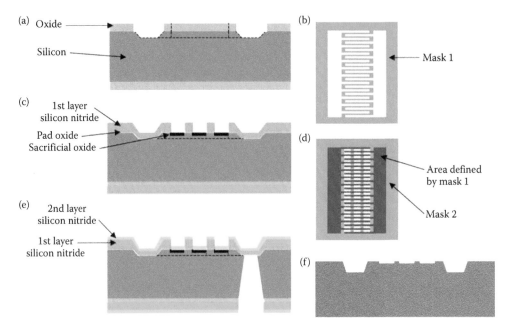

FIGURE 6.11 Nanochannel microchip fabrication: (a) Cross-sectional view demonstrating steps in the fabrication process. (b) Plan of mask 1, defining flow chambers and fingers. (c) Nanochannels and anchor points. (d) Plan of mask 2, defining nanochannels and anchor points. (e) Nanochannels protected by second layer of nitride and exit port (deep etch). (f) Complete bottom substrate fabrication. (With kind permission from Springer Science+Business Media: Lesinski, G. B. et al., 2005. *Biomed. Microdevices* 7(1): 71–79. Copyright 2005.)

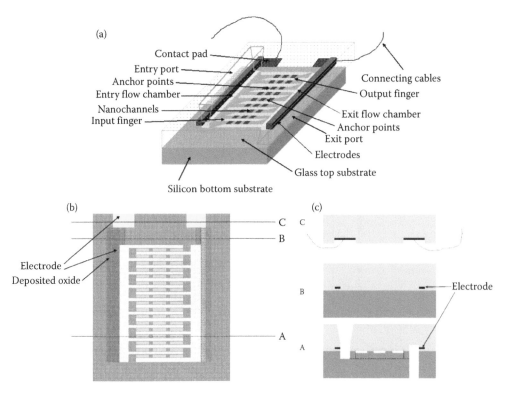

FIGURE 6.14 nDS2 Microchip: (a) a 3-D schematic view of the device, (b) a top view of the device. There are three cross-section locations marked as A, B, and C in this figure, cross-sectional views at these locations are shown in (c). (Reprinted from Sinha, P. M. 2005. Nanoengineered implantable devices for controlled drug delivery, Ph.D. Thesis, The Ohio State University. With permission.)

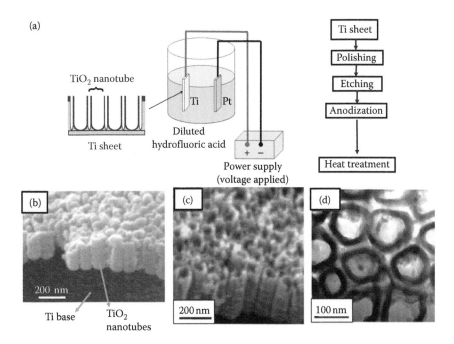

FIGURE 8.1 TiO$_2$ nanotube surface structuring. (a) Schematic illustration of electrochemical anodization and experimental flowchart to form TiO$_2$ nanotube arrays. (b) SEM image showing vertically aligned TiO$_2$ nanotube arrays on a Ti sheet. (c) Higher magnification SEM image. (d) Cross-sectional TEM image.

TiO$_2$ nanotube surface characteristics

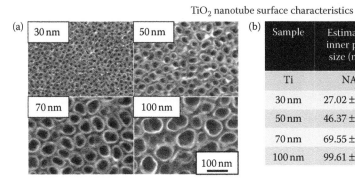

Sample	Estimated inner pore size (nm)	Roughness Ra (nm)	Contact angle (°)
Ti	NA	9.7	54 [ref. 22]
30 nm	27.02 ± 4.43	13.0	11
50 nm	46.37 ± 2.76	12.7	9
70 nm	69.55 ± 7.87	13.5	7
100 nm	99.61 ± 7.32	13.2	4

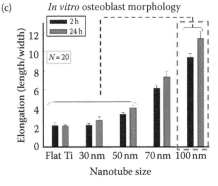

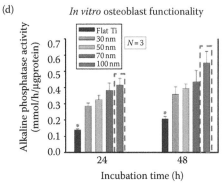

FIGURE 8.2 (a) SEM micrographs of self-aligned TiO$_2$ nanotubes with different diameters. The images show highly ordered nanotubes with four different pore sizes between 30 and 100 nm. (b) Table with pore size distribution ± standard deviation, average roughness (Ra) from atomic force microscopy measurements, and surface contact angle measurements for Ti and 30–100 nm TiO$_2$ nanotube surfaces. (c) Quantification of osteoblast elongation on the different sized nanotube surfaces. (d) Bone-building functionality represented by ALP activity of osteoblasts on the different sized nanotube surfaces. (Reprinted from Brammer, K. S. et al., 2009. *Acta Biomaterialia* 5(8): 3215–3212. Copyright 2009 with permission from Elsevier.)

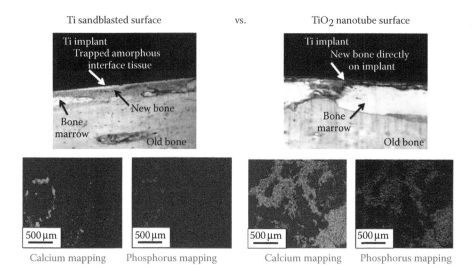

Ti sandblasted surface   vs.   TiO₂ nanotube surface

Calcium mapping   Phosphorus mapping   Calcium mapping   Phosphorus mapping

FIGURE 8.3 Comparative osseointegration at bone implant surface. Cross-sectional microscopy of implant–new bone interface by histology and bone mineralization mapping on sandblasted Ti implant versus TiO₂ nanotube surface implant. (From Bjursten, L. M. et al., 2010. *J Biomed Mater Res Part A* 1:92(3): 1218–24. Copyright Wiley-VCH Verlag GmbH & Co. KGaA. Reproduced with permission.)

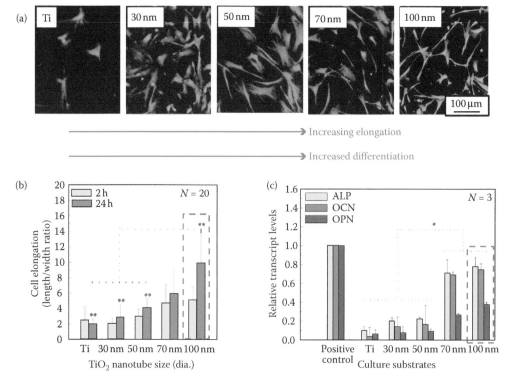

FIGURE 8.4 *In vitro* MSC response to different sized nanotube surfaces. (a) Morphological observation of cells by FDA live staining. MSCs increase in elongation with increasing nanotube diameter. (b) Quantification of MSC elongation. (c) Comparative bar graph showing osteogenic differentiation on the different sized nanotube surfaces evaluated by PCR relative transcription levels for the primary osteogenic markers (ALP, OCN, and OPN). (Adapted from Oh, S. et al. 2009. *Proc Natl Acad Sci USA* 106(7): 2130–5.)

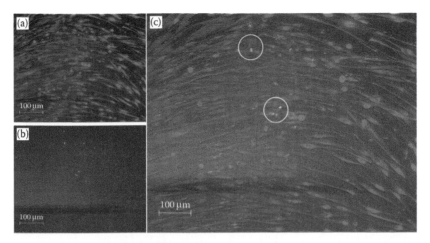

FIGURE 9.5 LIVE/DEAD cell assay analysis of cells exposed to 20 mg/mL PCL-L-DTH polyurethane film (a) dead cells, (b) live cells, and (c) combined image. Circles in yellow highlight representative dead cell nuclei.

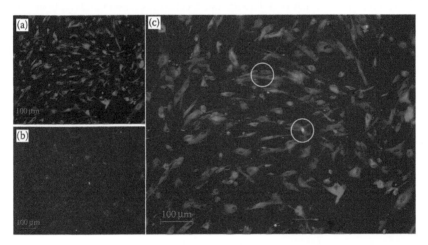

FIGURE 9.6 LIVE/DEAD cell assay analysis of cells exposed to 20 mg/mL PLGA film (a) dead cells, (b) live cells, and (c) combined image. Circles in yellow highlight representative dead cell nuclei.

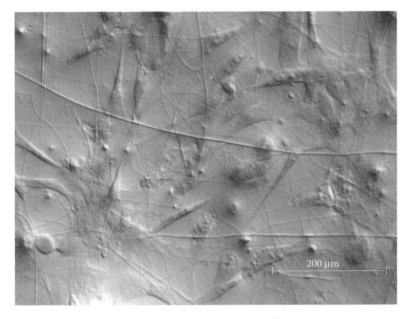

FIGURE 9.7 Attachment of human dermal fibroblasts to PCL-L-DTH fiber.

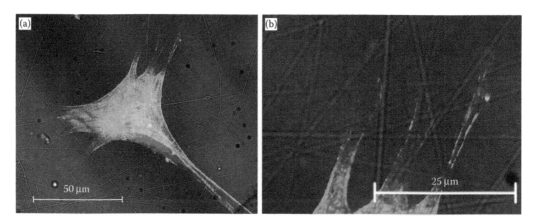

FIGURE 9.8 Vinculin immunofluorescence staining of human dermal fibroblast attachment to PCL-L-DTH fibers. Green color represents staining of actin using Alexa Fluor 488 phalloidin, blue represents Hoechst nuclear staining, and red represents anti-vinculin antibody conjugated with TRITC. (a) Image of a single cell and (b) close up of focal adhesion sites.

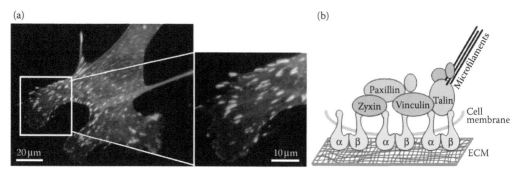

FIGURE 11.1 Cell–substratum adhesion. (a) Fluorescent microscope image of a single bovine capillary endothelial cell cultured on a smooth glass substrate. Cell was stained for vinculin (green) and F-actin (red). Focal adhesions (green) are located at the tips of stress fibers (inset image). (b) A simplified diagram of a focal adhesion that shows α and β integrins ligated to the extracellular matrix (ECM) and intracellular proteins that link integrins to the cytoskeleton.

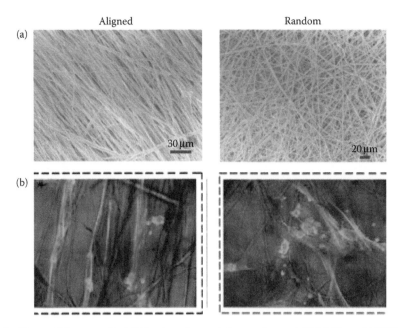

FIGURE 11.2 Human Schwann cells (hSC) cultured on poly(ε-caprolactone) (PCL) fibers. (a) SEM micrographs of PCL scaffolds for hSC culture. (b) Confocal fluorescent images of hSC on PCL scaffolds. Fluorescent-light images overlay. Green: actin cytosekelton, blue: DAPI. (Modified from Chew, S. Y. et al., 2008. *Biomaterials* 29 (6): 653–61. With permission.)

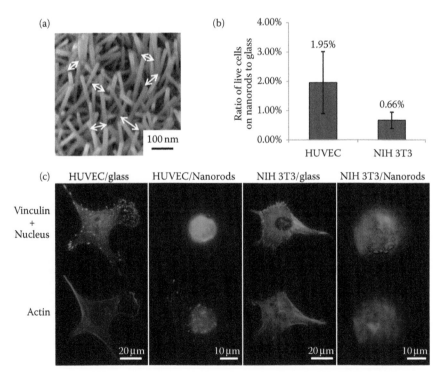

FIGURE 11.3 Human umbilical vein endothelial cells (HUVEC) and NIH 3T3 fibroblasts cultured on nanorods. (a) Scanning electron microscopy (SEM) image of nanorods on glass. White arrows indicate the spacing between nanorods which ranges from 80 to 100 nm. (b) The ratio of the number of live cells on nanorods to that on glass (*n* > 2500 for HUVECs, *n* > 1500 for NIH 3T3). Cells are considerably reduced in numbers on nanorods. Bar indicates SEM. (c) Fluorescent microscopic images of HUVEC and NIH 3T3 on glass and nanorods. HUVEC and NIH 3T3 on glass assemble focal adhesions stained with vinculin (green) and actin stress fibers (red). Nuclei were stained with DAPI (blue). HUVEC and NIH 3T3 on nanorods are unable to spread and assemble focal adhesions and stress fibers. (Modified from Lee, J. et al., 2009. *Biomaterials* 30 (27): 4488–93. With permission.)

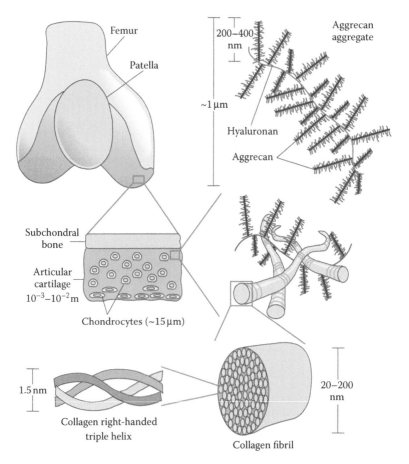

FIGURE 13.1 Structural hierarchy of articular cartilage. In the macroscale, articular cartilage spans about 0.5–15 cm. On the microscale, chondrocytes (around 15 μm in diameter) are the main components in articular cartilage. On the nanoscale, cartilage is composed of ECM proteoglycan aggregates embedded within collagen fibers. (Adapted from Mow, V. C., A. Ratcliffe, and A. R. Poole. 1992. *Biomaterials* 13(2): 67–97. Copyright 1991, Elsevier. With permission.)

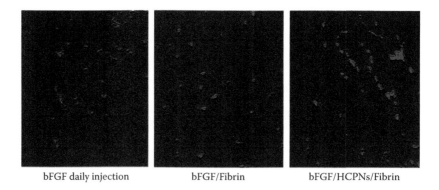

bFGF daily injection   bFGF/Fibrin   bFGF/HCPNs/Fibrin

FIGURE 13.3 Immunohistochemical analysis of mouse ischemic limbs 4 weeks after treatment with FGF loaded nanoparticles. The specimens were stained with cyanine-conjugated vWF antibodies, which bind specifically to endothelial cells. Note that the delivery of FGF through the heparin modified nanoparticles induces higher growth of endothelial cell when compared to FGF delivered in solution or through a fibrin gel. HCPNs = Heparin-conjugated PLGA nanospheres. (Reprinted from Jeon, O. et al. 2006. *Biomaterials* 27(8): 1598–607. Copyright 2006, Elsevier. With permission.)

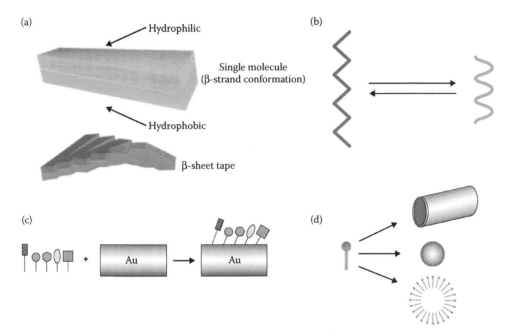

(a) Hydrophilic

Single molecule
(β-strand conformation)

Hydrophobic

β-sheet tape

(b)

(c)

Au + → Au

(d)

FIGURE 13.5 Various types of self-assembling peptide systems. (a) Amphiphilic peptides in β-strand conformation are chiral objects. As a consequence, they self-assemble into twisted tapes. (b) Helical dipolar peptides can undergo a conformational change between α-helix and β-sheet, much like a molecular switch. (c) Surface-binding peptides can form monolayers covalently bound to a surface. (d) Surfactant-like peptides can form vesicles and nanotubes. (Reprinted from Zhang, S. et al. 2002. *Current Opinion in Chemical Biology* 6(6): 865–71. Copyright 2002, Elsevier. With permission.)

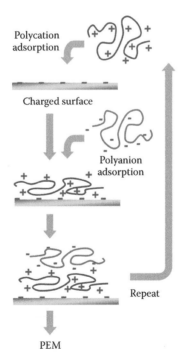

Polycation
adsorption

Charged surface

Polyanion
adsorption

Repeat

PEM

FIGURE 13.6 Construction of polyelectrolyte multilayers. A charged surface is exposed to a solution of an oppositely charged polyelectrolyte, resulting in polyelectrolyte adsorption and inversion of the surface charge. The charge inversion prevents additional adsorption of the polyelectrolyte, limiting the layer thickness. The surface is then rinsed and exposed to a polyelectrolyte with a charge opposite to that of the first polyelectrolyte. The surface charge is again inverted and the process can be repeated.

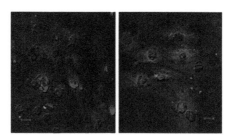

FIGURE 13.7 Expression of green fluorescence protein (GFP) of cells adhered on titanium surfaces 3 days after culture. (Left) Unmodified titanium surface with GFP plasmid vector delivered in solution with lipofectamine 2000. (Right) Titanium surface modified with chitosan/plasmid LBL assembly. The higher expression of GFP denotes a higher plasmid uptake by the cells. (Reprinted from Hu, Y. et al. 2009. *Biomaterials* 30(21): 3626–35. Copyright 2009, Elsevier. With permission.)

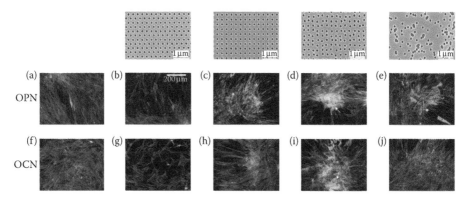

FIGURE 13.10 Osteopontin (OPN) and osteocalcin (OCN) staining of osteoprogenitor cells after 21 days of culture. The top row shows images of nanotopographies fabricated by EBL. All have 120 nm-diameter pits (100 nm deep, absolute or average 300 nm center-center spacing) with hexagonal, square, displaced square 50 (±50 nm from true center) and random placements. a–j, Osteoprogenitors cultured on the control (a,f), note the lack of positive OPN and OCN stain; HEX (b,g), note the loss of cell adhesion; SQ (c,h), note reduced cell numbers compared with the control, but some OPN and OCN positive cells; DSQ50 (d,i), note bone nodule formation (arrows); RAND (e,j), note good cell populations with cells expressing OPN and OCN. Actin = red, OPN/OCN = green. (Reprinted by permission from Macmillan Publishers LTD: Dalby, M. J. et al. 2007. *Nature Materials* 6(12): 997–1003. Copyright 2007.)

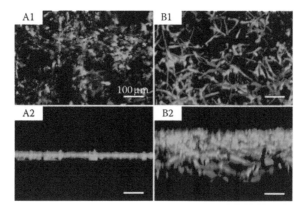

FIGURE 13.13 Reconstructed image of 3-D confocal micrographs of culturing on the different scaffolds consisting of different mix ratio of RADA16 1% (w/v) and PRG 1% (w/v) using calcein-AM staining. The bar represents 100 μm. A1 and A2: 10% of the 2-unit RGD binding sequence PRG and B1&B2: PRG 70%. A1 and B1 are vertical view and A2 and B2 are horizontal view. In the case of 10% PRG scaffold, the cells were attached on the surface of the scaffold, whereas the cells were migrated into the scaffold in the case of 70% PRG scaffold. There is a drastic cell migration into the scaffold with higher concentration of PRG motif. (Reprinted from Horii, A. et al. 2007. *PLoS ONE* 2(2): e190. doi:10.1371/journal.pone.0000190.)

11

Nanoscale Control of Cell–Substrate Adhesion

Jiyeon Lee
University of Florida

Nicole Clarke
University of Florida

Tanmay P. Lele
University of Florida

11.1 Introduction

Anchorage-dependent cells in the body require adhesion to the solid extracellular matrix (ECM) for normal function (Benzeev et al., 1980; Girard et al., 2007; Ingber, 2006; Re et al., 1994). The ECM consists of fibrous networks composed of proteins such as fibronectin, laminin, vitronectin, collagen, and elastin (Vakonakis et al., 2007). These structures provide physical and chemical signals at the nanometer length scale that control cell functions such as migration, proliferation, and apoptosis (Ingber, 1990; Girard et al., 2007; Stevens et al., 2005). The ECM in the body can be mimicked *in vitro* by fabricating materials that present defined chemical and physical signals to the cell (Chen et al., 1997; Clark et al., 1990; Flemming et al., 1999; Lo et al., 2000; Schnell et al., 2007). In particular, manipulating cell adhesion by fabricating material surfaces with nanoscale structures has emerged as a promising approach to control cell function both *in vivo* (Webster et al., 2000; Zhang et al., 2008) and *in vitro* (Dalby et al., 2008; Liliensiek et al., 2006; Sniadecki et al., 2006; Teixeira et al., 2006; Yim et al., 2005). Fabricating biomedical implants with nanostructured surfaces can allow the selective control of cellular interactions with the implant which is desirable for optimal implant performance. While it is clear that cells are exquisitely sensitive to nanostructured surfaces, the molecular mechanisms that determine this sensitivity are less clear. This chapter focuses on the current understanding of the mechanisms by which cells sense the nanoscale structure at the molecular level and how this understanding can be useful in developing novel antifouling materials.

11.2 Cell–Substratum Adhesion

Cell adhesion to the solid substratum occurs through specific binding interactions between transmembrane receptors called integrins and their ligands (e.g., fibronectin, collagen, laminin, and vitronectin)

(a)   (b)

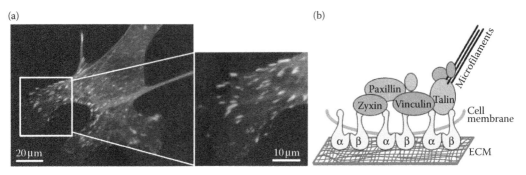

FIGURE 11.1   (See color insert following page 10-24.) Cell–substratum adhesion. (a) Fluorescent microscope image of a single bovine capillary endothelial cell cultured on a smooth glass substrate. Cell was stained for vinculin (green) and F-actin (red). Focal adhesions (green) are located at the tips of stress fibers (inset image). (b) A simplified diagram of a focal adhesion that shows α and β integrins ligated to the extracellular matrix (ECM) and intracellular proteins that link integrins to the cytoskeleton.

which are adsorbed on the substratum (Giancotti et al., 1999; Hynes, 1992, 2002). The integrin receptor is a heterodimer consisting of α and β subunits. In mammals, 18 α subunits and 8 β subunits have so far been discovered (Luo et al., 2007). The different subunits make it possible to form different types of integrin heterodimers which bind selectively to specific ligands. Many integrin receptors recognize arginine–glycine–aspartic acid (RGD) motifs which are present in ECM ligands such as fibronectin and vitronectin.

The ligation of integrin receptors causes a change in their conformation. This triggers the binding of cytoplasmic proteins such as talin to the cytoplasmic tails of integrins. Talin binding is thought to crosslink neighboring integrin receptors, giving rise to spatial clustering of ligated integrins (Nayal et al., 2004). The clustering of integrins causes the recruitment of several different types of proteins including enzymes like focal adhesion kinase and src kinase (Schlaepfer et al., 1994), adaptor molecules like paxillin (Brown et al., 2004) that are known to bind to several other proteins and α-actinin-1 (Otey et al., 2004), that directly link integrins and the actin cytoskeleton (Burridge et al., 1997; Hynes, 2002). The resulting multimolecular assembly of proteins is collectively called the focal adhesion. Focal adhesions roughly measure ~60 nm in thickness (Franz et al., 2005), and extend out a few square micrometers in the plane of the cell membrane (Figure 11.1). Tension generated through the action of the motor protein myosin as it walks along actin filaments is transmitted through connector proteins like α-actinin to integrins, and hence to the substrate-adsorbed ligands (Choquet et al., 1997; Hall et al., 2000; Kitamura et al., 1999; Wang et al., 1993). This connection between tensed actomyosin filaments (that are crosslinked further into tensed structures called stress fibers, see Figure 11.1) and focal adhesion proteins allows a continuous mechanical link between the inside of the cell and the external substratum. In this manner, the focal adhesion establishes a physical path for mechanical force transfer between the cell and the substratum. Importantly, focal adhesions are not static structures but dynamic multimolecular assemblies that start out as dot-like focal complexes at the leading edge of the motile cell, and eventually mature into focal adhesions (Zaidel-Bar et al., 2004; Zamir et al., 2001; Zimerman et al., 2004).

In addition to acting as locations where cellular tensile forces are in balance with compressive forces in the substrate, focal adhesions are also signaling complexes. For example, integrin ligation can trigger signaling cascades that control gene expression, differentiation, and apoptosis (DeMali et al., 2003). Interfering with the focal adhesion assembly controls the degree of cell spreading, cell shape, as well as cell fate (Huang et al., 1999). In fact, the control of focal adhesion assembly at the nanoscale is a key mechanism by which nanostructured surfaces control cell function.

11.3 Nanoscale Control of Cell–Substrate Adhesion

Evidence that focal adhesion assembly can be directly controlled at the nanometer scale has come from recent studies with gold nanodot arrays (Arnold et al., 2004; Cavalcanti-Adam et al., 2006, 2007; Girard et al., 2007; Huang et al., 2009; Walter et al., 2006). The approach relies on fabricating ordered arrays of nanodots, each with a diameter comparable to the size of a single integrin receptor (integrin receptors are roughly 5.6–7.2 nm in size (Erb et al., 1997) and the nanodots are 5–8 nm in diameter (Arnold et al., 2004). The nanodots are fabricated with diblock copolymer nanolithography, which allows precise control between nanodot spacing. An RGD peptide is conjugated to an organic molecule containing a thiol group that is bonded to the gold nanodot. The areas between the nanodots are passivated with adsorption of the linear poly(ethylene glycol) mPEG2000-urea polymer, which prevents any protein adsorption from serum. Owing to the size of the nanodot (5–8 nm), only one RGD peptide is presented per nanodot, and only one integrin receptor can be conjugated per nanodot. The systematic variation of nanodot spacing at the nanoscale therefore results in a control of the spacing between ligated integrins at the nanoscale.

This model system has been used to understand some key features of cell adhesion at the nanoscale. An important finding is that spacing larger than 70 nm cause a significant decrease in cell adhesion (Arnold et al., 2004). The number of attached osteoblasts on 73 nm nanodots was decreased by 80% compared with that on 28 nm nanodots. The cells were unable to assemble focal adhesions and stress fibers on 73 nm spaced nanodots. The dynamic turnover of focal adhesions was observed to be significantly higher on nanodots with spacing of 108 nm (Cavalcanti-Adam et al., 2007). The levels of the adhesion protein paxillin were found to be significantly decreased, and stress fiber formation and cell adhesion were decreased on the nanodots with spacing of 108 nm. These studies provide clear evidence that nanoscale presentation of ligands alters the focal adhesion assembly. It is hypothesized (Cavalcanti-Adam et al., 2007) that forcing ligated integrins to be more than 70 nm apart potentially prevents cross-linking on the cytoplasmic side and prevents adequate coupling between the actomyosin cytoskeleton and the substrate. This results in decreased adhesive forces on the substrate, a lack of cell spreading, and altered cell signaling.

The nanoscale topography of the surface can also profoundly control cell adhesion and cell migration, a process called contact guidance. The molecular mechanisms of how nanotopographical features alter cell adhesion are less clear. Multiple possibilities exist which are discussed below.

11.3.1 Protein Adsorption on Nanostructures

ECM protein adsorption can be substantially different on nanorough materials compared to smooth materials. Materials which are rough at the nanoscale display large changes in their surface hydrophilicity or hydrophobicity (Martines et al., 2005), which can potentially influence not only the amount of matrix protein adsorption, but also the conformation of the adsorbed protein. Interestingly, nanorough materials exhibit an increase in hydrophilicity if the corresponding smooth material is hydrophilic, and an increase in hydrophobicity if the corresponding smooth material is hydrophobic (Abdelsalam et al., 2005; Lau et al., 2003; Martines et al., 2005; Suh et al., 2005).

Webster et al. (2001) have shown that vitronectin adsorption is significantly enhanced on nanoscale alumina compared to conventional alumina. Vitronectin on nanoscale alumina was observed to be in a more unfolded structure, suggesting that binding motifs in the ligand may be more easily available on nanoscale alumina. The mechanism for increased vitronectin adsorption is less clear, but is attributable either to increased hydrophilicity of nanoscale alumina or increased adsorption of other molecules (such as calcium) that promote vitronectin adsorption (Webster et al., 2001). The adsorption of fibronectin has similarly been shown to increase with increased nanoscale roughness on composites made of carbon nanotubes and poly(carbonate) urethane (PCU) (Khang et al., 2007). The increased adsorption was shown to correlate with increased surface energy of the nanoscale structures. Fibronectin adsorption has also been shown to increase on titanium surfaces with increasing roughness at the nanoscale which is attributable to increased surface energy (Pegueroles et al., 2009).

Increasing hydrophobicity by creating nanorough surfaces has been proposed as an approach to create antifouling protein surfaces (Ainslie et al., 2005; Sun et al., 2005). For example, Fe–Co–Ni metal alloy nanowires are more hydrophobic than the corresponding smooth surface (Ainslie et al., 2005). Bovine serum albumin (BSA) adsorption on these nanowires decreased significantly compared to the flat surface. Superhydrophobic surfaces have also been created by grafting aligned carbon nanotubes with fluorinated PCU (Sun et al., 2005); abnormal platelet adhesion to these structures has been attributed to altered protein adsorption.

While these studies clearly indicate the importance of protein adsorption in cell-nanoscale interactions, considerable amount of work remains to be done for obtaining a clear atomic-level understanding of how protein adsorption is influenced by nanostructure.

11.3.2 Alterations in Focal Adhesion Assembly by Nanoscale Topography

As discussed in Section 11.2, the assembly of focal adhesions and the transfer of intracellular tension to the nanostructured material can be altered by nano-scale presentation of ligand molecules. In a similar manner, nano-scale topography could alter the assembly of focal adhesions. It has been shown, for example, that epithelial cells align parallel along nano-scale ridges of width 70 nm created on silicon substrates (Teixeira et al., 2003). Focal adhesions and stress fibers aligned parallel to the nano-scale ridges and the width of focal adhesions was observed to be controlled by the ridge width (Teixeira et al., 2003). Interestingly,

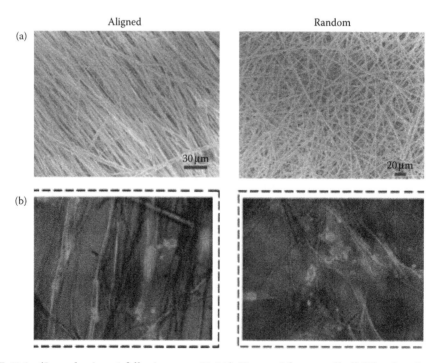

FIGURE 11.2 (See color insert following page 10-24.) Human Schwann cells (hSC) cultured on poly(ε-caprolactone) (PCL) fibers. (a) SEM micrographs of PCL scaffolds for hSC culture. (b) Confocal fluorescent images of hSC on PCL scaffolds. Fluorescent-light images overlay. Green: actin cytosekelton, blue: DAPI. (Modified from Chew, S. Y. et al., 2008. *Biomaterials* 29 (6): 653–61. With permission.)

cell and focal adhesion alignment could be made perpendicular to the nano-scale ridges by changing soluble factors in the culture medium, indicating an interplay between soluble signaling pathways and adhesion assembly at the nano-scale (Teixeira et al., 2006). Similarly, fibroblasts have been shown to align on the surface that presents nano-scale grooves (Loesberg et al., 2007; van Delft et al., 2008). Alignment was observed only when the depth of patterns was over 35 nm and the ridge widths were bigger than 100 nm (Loesberg et al., 2007; van Delft et al., 2008).

Electrospun nanofibers have been examined for creating cell aligning scaffolds (Chew et al., 2008; Lee et al., 2005). Human Schwann cells (hSC) cultured on aligned poly(ε-caprolactone) (PCL) fibers had aligned nuclei and stress fibers along the fiber axes (Figure 11.2a) (Chew et al., 2008). On random PCL fibers, cells were randomly oriented but still aligned along the random fiber axes (Figure 11.2b). Similarly, human ligament fibroblasts have been observed to align along electrospun pellethane (PU) nanofibers (Lee et al., 2005). These results clearly show that nano-scale topography guides cell alignment and elongation.

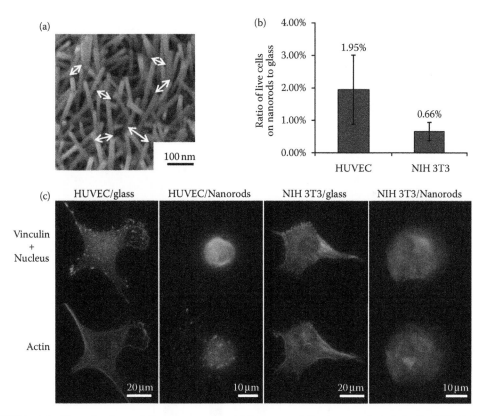

FIGURE 11.3 (See color insert following page 10-24.) Human umbilical vein endothelial cells (HUVEC) and NIH 3T3 fibroblasts cultured on nanorods. (a) Scanning electron microscopy (SEM) image of nanorods on glass. White arrows indicate the spacing between nanorods which ranges from 80 to 100 nm. (b) The ratio of the number of live cells on nanorods to that on glass ($n > 2500$ for HUVECs, $n > 1500$ for NIH 3T3). Cells are considerably reduced in numbers on nanorods. Bar indicates SEM. (c) Fluorescent microscopic images of HUVEC and NIH 3T3 on glass and nanorods. HUVEC and NIH 3T3 on glass assemble focal adhesions stained with vinculin (green) and actin stress fibers (red). Nuclei were stained with DAPI (blue). HUVEC and NIH 3T3 on nanorods are unable to spread and assemble focal adhesions and stress fibers. (Modified from Lee, J. et al., 2009. *Biomaterials* 30 (27): 4488–93. With permission.)

11.4 Nanostructured Surfaces for Antifouling Applications

As changing cell adhesion feeds back to change cell function, nanostructures can be used to guide cell fate (Berry et al., 2005; Washburn et al., 2004; Yim et al., 2007). An important application of tailoring the surface of biomedical implants is preventing mammalian cell adhesion to the implant surface. An example of this is antifouling tumor stents. Tumor stents are used to prevent the collapse of gastrointestinal, pancreatic, and biliary ducts that have tumors surgically removed from them. However, a persistent problem that interferes with normal stent function is the adhesion and growth of tumor cells on the stent surface (Dormann et al., 2004; Togawa et al., 2008). As the stent blockage increases morbidity and mortality in patients, there is a critical need for strategies for preventing tumor cell adhesion to the stent surface. Similarly, preventing macrophage adhesion to titanium surfaces is crucial for the success of bone prosthesis (Refai et al., 2004). Platelet adhesion and subsequent clogging of cardiovascular stents is another problem that needs antifouling materials (Peppas et al., 1994; Sun et al., 2005).

A class of nanostructures that shows promise for reducing mammalian cell adhesion is a surface covered with upright nanoscale cylinders, variously referred to as nanorods, nanoposts, and nanoislands (Choi et al., 2007; Dalby et al., 2005, 2006; Lee et al., 2008, 2009). We have recently reported nanorods as an effective antifouling surface (Lee et al., 2008, 2009). The approach is to crystallize ZnO nanorods onto surfaces at low temperature (~60°C). The advantage of crystallizing nanorods is that the coating can be fabricated on temperature-sensitive materials such as plastic. These nanorods are then coated with a nanothin silicon dioxide (SiO_2) layer to prevent ZnO from leaching into the culture media (Zn ions are known to be toxic to cells) (Brinkman et al., 2008; Lin et al., 2009). As shown in Figure 11.3a, nanorods were 50 nm in diameter, 500 nm in height, and spaced at 80–100 nm spacing. The adhesion and viability of endothelial cells and fibroblasts was significantly decreased on SiO_2-coated nanorods

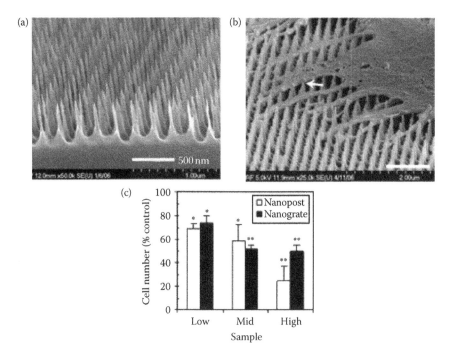

FIGURE 11.4 Human foreskin fibroblasts on nanoposts. (a) SEM images of the 3D sharp-tip nanotopography samples of silicon. (b) Filopodial interactions with 3D sharp-tip nanotopography. The scale bar is 1 μm. (c) Cell numbers are reduced on nanoposts compared to smooth substrates. (Modified from Choi, C. H. et al., 2007. *Biomaterials* 28 (9): 1672–79. With permission.)

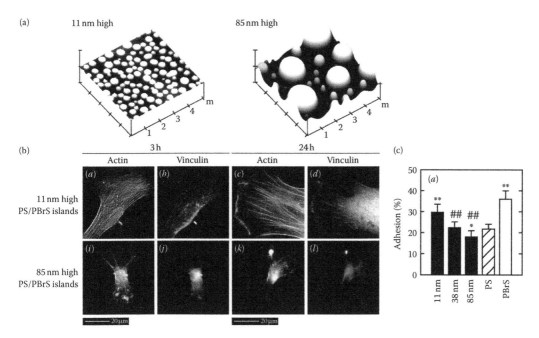

FIGURE 11.5 Human fetal osteoblasts (hFOB) on nanoislands. (a) AFM images of PS/PBrS polymer-demixed nanotopographies with islands of height 11 nm and 85 nm. All images are shown at the same scale (5×5 μm^2 size with z-scale of 150 nm per division). (b) Actin and vinculin double labeled immunofluorescence images of hFOB cells cultured for 3 and 24 h on nanoislands. Distinct actin stress fibers and vinculin plaques are observed on 11 nm high nanoisland surfaces, while more diffuse actin and vinculin is observed on 85 nm nanoislands. (c) hFOB cell adhesion after 3 h of culture on nanoislands. Cell adhesion was greater on surfaces with smaller islands. (Modified from Lim, J. Y. et al., 2005. *J R Soc Interface* 2 (2): 97–108. With permission.)

(Figure 11.3b) with viable cell numbers decreased nearly 50-fold compared to those on the flat glass substrate. Cells were unable to assemble focal adhesion and stress fibers on nanorods (Figure 11.3c). By culturing cells in media that was incubated for up to 7 days with the nanorods, we confirmed that the cell death was not due to toxicity of unknown dissolving material from the nanorods (Lee et al., 2009). Our results suggest that densely packed nanorods have an excellent antifouling potential by virtue of their topology.

On similar lines, a recent paper showed that fibroblast numbers were reduced to approximately 30% on needle-like silicon nanoposts compared to the smooth substrate (Figure 11.4c; see Choi et al., 2007). The nanoposts have sharp tips, 500–600 nm height and less than 10 nm diameter (Figure 11.4a). Cells on nanoposts extended the filopodia structure along the sharp tips (Figure 11.4b), and spread much less than cells on the smooth surface. The authors of this study also suggest that upright nanoposts may be useful as an antifouling surface (Choi et al., 2007).

Other studies have demonstrated that nanoscale island structures can reduce cell adhesion (Dalby et al., 2005, 2006; Lim et al., 2005). These studies showed that the dimension of the nanoisland plays an important role in modulating cell adhesion. The fibroblast spreading area decreased by nearly two-fold as the height of the nanoislands was increased from 10 to 50 nm and the diameter was increased from 31 to 99 nm (Dalby et al., 2003). Focal adhesions were observed to decrease with an increase in the height and diameter of the nanoislands (Lim et al., 2005). Similarly, in osteoblasts, clear stress fibers and focal adhesions were not observed on 85 nm height nanoislands (Figure 11.5a and b). Cell numbers on nanoislands with height 85 nm were reduced by ~67% compared to cells on nanoislands with height 13 nm (Figure 11.5c). Similarly, human endothelial cells on 13 nm height and 31 nm diameter nanoislands had well-spread morphology and well-developed stress fibers compared to islands of 95 nm height and 145 nm diameter (Dalby et al., 2002). Aligned and densely packed carbon nanotubes have also been reported as an excellent antifouling surface toward platelet adhesion (Sun et al., 2005). Few platelets could adhere to fluorinated PCU treated carbon nanotubes (these are superhydrophobic films which potentially interfere with ECM protein adsorption). Moreover, the activation of platelets was decreased by 50% on nanotubes.

The above studies offer strong support to the hypothesis that upright cylindrical structures with nanoscale dimensions can be used to decrease cell adhesion. The mechanisms of how this may occur at the molecular scale are less clear. As discussed before, altered matrix protein adsorption may be an important factor in determining cell response. Other possibilities include the disruption of integrin clustering and lack of focal adhesion assembly, due to interligand spacing that may be larger than 80 nm—this response may be particularly significant for the randomly oriented nanorods which do not allow any flat areas for adhesion owing to their relatively dense structure. Indeed, when the distances between nanowires are on the micron scale, cells can survive and proliferate for over a week (Kim et al., 2007).

11.5 Conclusion

Cells are sensitive to the nanostructure on the surface of the substratum. The mechanisms of how cells sense nanostructure are less clear. ECM ligands on a nanorough material could influence the degree of integrin clustering by virtue of their three-dimensional presentation. This could feedback to regulate cell tension, cell shape, and hence cell fate. Such effects in combination with altered matrix protein conformation or local surface concentration on nanorough materials could alter the adhesion assembly. Parsing out the degree to which these factors influence cell adhesion remains a formidable challenge, but is the key to a clear understanding of cell sensing of nanostructure. Such understanding can greatly promote the rational design of nanostructured biomedical implants for applications such as the development of antifouling stents.

References

Abdelsalam, M. E., P. N. Bartlett, T. Kelf, and J. Baumberg, 2005. Wetting of regularly structured gold surfaces. *Langmuir* 21 (5): 1753–57.

Ainslie, K. M., G. Sharma, M. A. Dyer, C. A. Grimes, and M. V. Pishko, 2005. Attenuation of protein adsorption on static and oscillating magnetostrictive nanowires. *Nano Lett* 5 (9): 1852–6.

Arnold, M., E. A. Cavalcanti-Adam, R. Glass, J. Blummel, W. Eck, M. Kantlehner, H. Kessler, and J. P. Spatz, 2004. Activation of integrin function by nanopatterned adhesive interfaces. *ChemPhysChem* 5 (3): 383–8.

Benzeev, A., S. R. Farmer, and S. Penman, 1980. Protein-synthesis requires cell-surface contact while nuclear events respond to cell-shape in anchorage-dependent fibroblasts. *Cell* 21 (2): 365–72.

Berry, C. C., M. J. Dalby, D. McCloy, and S. Affrossman, 2005. The fibroblast response to tubes exhibiting internal nanotopography. *Biomaterials* 26 (24): 4985–92.

Brinkman, S. F., and W. D. Johnston, 2008. Acute toxicity of aqueous copper, cadmium, and zinc to the mayfly. *Rhithrogena Hageni. Arch Environ Contam Toxicol* 54 (3): 466–72.

Brown, M. C., and C. E. Turner, 2004. Paxillin: Adapting to change. *Physiol Rev* 84 (4): 1315–39.

Burridge, K., M. ChrzanowskaWodnicka, and C. L. Zhong, 1997. Focal adhesion assembly. *Trends Cell Biol* 7 (9): 342–47.

Cavalcanti-Adam, E. A., A. Micoulet, J. Blummel, J. Auernheimer, H. Kessler, and J. P. Spatz, 2006. Lateral spacing of integrin ligands influences cell spreading and focal adhesion assembly. *Eur. J Cell Biol* 85 (3–4): 219–24.

Cavalcanti-Adam, E. A., T. Volberg, A. Micoulet, H. Kessler, B. Geiger, and J. P. Spatz, 2007. Cell spreading and focal adhesion dynamics are regulated by spacing of integrin ligands. *Biophys J* 92 (8): 2964–74.

Chen, C. S., M. Mrksich, S. Huang, G. M. Whitesides, and D. E. Ingber, 1997. Geometric control of cell life and death. *Science* 276 (5317): 1425–8.

Chew, S. Y., R. Mi, A. Hoke, and K. W. Leong, 2008. The effect of the alignment of electrospun fibrous scaffolds on Schwann cell maturation. *Biomaterials* 29 (6): 653–61.

Choi, C. H., S. H. Hagvall, B. M. Wu, J. C. Y, 2007. Dunn, R. E. Beygui, and C. J. Kim. Cell interaction with three-dimensional sharp-tip nanotopography. *Biomaterials* 28 (9): 1672–79.

Choquet, D., D. P. Felsenfeld, and M. P. Sheetz, 1997. Extracellular matrix rigidity causes strengthening of integrin-cytoskeleton linkages. *Cell* 88 (1): 39–48.

Clark, P., P. Connolly, A. S. Curtis, J. A. Dow, and C. D. Wilkinson, 1990. Topographical control of cell behaviour: Ii. Multiple grooved substrata. *Development* 108 (4): 635–44.

Dalby, M. J., N. Gadegaard, and C. D. Wilkinson, 2008. The response of fibroblasts to hexagonal nano-topography fabricated by electron beam lithography. *J Biomed Mater Res A* 84 (4): 973–9.

Dalby, M. J., D. McCloy, M. Robertson, H. Agheli, D. Sutherland, S. Affrossman, and R. O. Oreffo, 2006. Osteoprogenitor response to emi-ordered and random nanotopographies. *Biomaterials* 27 (15): 2980–7.

Dalby, M. J., M. O. Riehle, H. Johnstone, S. Affrossman, and A. S. Curtis, 2002. In vitro reaction of endothelial cells to polymer demixed nanotopography. *Biomaterials* 23 (14): 2945–54.

Dalby, M. J., M. O. Riehle, H. J. Johnstone, S. Affrossman, and A. S. Curtis, 2003. Nonadhesive nanotopography: Fibroblast response to poly(N-butyl methacrylate)-poly(styrene) demixed surface features. *J Biomed Mater Res A* 67 (3): 1025–32.

Dalby, M. J., M. O. Riehle, D. S. Sutherland, H. Agheli, and A. S. Curtis, 2005. Morphological and microarray analysis of human fibroblasts cultured on nanocolumns produced by colloidal lithography. *Eur Cell Mater* 9: 1–8; discussion 8.

DeMali, K. A., K. Wennerberg, and K. Burridge, 2003. Integrin signaling to the actin cytoskeleton. *Curr Opin Cell Biol* 15 (5): 572–82.

Dormann, A., S. Meisner, N. Verin, and A. W. Lang, 2004. Self-expanding metal stents for gastroduodenal malignancies: Systematic review of their clinical effectiveness. *Endoscopy* 36 (6): 543–50.

Erb, E. M., K. Tangemann, B. Bohrmann, B. Muller, and J. Engel, 1997. Integrin alphaiib beta3 reconstituted into lipid bilayers is nonclustered in its activated state but clusters after fibrinogen binding. *Biochemistry* 36 (24): 7395–402.

Flemming, R. G., C. J. Murphy, G. A. Abrams, S. L. Goodman, and P. F. Nealey, 1999. Effects of synthetic micro- and nano-structured surfaces on cell behavior. *Biomaterials* 20 (6): 573–88.

Franz, C. M., and D. J. Muller, 2005. Analyzing focal adhesion structure by atomic force microscopy. *J Cell Sci* 118 (Pt 22): 5315–23.

Giancotti, F. G., and E. Ruoslahti, 1999. Transduction—integrin signaling. *Science* 285 (5430): 1028–32.

Girard, P. P., E. A. Cavalcanti-Adam, R. Kemkemer, and J. P. Spatz, 2007. Cellular chemomechanics at interfaces: Sensing, integration and response. *Soft Matter* 3 (3): 307–26.

Hall, A., and C. D. Nobes, 2000. Rho Gtpases: Molecular switches that control the organization and dynamics of the actin cytoskeleton. *Philos Trans R Soc B—Biol Sci* 355 (1399): 965–70.

Huang, J. H., S. V. Grater, F. Corbellinl, S. Rinck, E. Bock, R. Kemkemer, H. Kessler, J. D. Ding, and J. P. Spatz, 2009. Impact of order and disorder in Rgd nanopatterns on cell adhesion. *Nano Letters* 9 (3): 1111–16.

Huang, S., and D. E. Ingber, 1999. The structural and mechanical complexity of cell-growth control. *Nat Cell Biol* 1 (5): E131–8.

Hynes, R. O, 1992. Integrins—versatility, modulation, and signaling in cell-adhesion. *Cell* 69 (1): 11–25.

Hynes, R. O, 2002. Integrins: Bidirectional, allosteric signaling machines. *Cell* 110 (6): 673–87.

Ingber, D. E, 2006. Cellular mechanotransduction: Putting all the pieces together again. *FASEB J* 20 (7): 811–27.

Ingber, D. E, 1990. Fibronectin controls capillary endothelial cell growth by modulating cell shape. *Proc Natl Acad Sci USA* 87 (9) : 3579–83.

Khang, D., S. Y. Kim, P. Liu-Snyder, G. T. Palmore, S. M. Durbin, and T. J. Webster, 2007. Enhanced fibronectin adsorption on carbon nanotube/poly(carbonate) urethane: Independent role of surface nano-roughness and associated surface energy. *Biomaterials* 28 (32): 4756–68.

Kim, W., J. K. Ng, M. E. Kunitake, B. R. Conklin, and P. Yang, 2007. Interfacing silicon nanowires with mammalian cells. *J Am Chem Soc* 129 (23): 7228–9.

Kitamura, K., M. Tokunaga, A. H. Iwane, and T. Yanagida, 1999. A single myosin head moves along an actin filament with regular steps of 5.3 nanometres. *Nature* 397 (6715) : 129–34.

Lau, K. K. S., J. Bico, K. B. K. Teo, M. Chhowalla, G. A. J. Amaratunga, W. I. Milne, G. H. McKinley, and K. K. Gleason, 2003. Superhydrophobic carbon nanotube forests. *Nano Letters* 3 (12): 1701–05.

Lee, C. H., H. J. Shin, I. H. Cho, Y. M. Kang, I. A. Kim, K. D. Park, and J. W. Shin, 2005. Nanofiber alignment and direction of mechanical strain affect the ECM production of human ACL fibroblast. *Biomaterials* 26 (11): 1261–70.

Lee, J., B. H. Chu, K. H. Chen, F. Ren, and T. P. Lele, 2009. Randomly oriented, upright SiO2 coated nanorods for reduced adhesion of mammalian cells. *Biomaterials* 30 (27): 4488–93.

Lee, J., B. S. Kang, B. Hicks, T. F. Chancellor, Jr., B. H. Chu, H. T. Wang, B. G. Keselowsky, F. Ren, and T. P. Lele, 2008. The control of cell adhesion and viability by zinc oxide nanorods. *Biomaterials* 29 (27): 3743–9.

Liliensiek, S. J., S. Campbell, P. F. Nealey, and C. J. Murphy, 2006. The scale of substratum topographic features modulates proliferation of corneal epithelial cells and corneal fibroblasts. *J Biomed Mater Res A* 79 (1): 185–92.

Lim, J. Y., J. C. Hansen, C. A. Siedlecki, J. Runt, and H. J. Donahue, 2005. Human foetal osteoblastic cell response to polymer-demixed nanotopographic interfaces. *J R Soc Interface* 2 (2): 97–108.

Lin, W. S., Y. Xu, C. C. Huang, Y. F. Ma, K. B. Shannon, D. R. Chen, and Y. W. Huang, 2009. Toxicity of nano- and micro-sized Zno particles in human lung epithelial cells. *J Nanoparticle Res* 11 (1): 25–39.

Lo, C. M., H. B. Wang, M. Dembo, and Y. L. Wang, 2000. Cell movement is guided by the rigidity of the substrate. *Biophys J* 79 (1): 144–52.

Loesberg, W. A., J. te Riet, F. C. M. J. M. van Delft, P. Schon, C. G. Figdor, S. Speller, J. J. W. A. van Loon, X. F. Walboomers, and J. A. Jansen, 2007. The threshold at which substrate nanogroove dimensions may influence fibroblast alignment and adhesion. *Biomaterials* 28 (27): 3944–51.

Luo, B. H., C. V. Carman, and T. A. Springer. Structural basis of integrin regulation and signaling. *Annu Rev Immunol* 25 (2007): 619–47.

Martines, E., K. Seunarine, H. Morgan, N. Gadegaard, C. D. W, 2005. Wilkinson, and M. O. Riehle. Superhydrophobicity and superhydrophilicity of regular nanopatterns. *Nano Letters* 5 (10): 2097–103.

Nayal, A., D. J. Webb, and A. F. Horwitz, 2004. Talin: An emerging focal point of adhesion dynamics. *Curr Opin Cell Biol* 16 (1): 94–8.

Otey, C. A., and O. Carpen, 2004. Alpha-actinin revisited: A fresh look at an old player. *Cell Motil Cytoskeleton* 58 (2): 104–11.

Pegueroles, M., C. Aparicio, M. Bosio, E. Engel, F. J. Gil, J. A. Planell, and G. Altankov, 2010. Spatial organization of osteoblast fibronectin matrix on titanium surfaces: Effects of roughness, chemical heterogeneity and surface energy. *Acta Biomater* 6 (1): 281-301.

Peppas, N. A., and R. Langer, 1994. New challenges in biomaterials. *Science* 263 (5154): 1715–20.

Re, F., A. Zanetti, M. Sironi, N. Polentarutti, L. Lanfrancone, E. Dejana, and F. Colotta, 1994. Inhibition of anchorage-dependent cell spreading triggers apoptosis in cultured human endothelial cells. *J Cell Biol* 127 (2): 537–46.

Refai, A. K., M. Textor, D. M. Brunette, and J. D. Waterfield, 2004. Effect of titanium surface topography on macrophage activation and secretion of proinflammatory cytokines and chemokines. *J Biomed Mater Res A* 70 (2): 194–205.

Schlaepfer, D. D., S. K. Hanks, T. Hunter, and P. van der Geer, 1994. Integrin-mediated signal transduction linked to Ras pathway by Grb2 binding to focal adhesion kinase. *Nature* 372 (6508): 786–91.

Schnell, E., K. Klinkhammer, S. Balzer, G. Brook, D. Klee, P. Dalton, and J. Mey, 2007. Guidance of glial cell. Migration and axonal growth on electrospun nanofibers of poly-epsilon-caprolactone and a collagen/poly-epsilon-caprolactone blend. *Biomaterials* 28 (19): 3012–25.

Sniadecki, N. J., R. A. Desai, S. A. Ruiz, and C. S. Chen, 2006. Nanotechnology for cell–substrate interactions. *Ann Biomed Eng* 34 (1): 59–74.

Stevens, M. M., and J. H. George, 2005. Exploring and engineering the cell surface interface. *Science* 310 (5751): 1135–8.

Suh, K. Y., and S. Jon, 2005. Control over wettability of polyethylene glycol surfaces using capillary lithography. *Langmuir* 21 (15): 6836–41.

Sun, T., H. Tan, D. Han, Q. Fu, and L. Jiang, 2005. No platelet can adhere–largely improved blood compatibility on nanostructured superhydrophobic surfaces. *Small* 1 (10): 959–63.

Teixeira, A. I., G. A. Abrams, P. J. Bertics, C. J. Murphy, and P. F. Nealey, 2003. Epithelial contact guidance on well-defined micro- and nanostructured substrates. *J Cell Sci* 116 (10): 1881–92.

Teixeira, A. I., G. A. McKie, J. D. Foley, P. J. Bertics, P. F. Nealey, and C. J. Murphy, 2006. The effect of environmental factors on the response of human corneal epithelial cells to nanoscale substrate topography. *Biomaterials* 27 (21): 3945–54.

Togawa, O., T. Kawabe, H. Isayama, Y. Nakai, T. Sasaki, T. Arizumi, S. Matsubara, et al., 2008. Management of occluded uncovered metallic stents in patients with malignant distal biliary obstructions using covered metallic stents. *Journal of Clinical Gastroenterology* 42 (5): 546–49.

Vakonakis, I., and I. D. Campbell, 2007. Extracellular matrix: From atomic resolution to ultrastructure. *Curr Opin Cell Biol* 19 (5): 578–83.

van Delft, F. C. M. J., F. C. van den Heuvel, W. A. Loesberg, J. te Riet, P. Schon, C. G. Figdor, S. Speller, J. J. W. A. van Loon, X. F. Walboomers, and J. A. Jansen, 2008. Manufacturing substrate nano-grooves for studying cell alignment and adhesion. *Microelectronic Engineering* 85 (5–6): 1362–66.

Walter, N., C. Selhuber, H. Kessler, and J. P. Spatz, 2006. Cellular unbinding forces of initial adhesion processes on nanopatterned surfaces probed with magnetic tweezers. *Nano Letters* 6 (3): 398–402.

Wang, N., J. P. Butler, and D. E. Ingber, 1993. Mechanotransduction across the cell surface and through the cytoskeleton. *Science* 260 (5111): 1124–7.

Washburn, N. R., K. M. Yamada, C. G. Simon, Jr., S. B. Kennedy, and E. J. Amis, 2004. High-throughput investigation of osteoblast response to polymer crystallinity: Influence of nanometer-scale roughness on proliferation. *Biomaterials* 25 (7–8): 1215–24.

Webster, T. J., C. Ergun, R. H. Doremus, R. W. Siegel, and R. Bizios, 2000. Specific proteins mediate enhanced osteoblast adhesion on nanophase ceramics. *J Biomed Mater Res* 51 (3): 475–83.

Webster, T. J., L. S. Schadler, R. W. Siegel, and R. Bizios, 2001. Mechanisms of enhanced osteoblast adhesion on nanophase alumina involve vitronectin. *Tissue Eng* 7 (3): 291–301.

Yim, E. K., S. W. Pang, and K. W. Leong, 2007. Synthetic nanostructures inducing differentiation of human mesenchymal stem cells into neuronal lineage. *Exp Cell Res* 313 (9): 1820–9.

Yim, E. K., R. M. Reano, S. W. Pang, A. F. Yee, C. S. Chen, and K. W. Leong, 2005. Nanopattern-induced changes in morphology and motility of smooth muscle cells. *Biomaterials* 26 (26): 5405–13.

Zaidel-Bar, R., M. Cohen, L. Addadi, and B. Geiger, 2004. Hierarchical assembly of cell–matrix adhesion complexes. *Biochem Soc Trans* 32 (Pt 3): 416–20.

Zamir, E., and B. Geiger, 2001. Molecular complexity and dynamics of cell–matrix adhesions. *J Cell Sci* 114 (Pt 20): 3583–90.

Zhang, L., Y. Chen, J. Rodriguez, H. Fenniri, and T. J. Webster, 2008. Biomimetic helical rosette nanotubes and nanocrystalline hydroxyapatite coatings on titanium for improving orthopedic implants. *Int J Nanomedicine* 3 (3): 323–33.

Zimerman, B., T. Volberg, and B. Geiger, 2004. Early molecular events in the assembly of the focal adhesion-stress fiber complex during fibroblast spreading. *Cell Motil Cytoskeleton* 58 (3): 143–59.

12

Nanofibrous Materials for Vascular Tissue Engineering and Regeneration

Wei Tan
University of Colorado at Boulder

Walter Bonani
University of Colorado at Boulder

Krishna Madhavan
University of Colorado at Boulder

12.1 Needs for Biodegradable Nanofibrous Vascular Graft Implants

For almost half a century, synthetic vascular grafts have been an integral tool of vascular surgery. Although impressive success of these grafts has been made in aortic and iliac surgery, smaller diameter (≤6 mm) grafts has been a symbol for the limitations of modern biotechnology, because their long-term failure rates are still high. Small-diameter vascular grafts are used as medical implants for a number of diseases. Some examples of graft implants are coronary or periphery artery bypass grafts, pediatric vascular shunts, and vascular access grafts.

The most common causes for the poor performance of small-diameter grafts are surface thrombogenicity and intimal hyperplasia (IH). Thrombogenicity and IH are mainly mediated by the denude of endothelium and lack of control over cell growth, respectively. The exposition of a bare graft surface to blood flow results rapidly in a deposition of blood proteins on the luminal surface, activating platelets and leading to thrombus formation via the intrinsic coagulation pathway and ultimately to vessel occlusion. Also, activated platelets secrete molecules such as platelet-derived growth factor (PDGF) which is responsible for the proliferation and migration of smooth muscle cells (SMC) from the media into the intima leading to IH. IH narrows the vessel lumen decreasing blood flow to the point that it may in turn promote local thrombosis. Intima hyperplasia can also be induced by flow turbulence at the graft–vessel junction, due to the mismatched mechanical compliance between the graft. Zilla et al. have provided insightful reviews on the problems caused by contemporary grafting materials and underlying mechanisms. It is generally agreed that efforts to improve the graft should be made on the formation of physiological vascular tissues including functional endothelium, smooth muscle, and connective layers around the vascular graft. The tissue structure ensure mimetic ensure mimetic biological and mechanical functioning of the graft and allow it to be better integrated with native blood vessels.

Before discussing the development of new materials, it seems paramount to understand the limitations in the contemporary grafting materials. The materials and structures of contemporary grafts, made of polytetrafluoroethylene (PTFE), Dacron and polyurethane (PU), provide limited capability of endothelium regeneration and tissue ingrowth. Currently, the PTFE grafts occupy the majority of the vascular graft market, due to better clinical performances. The PTFE grafts are characterized by a typical node-and-fiber structure consisting of circumferentially aligned, irregular-shaped solid membranes (called "nodes"), and a dense meshwork of microfibrils stretching between the nodes. High porosity PTFE grafts with continual interfibrillar space allows tissue ingrowth and transmural capillarization, and have been quite successful in the replacement of blood vessels. Different from the structure of PTFE grafts, Dacron grafts consist of polyester fibers, which are bundled into multifilament yarns that are either woven or knitted into a fabric. This rigid structure limits liquid permeation and capillary penetration. Lack of good tissue ingrowth and regeneration in the grafts makes grafts more prone to ongoing thrombogenity and intima hyperplasia. For instance, 2 weeks after implantation, the fibrin layer developed on both PTFE and Dacron grafts. PTFE grafts had a thickness of the surface thrombus about 10–20 μm, 1/8 to 1/4 of that on Dacron grafts. PU grafts, less-often used grafts, have either a fibrillar or foamy structure. They have the advantage of being more elastic than PTFE and Dacron, but the limited tissue ingrowth in PU grafts have been found even though many efforts have been made to increase the porosity.

During the past few decades, many efforts have been made to improve the performance of vascular grafts mainly through the attempts that modify the structure and surface of the contemporary graft materials. These attempts include: (1) increasing structural porosity; (2) increasing mechanical compliance; (3) pre-endothelialization; and (4) incorporating antithrombotic molecules on the surface. Impressive advancement on these synthetic vascular grafts has been made to improve graft patency. However, as commented by Zilla et al., these graft materials have structure-related limitations to regenerating vascular tissue both on the surface and in the transmural space. For example, structural porosity is often ranked above material properties for synthetic grafts research and has been significantly altered in the grafting materials to increase the ingrowth of tissues and capillaries, but till now, biologically and mechanically functional smooth muscle or connective tissues are not yet capable of regeneration in the grafts. The nondegradable nature of the materials restricts the remodeling and regeneration capability of media and adventitia. Another example is the attempt to modify the graft surface with protein lining, heparin incorporation, or polymer surface chemistry, which reduces thrombosis and IH but does little to improve long-term patency of small arterial grafts. Lack of confluent, functional endothelium in most part of the grafts is still observed and attributed to the ongoing thrombogenity.

Considering the important role that physiological tissue formation on or around the grafts plays in the long-term patency of small-diameter vascular grafts, a more recent research thrust is to develop various tissue engineering approaches which allow tissue formation to spontaneously occur *in vitro* or *in vivo* and eventually replace the grafts. These approaches, in particular approaches using biodegradable nanofibrous materials, would potentially make significant inroads in the future vascular implants.

Recent developments in nanofiber fabrication technology provide tremendous opportunities to improve vascular implant performances, because diverse fabrication methods and functionalization strategies allow one to design optimal material properties and environments for desired short-term and long-term performances that meet the needs of a specific treatment. Specifically, nanofiber scaffolding materials offer a number of advantages for vascular grafting applications. First, the nanofibers mimic the nanostructure of the extracellular matrix (ECM) of natural tissues. Cells live in a nanofeatured ECM environment. They attach and organize better around fibers with diameters much smaller than the cell diameter (>5 μm). It is found that nanometric surface topography with a high surface area-to-volume ratio attracts more endothelial cells (EC) and promotes their growth, thus, accelerating the reformation of an endothelium to prohibit thrombosis of the artery. Second, controllable porosity and interconnected pores together with biodegradable property allow the materials to have large and ever increasing space for SMCs to grow, migrate, and fulfil regeneration and for better integration of the host tissue in the long-term run. Third, the surface chemistry of nanofibers can easily be modified. Due to the large surface-volume ratio, the functional molecules integrated on the surface can better guide cell remodeling and tissue regeneration. Fourth, new fabrication approaches have been developed to impregnate DNA, drugs, growth factors, or other bioactive molecules in the nanofibers and slowly release from the nanofibrous scaffolds for local delivery; thus, signaling molecules that provide appropriate spatiotemporal cues to cells may be precisely programmed for the long-term performance. Finally, with the developed nanomanufacturing and composite engineering approaches, it is possible to tune mechanical compliance, material degradation, and surface properties to the needs of tissue regeneration.

12.2 Fabrication Techniques to Produce Nanofibrous Vascular Grafts

Nanofibrous materials are materials composed of high-aspect-ratio nanofibers with diameter in nanoscale (1–100 nm) and length in microscale (1–100 μm). They can be made from synthetic polymer or natural-derived polymer. A variety of synthetic degradable polymer nanofibers, including poly(ε-caprolactone) (PCL), poly(lactic acid) (PLA), poly(glycolic acid) (PGA), and poly(lactic-*co*-glycolic acid) (PLGA) and poly(ethylene) oxide (PEO), have been explored for vascular application. Naturally derived materials are often structural proteins derived from the ECM of natural tissues, or biopolymers from insects or shellfish such as silk-fibroin and chitosan. The last decade has seen great development in nanofiber fabrication techniques for biomedical applications, particularly tissue engineering and drug delivery. Table 12.1 has listed comparisons among some fabrication techniques including electrospinning, self-assembly, phase separation, template synthesis, and drawing. Besides these general techniques, ECM-based nanofibrous materials for vascular grafts can be obtained by decellularizing vascular tissues or inducing vascular cells to produce and build up the materials *in vitro*.

12.2.1 Fabrication Techniques for Nanofibrous Materials

12.2.1.1 Electrospinning

Electrospinning is the most widely used method to generate nanofibers. The electrospinning process can be manipulated by a number of variables for the desired morphology and property of nanofibers. These variables include solution characteristics, process variables, and environmental parameters. Polymer solution characteristics, such as polymer molecular weight, concentration, solution viscosity, solution charge density, conductivity, dielectric constant, and surface tension, are often difficult to isolate, since varying one generally affect the others. Process or system variables include flow-rate, field voltage, distance between the tip and collector, needle tip design and placement, and collector composition and geometry. Environmental parameters, such as environmental temperature, humidity, and atmosphere, are as important but less often explored. A general understanding of these parameters, allows one to set up a process to produce defect-free fibers with controllable nanofiber morphology. When electrospinning parameters are optimized, the obtained fiber diameters should have a narrow

TABLE 12.1   Comparisons among Different Nanofiber Techniques

Technique	Diameter of Nanofibers	Advantages	Disadvantages
Electrospinning	3 nm to several micrometers	Easy and inexpensive setup Flexibility of the process for a variety of materials for various compositions, topographies, fiber diameters, and alignment	Porosity of the net is usually too small for a large number of cells to invade and regenerate the tissue Difficult to reproduce some conditions and thus results can vary considerably in different environments
		Yield continuous nanofibers with interconnected pores	
		Relatively easy to scale from lab to industrial production	
		Nanofibers can be designed to have slow release of biomolecules and be versatile in controlling the release	
Self-assembly	A few to a hundred nanometer	Self-assembly process is mild and thus can incorporate cells during the process	Self-assembled materials are often mechanically weak
		Multifunctional peptide sequences can be incorporated into the artificial peptide	An extremely elaborate technique with low productivity
			Slow process
Phase separation	50–500 nm	Relatively simple procedure and the requirements for the equipment are not high	Long fabrication time
		Produce microporous foams	
		The simultaneous presence of nano- and macro-architecture can be beneficial in terms of cell response at the nanofiber level, and in terms of cell distribution and tissue architecture at the macroporosity level	
Template synthesis	A few to hundred nanometer	Suitable for surface modifications of biomaterials	Do not result in continuous fibers
Drawing	A few nanometer to micrometers	Simple and easy to setup	Only using viscoelastic materials that can withstand applied stresses can be used. This limits its application

distribution. Also, the porosity of electrospun materials can be altered by changing the void spaces lying between the fibers through varying the mean fiber diameter, the diameter distribution, and the degree of fiber packing. Electrospun nanofiber matrices are characterized by ultrafine continuous fibers, interconnected pores, high porosity, and variable pore-size distribution similar to the dimensions of basement membranes. Those matrices present a dynamic system in which the pore size and shape can change when compared to other rigid porous structures. Detailed information regarding fiber fabrication and parameter control is given by two books *Polymeric Nanofibers* edited by Reneker and Fong and *Science and Technology of Polymeric Nanofibers* by Anthony L. Andrady, and detailed reviews on the topic of electrospinning for tissue engineering are given by several groups.

Electrospinning of synthetic fibers and protein fibers have been demonstrated for vascular applications. Electrospun synthetic polymers such as PCL and PLGA have successfully been applied to engineer vascular tissues. Electrospinning of natural-derived biopolymers such as collagen, elastin, silk fibroin, chitosan, and fibrinogen have also been developed for vascular engineering. In particular, elastin and its derived molecules are believed to be an integral part of vascular grafting materials, due to their elasticity and significant biological functions. Elastin, tropoelastin, elastin peptides, or elastic-mimetic proteins have been electrospun alone or together with other biological or synthetic polymers.

A particularly interesting and promising area of electrospinning is creating composite scaffolds with mixed nanofibers or with a blended composition of polymers in the nanofiber. The benefit of scaffolds formed with a combination of different polymers is in the possibility of synergizing the favorable characteristics of each individual component to obtain a composite with superior mechanical and/or biological properties required for vascular grafts. Nanofibers with different physical or biological properties, such as hydrophobic/hydrophilic fibers, fibers with different degradation rates, and synthetic/biological fibers, can be combined to form hybrid fibers with desired properties. The hydrophilic/hydrophobic characteristic is a critical factor that affects protein adhesion thus influencing blot clotting formation and cell adhesion. It also affects biomolecule release and mechanical properties. Therefore, a composite made of hydrophobic and hydrophilic polymers can combine superior mechanical properties, better hydrolytic resistance, and better thrombo-resistance which hydrophobic polymers provide with higher molecule incorporation potential provided by hydrophilic polymers. Using fiber composites with a polymer that degrades faster than the other can increase the porosity for tissue ingrowth. This was shown with the spinning of PCL and gelatin solutions. Recent studies have also shown the increasing use of a blend of natural and synthetic polymers to form a biohybrid scaffold. Synthetic biodegradable polymers often are stronger than natural-derived polymers, while biopolymers are more compatible *in vivo* and rich in biological signals. A blend of a synthetic polymer PLGA, gelatin, and α-elastin was electrospun to obtain a solid–gel multicomponent material, with the synthetic polymer acting as a solid fibrous backbone and a protein cross-linked gel acting as a promoter for cell adhesion and growth. As a result, different cells simultaneously attached, migrated, and proliferated within the multicomponent scaffolds. Huang et al., demonstrated a great combination of biological and mechanical properties presented by the collagen/PEO electrospun nanofibers; the mechanical strength of the nanofiber system was significantly increased, due to a high number of intermolecular interactions. Zhang et al., developed gelatin/PCL composite fibrous scaffolds which improved the mechanical strength and wettability and promoted cell attachment, growth, and migration.

There are two general approaches to fabricate electrospun nanofiber composites with mixed nanofibers. By sequentially spinning different polymer solutions, a scaffold with layers can be created. Boland et al. have demonstrated a multilayered scaffold of collagen type-I and type-III and elastin, and they showed SMC infiltration into the scaffold when cultured in a rotary culture system. Yarin et al. developed PLA/PCL bilayer tubular scaffolds which have concentric outer layers of circumferentially oriented PLA fibers analogous to the tunica media layer and concentric inner layers of randomly oriented PCL fibers representing the elastic lamina and tunica intima layers. The bilayer scaffolds were strong and compliant necessary for vessel substitutes, and promoted cell attachment, spreading, and proliferation. Alternatively, two or more polymer solutions can be spun concurrently, resulting in a scaffold with mixed types of fibers. This approach has been used to fabricate hydrophobic/hydrophilic mixed nanofibers.

12.2.1.2 Molecular Self-Assembly

Self-assembly is a process in which molecular components are spontaneously organized into ordered patterns or stable structures of greater complexity under thermodynamical equilibrium conditions, through weak noncovalent bonds such as hydrogen bond, ionic bonds, Van der Waals forces, and/or hydrophobic interactions. The self-assembly strategy is widely used in native tissues for the development of complex and multifunctional structures. Many unique performances of natural materials emerge from a precise hierarchical self-assembled organization. Collagen, elastin, and fibrin fibers provide natural examples of self-assembly. The collagen molecule (tropo-collagen) consists of three peptide chains which self-assemble into a triple-helical structure. Also electrostatic and hydrophobic interactions between tropo-collagen molecules further assemble the triple-helixes into microfibrils. Collagen fibrils can also be reconstituted *in vitro* by self-assembly with proper pH, temperature, and ion strength. Self-assembly into nanofibers is also well known to elastin, and was observed *in vitro* with tropoelastin, tropoelastin fragments, and synthetic elastin block polymers. Upon heating, these molecules coacervate due to hydrophobic interactions. Fibrin gel, self-assembled *in vitro* from the mixture of thrombin and fibrinogen, is yet another type of natural material that has been used extensively in vascular tissue engineering.

Another nanofiber fabrication method, a synthetic peptide-amphiphile (PA) self-assembly system was first developed by Berndt et al. who were able to produce thermally stable protein structures based on the mimetic PA system. The PA consisted of two parts; a hydrophobic dialkyl chain and a hydrophilic N-α amino group peptide chain. The peptide chain was derived from the ECM collagen ligand sequence. The thermal stability of the PAs was later improved by Yu et al. who used an alkyl chain with up to 16 carbon-atoms instead of a dialkyl chain. Yu et al. also demonstrated the formation of 3D triple helix from the new PAs, a structure similar to natural ECM. The PAs can also assemble themselves into nanofibrous scaffolds by forming micelles, vesicles, or tubules. More recently, Stupp et al. designed di- and tri-block PAs that self-assembled into a rod-like architecture. They also introduced different methods such as pH control, drying-on surface or divalent ion to induce the self-assembly process.

As self-assembly is based on noncovalent bonds formed by highly defined polypeptides or proteins with a propensity to self-aggregate, it results in mechanically weak biomaterials. Thus, it is not suitable to fabricate supporting materials directly used for *in vivo* regeneration without cross-linking. Often, self-assembly is used to obtain surface coatings for biomaterials to improve biocompatibility. More often, it is used for *in vitro* regeneration. Self-assembled nanofibers provide cells with a 3D hydrated environment which mimics *in vivo* environments. Also, as self-assembly can spontaneously occur in mild conditions, cells can be incorporated during the self-assembly. Of particular interest are the cell-driven remodeling events *in vitro* that result in the requisite structure and mechanical properties needed for proper function *in vitro*.

A particularly interesting and promising characteristic of self-assembled materials is the possibility of increasing specific biological activity to enhance biomaterial function. Molecular self-assembly provides an innovative way to design and produce novel materials, as it provides the basis for important manufacturing techniques at multiple levels (nano–micro–macro). One promising generation of biomaterials is to mimic the structure and characteristics of native ECM, such as fibrillar structure, viscoelasticity, cell adhesion domains, growth factor binding, and proteolytic sensitivity. Such materials are attractive because, in principle, their properties can be readily controlled while mimicking many of the critical biological functions of the native ECM, which are largely lacking from synthetic polymers. As the native ECM, specifically designed materials may eventually exhibit great hierarchical complexity and multifunctionality.

12.2.1.3 Phase Separation

Ma and Zhang have demonstrated a couple of phase separation methods which can be used to fabricate synthetic nanofibers. One of the methods involves multiple steps, including dissolution of the polymer, liquid–liquid phase separation, polymer gelation at low temperature, solvent extraction, freezing, and freeze-drying under vacuum. Another method involved thermally induced 3D network formation at high temperature with macroporosity generators using porogens like sugar and salt, followed by thermal-phase separation and removal of porogens with water. Both methods have produced highly porous materials. The porous morphology of the nanofibrous foams is dependent on the gelation temperature, polymer concentration, thermal annealing temperature, solvent extraction, and freezing temperatures. Woo et al., demonstrated that a synthetic ECM made with phase-separated nanofibers improved cell adhesion and protein adsorption, particularly fibronectin and collagen, because of the high porosity of the 3D network in the macroscale and microscale.

12.2.1.4 Template Synthesis

Template synthesis uses a template to synthesize nanofibers. An aluminum oxide membrane is used as a template to fabricate aligned polyacrylonitrile fibers. A solution of the polymer is forced through the membrane with the cylindrical column for nanofiber synthesis, using the pressure developed by a column of water above the polymer solution. Once the nanofibers come out of the cylindrical channels inside the membrane, they are passed through a solidification solution. The diameter of fibers can be controlled by varying the diameter of the cylindrical channels inside the membrane. More recently, aligned arrays of biodegradable PCL nanofibers and nanowires have been fabricated by the template synthesis method. The method is potentially useful in the preparation of scaffolds with highly porous surface for tissue engineering implants.

12.2.1.5 Drawing

Nain et al., showed that nanofibers can be drawn from a droplet using a micropipette tip. The polymer solution is drawn into a micropipette, which is followed by moving the substrate to come in contact with the polymer droplet at the end of the micropipette. Then, the micropipette stage is moved vertically at a constant speed and stopped at a predetermined height. Subsequently, the stage is moved at a constant speed drawing a nanofiber which is formed due to the evaporation of the solvent. Finally, the droplet is released onto the substrate forming nanofibers in-between two drops of the polymer. The authors also developed another drawing method to fabricate nanofibers. The method used the indenter probe in an atomic force microscope to draw fibers out of the polymer droplets placed on the substrate.

12.2.2 Techniques to Acquire Extracellular Matrix (ECM) Nanofibers with Natural Tissue Structure

Besides the above techniques that have been developed to fabricate synthetic and naturally derived nanofibers, ECM nanofibers can also be acquired by decellularizing native arteries or produced with *in vitro* vascular cell culture techniques. These methods result in ECM nanofibrous materials simulating the structure of native arteries.

Decellarized blood vessels obtained from rat aorta, porcine carotid arteries, or veins of canine origin have been tested as grafting materials in the animal models. To produce a biocompatible biological graft, antigen reduction with preservation of the matrix for remodeling is necessary. The removal of cells theoretically reduces the immunologic response by the recipient and leaves the 3D architecture of the vessel for remodeling. It is hoped that migration of the recipient's vascular cells into the matrix might eventually render the graft indistinguishable from native vessels. The apparent advantage of decellularized constructs is that the structural design of the tissue is preserved, but the drawbacks are that it is difficult to obtain highly purified preparations and the results vary greatly from batch to batch. Also, decellularization generally produces weaker tissues so that subsequent cross-linking is needed to make the materials stronger and stiffer. In addition, though studies have shown that the materials are inflammation-resistant and inhibit SMC proliferation, calcification is a problem accompanying the decelluarized arteries.

Another widely adopted approach is to allow cells to synthesize and assemble its own ECM nanofibers. Culturing monolayers of fibroblasts and SMCs in medium enriched in ascorbic acid or other growth-stimulating factors and/or in a mechanically dynamic environment induce large production of ECM nanofiber components, such as collagen and elastin fibers. The cell culture can take place in different substrate environments, for example: (1) on a flat plate to form cell sheet; (2) in collagen or fibrin gel-based environment; or (3) on degradable scaffold grafts. The ECM produced by the vascular cells is complex and combines to provide biomechanical properties of the engineered vessels. The stimulation of cells to form collagen and elastin, translating to mechanical strength and mimetic elasticity, can be enhanced by the substrate environment as well as the biomechanical and biochemical environments.

12.3 Design Strategies of Nanofiber Constructs for Vascular Tissue Regeneration

12.3.1 Nanofibrous Vascular Constructs for *In Vitro* or *In Vivo* Tissue Regeneration

Engineering blood vessels or vascular tissue regeneration has been investigated following two different principal approaches: *in vitro* tissue regeneration and *in vivo* tissue regeneration. *In vitro* tissue regeneration often starts with the expansion of autologous cells by cell culture, and then organizes cells on a scaffold and performs continuous culture in a specifically designed bioreactor to produce an engineered functional tissue similar to the native one. It is clear that this approach consists of a time-consuming and expensive series of steps that may require a few weeks or even months to build up robust engineered arteries for implantation. Scale-up the *in vitro* process is also problematic due to large variations in autologous cells. These reasons make this approach difficult in many clinical practices, particularly in the cases of acute diseases.

For *in vivo* tissue regeneration, a scaffold is directly implanted either in the site of injury or in another location (i.e., body cavities, under the skin). In this case, the patient's body itself produces the new tissues, by invading the scaffold with cells, remodeling, and sometimes replacing it over the time. If the scaffold is implanted directly as a vascular substitute, it needs to act as a suitable substrate for vascular cell ingrowth and tissue regeneration. On the other hand, the scaffold has to accomplish the functions of a blood vessel, such as withstanding intraluminal pressure and aggressive physiological environment. Degradation kinetics and decrease in the mechanical properties of the synthetic degradable scaffold need to be carefully controlled so that the structural integrity of the vessel is preserved until the new tissue is formed. Ideally, the scaffold should degrade with the same rate at which tissue grows, transferring gradually mechanical loads to the developing tissue. Highly cross-linked biological scaffolds, or slowly degradable semicrystalline polymers, such as PCL and PLA, are selected for this application.

In spite of the differences, the *in vitro* and *in vivo* regeneration approaches to vascular grafting implants share some common design requirements for nanofiber-based scaffolds. The scaffold should not only provide appropriate nanoscale and microscale structure and degradation rates for cell activity and tissue regeneration, but also provide signals or signaling mechanisms for cell attachment, migration, differentiation, and remodeling. To meet these requirements, recent studies have investigated design and fabrication strategies to better integrate cells.

12.3.2 Cell Source and Signaling Mechanisms Involved in Vascular Tissue Regeneration

As reviewed in Section 12.1, an ideal vascular graft should achieve regeneration of a biomimetic blood vessel, which include regeneration of functional endothelium and smooth muscle media layer. To achieve this goal, appropriate cell types should be used. The cell type chosen for tissue regeneration largely determines the design of molecule signals in the scaffold. Blood vessels are characterized by a concentric layered structure, with each layer being distinct in its cell and protein composition. The innermost layer, called the intima, consists of EC. Beneath the EC is a layer of basement membrane enriched in collagen IV and laminin, followed by a fenestrated but acellular layer of elastin called the internal elastic lamina. The muscular layer of the artery, called the media, consists of SMCs and collagen and elastin as well as proteoglycans and other proteins. The outermost layer, called the adventitia, consists of fibroblasts, connective tissue, and vasa vasorum capillaries.

The traditional cells used for tissue regeneration are vascular EC, SMC, and fibroblasts. EC presents a nonthrombogenic layer, a signal to the muscular layer, and prevents inflammation by releasing molecular factors necessary for antiplatelet, vasoregulation, and anti-inflammatory actions; SMC have the ability to regulate endothelial functions and contract in response to hemodynamic conditions; fibroblasts synthesize the ECM nanofibers which are responsible for mechanical integrity. L'Heureux cultured fibroblasts to form ECM sheets and repeatedly rolled these sheets around a mandrel to obtain mechanically strong engineered vascular tissue. More frequently, autologous vascular ECs and SMCs are used for vascular regeneration. Studies have repeatedly shown that endothelial seeding and tissue engineering approaches can reduce thromogenicity, reduce infection, and improve graft patency. Since ECs have only limited capacity of regenerating *in vivo*, re-endothelialization of the large graft surface areas encountered clinically exceeds the normal ingrowth capacity of ECs from the adjacent vascular surfaces. A generally used method for improving EC seeding is to place high-density cells on the graft surface *in vitro*. Approaches to obtain EC for seeding include harvesting autologous venous EC in sufficient quantity or in small quantity followed by expansion *in vitro*, harvesting microvascular EC, genetically engineered EC, and the precursor cells from bone marrow or circulating blood. The latter two approaches are emerging, exciting techniques in recent years. To enable EC to anchor more securely to the surface, the graft surface is often precoated with adhesive molecules such as fibrin, gelatin, laminin, fibronectin, or collagen. The impregnation of vascular grafts with bioactive factors has also been used to promote the adherence and growth of ECs on the graft surface. These include fibrin/FGF/heparin complex, FGF1/heparin bFGF/heparin, VPF/VEGF, and plasmid DNA encoding VEGF. With regard to SMC, difficulties have centered around the contraction of SMC on substrates, along with culture difficulties due to the early senescence of SMC. Though numerous studies used autologous EC, SMC, and fibroblasts, the limitations of using these autologous vascular cells include the limited regenerative capacity of these cells in aged and/or diseased persons and the cell availability in emergency situations.

The ideal EC and SMC source is easily and rapidly harvestable cells in numbers large enough for immediate high-density vascular graft seeding. Such a source does not currently exist for clinical studies. Due to the restrictions of clinically using vascular cells, more recent studies started to employ progenitors or stem cells including endothelial progenitor cells (EPC), mesenchymal stem cells (MSC), and embryonic stem cells (ESC) as alternative cell sources. However, these cell types require more defined molecular signaling environments for recruitment and controlled differentiation. EPC are found within the bone marrow as well as the blood stream expressing Flk-1, CD133, and CD34. EPC can be differentiated into vascular EC or SMC *in vivo* or *in vitro*. They were also found to aid in the process of vasculogenesis. Griese et al., have demonstrated that the EPC transplantation plays an active role in re-establishing the endothelial integrity and the inhibition of IH. They have also reported that up to 60% of the vascular graft was endothelialized in 4 weeks *in vivo*, and the grafts also exhibited contractile activity and patency in 5 months. The limitations of using EPC, however, are *ex vivo* expansion time, difficulty in purifying and culturing EPCs, and change of the phenotype during culture. Recent studies also seeded MSC on the scaffold for vascular tissue engineering. Reports have suggested that the graft surfaces seeded with MSC are thrombo-resistant. Also, molecular factors such as VEGF can guide MSC to differentiate into EC-like cells, and factors such as TGF-β stimulates MSC differentiation into SMC-like cells. Derived from the inner cell mass of the blastocyst, ESC have the highest pluripotency and indefinite renewal capacity and can give rise to all somatic lineages including vascular cell types. ESC can differentiate into vascular CD31 EC *in vitro*, and aid in the formation of vasculature *in vivo*. Signaling chemicals such as VEGF and PDGF stimulate ESC to differentiate into EC and SMC, respectively. Several limitations are also acknowledged in the use of ESC. These include acquired immunogenicity after differentiation.

12.3.3 Design Strategies for Nanofibrous Constructs: The Impact of "Nano"-Effects

Due to the fact that tissue function is dependent on cell and structure, it is necessary to define cell environment and recreate the appropriate tissue nanoarchitecture and microarchitecture, a major component of which is the ECM. The ECM structure has implications for both the mechanical performance of the tissue and the maintenance of an appropriate local environment for cellular activity. Nanofibers are important building blocks for the fabrication of vascular equivalents. Design considerations for a nanofibrous vascular graft include its mechanical scaffolding function, mimetic vessel architecture at a nanoscale and microscale, and its interaction with cells, particularly for stem or progenitor cells, interaction at the subcellular level as to transform them into functional EC and/or SMC for the endothelium formation and/or smooth muscle regeneration. For nanofiber-cell interactions at the subcellular level, cell molecular signaling mechanisms to bring about specific cell behaviors should be considered. The use of nanofibers as small units to incorporate bioactive molecules and to build up larger functional structures with complexity offer great potential for constructing smart biomimetic blood vessels with novel functionalities.

12.3.3.1 Mechanical Scaffolding Function

Mechanical properties are essential for vascular grafts, because the grafts must withstand transluminal pressure and need to match arterial compliance to avoid flow disturbance around anastomosis, which leads to an inflammatory milieu in cells. Both strength and elasticity should be considered in the design of scaffolds. The nanofibrous scaffold prepared by self-assembly is often mechanically weak, thus requiring cross-linking or some other reinforcing method. The nanofibrous scaffold prepared by electrospinning is often a strong scaffold, and electrospinning provides the capability of tuning strength and elasticity with several fabrication parameters. These include nanostructural factors such as fiber alignment, crystallinity, microstructural factors such as porosity, and macroscopic features such as thickness and delamination.

For vascular grafts, the directional bias of fibers with respect to the tubular axis is desired to mimetically obtain an anisotropic mechanical property and to improve burst strength. Toward this, aligned nanofibrous scaffolds have been successfully produced.

Besides the anisotropic mechanical property, in recognition of the complex mechanical behavior of native tissues, more emphasis is placed on characterizing the viscoelastic nature of the constructs that are produced. In particular, the incorporation of elastin or elastin-mimetic peptides into the scaffolding matrix has become an important goal to enhance construct recoil and prevent aneurysm formation. The movement of the field toward mimicking more specialized features of vascular tissue is exciting, although the recapitulation of native tissue mechanics and contractility is an ambitious endpoint. However, it is not clear how close to native mechanical properties a blood vessel construct must have for effective therapy.

12.3.3.2 Topographical Effect of Nanofibers

The remarkable nanotopographic features of nanofiber scaffolds provide cells the necessary physical cues similar to the nanotopographical features of the natural ECM, thus enhancing cell-scaffold interactions. It has long been known that surface topography affects a variety of cell behaviors. Topographical features have direct effects on cell adhesion, alignment, migration, cytoskeleton protein production, and differentiation, all independent of surface biochemistry. More recently, it was shown that nanotopography, rather than microtopography, was ideal for vascular cells, particularly ECs, as they naturally live in a nanoenvironment. Buttiglieri et al., showed that nanotextured surfaces ensured a higher confluent surface of EC compared to flat cultured dishes and the cells emitted pseudopodia with focal contacts. As cell adhesion on synthetic materials is mediated by absorbed proteins on the surface, the mechanism that nanofibrous surfaces enhance cell adhesion may be caused by increased protein adsorption. To that end, the high surface-to-volume ratio in nanofibrous materials has been demonstrated to induce a higher cell adhesion by increasing the adsorption of plasma proteins such as vitronectin and fibronectin, which facilitate interactions of cell adhesion proteins. This effect has further been shown to be affected by the nanofiber size. In addition to cell adhesion, the nanotopography of fibrous scaffold constructs also affect other cell behaviors including differentiation and remodeling. Bondar et al., have shown that EC attaching to nanofibrous silk-fibroin resulted in the formation of a differentiated and interconnected endothelial layer. Also, it was shown that cells spread to absorbed proteins at multiple focal points of nanofibers. As the fiber diameters of nanofiber scaffolds are orders of magnitude smaller than the size of cells, cells are able to organize around the fibers. However, cell movement and aggregation appear to be slightly restricted by the *nanofiber* surface *topography* as compared to film surface.

Aligned nanofibers, in comparison to randomly oriented fibers, play a critical role in controlling cell shape, regulating physiological function, and defining organ architecture. Aligned nanofibers provide specific signals to vascular cells. A direct influence of aligned nanofibers is cell alignment which in turn affects differentiation and proliferation. Mo et al., developed an aligned biodegradable PLLA-CL nanofibrous scaffold using a rotating collector disk for the collection of aligned electrospun nanofibers. The resultant materials not only provided structural integrity and mechanical properties comparable to human coronary artery that sustain high pressure of the circulatory system, but also formed a well-defined architecture for enhanced adhesion and proliferation of both EC and SMC. Aligned fibers also maintained vasoactivity. Xu et al., demonstrated SMC contractile phenotype, cytoskeleton organization, and migration along the nanofibers. These aligned nanofibrous tubular scaffolds could be useful in engineering blood vessels.

12.3.3.3 Integration of Molecules and Cells in the Nanofibrous Scaffold

In addition to the mechanical scaffolding function and topographical effect, nanofibers can be physically or chemically modified to fulfil different requirements imposed on the future vascular grafts, and control the cell-matrix interactions to enhance the bioactivity of vascular implants or engineered tissues. Also, nanofibers can serve as a molecular delivery system in the scaffold, providing bioactive factors for cell function and tissue regeneration, or preventing infection, inflammation, or thrombosis while tissue regeneration occurs. The high surface-volume ratio of nanofibers allows efficient delivery of molecules. Important issues around the molecular incorporation include the local delivery, temporal release, concentration, and bioactivity of molecules upon release.

Diverse molecules and peptide sequences have been attempted to incorporate into vascular grafts or engineered vascular tissues. These include (1) molecules that reduce thrombogenicity; (2) molecules such as growth factors and DNA that affect cell behaviors; and (3) drugs such as antibiotics and anti-inflammatory drugs that influence the grafting performance. The incorporation of molecules which affect thrombogenicity by reducing platelet adherence has been shown to enhance the patency of vascular grafts for a long time. Anticoagulation factors such as heparin prevent not only thrombosis but also IH through inhibition of arterial SMC proliferation *in vitro* and *in vivo*. The incorporation of molecules which affect cell function and tissue regeneration must be designed to target at specific cell physiology process, dependent on cell type and cell differentiating state. Thus, an in-depth understanding of vascular cell biology and/or stem cell biology, particularly cell signaling, is important for the incorporation of the right molecular signals at the right location and time. Signaling molecules that enhance EC adhesion and reduce SMC migration are used, because endothelial denudation and an abnormal migration of vascular media SMCs into the intima are major causes of graft failure. Cell adhesion is often enhanced by the matrix surface molecules interacting with the cell receptors such as integrins through ligand-receptor binding at the cell–ECM interface. Adhesion sequences or functional domains derived from ECM components (collagen, fibronectin, fibrinogen, or vitronectin), for example Arg-Gly-Asp peptide (RGD), Tyr-Ile-Gly-Ser-Arg peptide (YIGSR), and Ile-Lys-Val-Ala-Val peptide (IKVAV), can be incorporated on the surface. This has been used to accelerate endothelialization. Functionalized vascular grafts can also target several biological processes to promote *in situ* endothelialization with EPCs or stem cells through: (1) encouraging cell-specific (circulating EPCs or stem cells) homing to the vascular graft site by providing cell-specific adhesion peptides on the graft; (2) promoting cell immobilization; (3) directing the differentiation and proliferation of the cells after their adhesion in order to rapidly form a mature, functioning endothelium capable of self-repair.

Designing bioinspired vascular grafting materials through nanofiber fabrication techniques, such as electrospinning, molecular self-assembly, and phase separation, is an emerging field. To enhance the biomimicry of nanofibrous scaffolds, multifunctional nanofibers should be made by combining the bioactive surface with spatiotemporal release of functional molecules and drugs. This is being explored by the following techniques: (1) modifying the surface of nanofibers; (2) incorporating bioactive molecules in the nanofibers and achieving spatiotemporal control over the molecule release; (3) incorporating cells during the fiber-formation process; and (4) forming composite nanofibers that combine the different mechanical, bioactive, and degradable properties of component materials (discussed in Section 12.2.1).

12.3.3.3.1 Surface Functionalization and Surface Effects

Due to the extremely large surface-to-volume ratio of nanofibers, functionalization of the nanofiber surface or modification of molecular sequences presented on the nanofiber surface can make nanofibrous materials highly bioactive. Surface functionalization and molecular chain modification provide opportunities to effectively modify specific nanofiber functions such as enhanced solubility, biocompatibility, and biorecognition. The percentage of the polymer chain presenting functional groups or molecular sequences on the fiber surface was roughly estimated as $100\pi d/D$, where d and D represented the diameters of the polymer chain and the fiber, respectively. Thus, reducing the fiber diameter could proportionally increase the ratio of the exposed polymer chains together with its functional groups.

Different nanofiber fabrication approaches provide means of surface functionalization. For electrospun or phase-separated nanofibrous materials, the general techniques to create surface-immobilized chemical groups include physical adsorption of the molecules on the nanofibers, and covalent linking of the molecules via peptide bond formation through primary carboxylic acid or amine moieties. For example, gelatin grafting on polyethylene terephthalate (PET) increased the hydrophilicity of the scaffold which enabled EC to adopt a well-spread polygonal-shaped morphology and upregulate the adhesion proteins. In the self-assembled PA system, surface functionalization can be easily achieved through the design of a PA system with functional peptides. For example, nanofibers produced with cellular activation sequences have shown encouraging cell response. Also, a new technique, the biomimetic molecular biomimetic imprinting technique, may introduce new molecules on nanofibrous materials.

12.3.3.3.2 Incorporation and Spatiotemporal Release Control of Molecules in Nanofibers

Polymeric nanofibers can act as controlled-release carriers for a variety of bioactive molecules including antibiotics, proteins (such as growth factors), DNA, drugs, and other small biomolecules. While these factors are traditionally delivered homogeneously *in vitro* or *in vivo*, temporal and spatial control over their delivery is an understood requirement for biomimetic repair and regeneration. The incorporation of growth factors or drugs can be encapsulated or impregnated in the nanofibers. This is often achieved by the electrospinning fabrication method.

Delivering bioactive or pharmaceutical molecules with electrospun nanofibers was first attempted by simply mixing the molecules in the electrospinning polymer solution. Nanofibers loaded with bioactive molecules were made by dispersing the molecules in an amorphous state to facilitate the drug dissolution. The release of molecules can be designed to facilitate immediate or delayed dissolution, depending on the polymer carrier used. The nanofibrous molecule–carrier complex is closely associated with the solubility and compatibility of the molecule in the polymer solution as well as the processing conditions. Several possible interaction modes between the molecule and the polymer carrier result in different nanostructures. These modes are: (1) biomolecules that are not soluble in the polymer solution form tiny particles and attach onto the surface of the nanofiber carriers; (2) the mixture of biomolecule and polymer solution forms an emulsion and the encapsulation of the biomolecule with the emulsion is due to phase separation of the solution during the electrospinning process; and (3) a blend of them is integrated into uniform composite nanofibers either by wrapping or mixing evenly, due to good compatibility. The molecule–polymer interaction determines the nanofiber structure and the release behavior: the first mode likely results in initial burst release, the second mode likely results in nanofibers with a layered or so-called core-sheath structure showing stepwise release, and the third mode should result in more gradual release. In addition to the interaction modes, several approaches have been developed to modify the release kinetics of molecules by using polymer blend to improve the compatibility with biomolecules. One approach is to use a blend of hydrophobic and hydrophilic polymers in the scaffolds. The hydrophobic polymer such as PCL, PLGA, and PLLA, can act like a shield for the hydrophilic polymer such as dextran and chitosan, reducing the water intake and the hydrolytic degradation rate. This is an advantage, because the burst effect is a problem for many hydrophilic biological molecules as the loaded molecules tend to segregate on the nanofibers surface and are immediately available. Another example is that Casper et al. incorporated heparin into nanofibers of PEO and PLGA by mixing it directly into the spinning solution. As PEO assisted the incorporation of heparin in the solution, heparin retention in the nanofibers of PEO and PLGA was improved compared to that in the PLGA nanofibers. Thus, the uniform distribution of heparin was shown in the fibers and over the thickness of the scaffold. This could in turn allow slower release of factors that bind to heparin. With a uniform distribution, different release rates may be obtained by simply varying the fiber diameter or loading dosage. As a high permeability and interconnected pore structure of nanofibrous materials facilitates the exchange of growth medium and the removal of metabolic wastes, the biological molecules are made available as a consequence of the degradation of the scaffold, and release via diffusive mechanisms is neglected. Another approach to achieving slow release involves the post-electrospinning coating of molecule-loaded fibers. Coating with hydrophobic poly(p-xylylene) of poly(vinyl alcohol) nanofibers was found to lead to a significant retardation of the release of contained molecules. Control of release at prolonged time intervals can be achieved by controlling water permeability of the coating polymer. Additionally, it is noted that molecule loading may change the polymer behavior. The incorporation may influence the nanofiber formation because of an increase in ionic charges in the polymer solution. Li et al. incorporated proteinase K into a copolymer PEG/PLA, showing a significant increase in the rate of polymer degradation. Luong-Van et al. showed that fiber diameter was dependent on the concentration of heparin, and Zeng et al., demonstrated that the addition of various surfactants reduced the diameter and distribution of electrospun nanofibers.

A more advanced approach to achieve molecular encapsulation with electrospinning is the coaxial electrospinning method. In this case, the nanofibers assume a core/sheath structure. The coaxial electrospinning uses two concentric needles, one inside the other; each needle is fed with different polymer solutions. The outer needle originates the sheath and the inner one produces the core. When the bioactive molecule is incorporated with the polymer in the core, its release is limited by the presence of an impermeable or a less permeable sheath. Thus, the shell functions as a release control mechanism. The release rate of bioactive molecule can further be regulated on the basis of nanofiber core-shell thickness. The process has a higher efficiency than traditionally used methods for encapsulation.

In addition to temporal control over the molecule release, spatial control over the release is important for delivering the right signals to the right cells for the regeneration of a specific tissue. For instance, the local delivery of heparin in the region close to lumen is necessary for vascular grafts, because heparin reduces thrombosis and increases endothelial proliferation, but it inhibits SMC migration and ingrowth thus preventing the regeneration of the media layer if uniformly distributed in a vascular scaffold. Also, transforming growth factors that are responsible for SMC differentiation and collagen secretion signals EC apoptosis. Another example is that stem cells or progenitor cells have differentiation plasticity (capable of differentiating into different types of vascular cells), and therefore locally guiding their differentiation to a certain type (i.e., EC or SMC) helps the formation of biomimetic vascular tissues.

Often, spatial control and temporal control over the molecule release are needed simultaneously to optimize the performances of vascular grafts. For instance, the delivery of potent angiogenic proteins or genes that promote EC-specific mitogenesis or chemotaxis is desired to be upon vascular graft surfaces at the beginning of implantation. FGF, notably FGF-1 and FGF-2, have potent angiogenic, mitogenic, and chemotactic activity on vascular cells. As the delivery of FGF helps to locally direct intimal regeneration and long-term release of FGF can cause an overgrowth of intima or IH response, a delivery system that provides predictable local release meanwhile preserving the bioactivity over a specific interval of time is required. Core-shell nanofibers have been successfully designed to release desired bioactive molecules at therapeutic concentrations in both a spatial and temporal pattern.

12.3.3.3.3 Cell Encapsulation in Nanofibrous Scaffolds

In addition to molecule incorporation, many studies have worked on directly incorporating cells in the nanofibrous constructs. The advantage is that a uniform cell distribution can be achieved throughout the constructs. A widely used vascular tissue engineering method is to incorporate cells in collagen or fibrin before inducing them to self-assemble into nanofibers. Cells were also encapsulated *in vitro* within a 3D network of epitope containing PA nanofibers prepared by self-assembly. It is also possible to incorporate cells with electrospun nanofibers. Electrospinning of living cells with or without polymer nanofibers has been shown by Jayasinghe et al.

12.3.3.4 Hierarchical Structural Effects

Successful orchestration of the molecular factors is likely to require greater complexity than the nanofiber design alone, and is likely to involve hierarchical structure and molecules incorporated at the hierarchical structure. Nanofiber matrices encapsulated with suitable bioactive molecules provide cells with necessary chemical cues in nanoscale environments. Because of the size of vascular cells (>5 μm), microporous structures are also needed for cell migration and tissue ingrowth. This is not much of an issue to self-assembled or phase-separated nanofibrous scaffolds, as they can provide a flexible structure or a microstructure. Nanofibrous scaffolds fabricated by electrospinning result in high porosity with connected interfibrillar space, but one limitation of traditional electrospun materials is that the pore size is too small for a large number of cells to penetrate and migrate *in vitro*. Several approaches that introduce microscale or macro scale pores have been developed. One approach is to add porogens in the electrospinning solution. For instance, Buttafoco et al., electrospun collagen on soluble type I collagen and soluble elastin in 10 mM HCl with PEO and NaCl. PEO and NaCl were fully leached out after crosslinking. The resultant structure is characterized by nanoscale and microscale structures or dual structures. Another approach is to fabricate nanofiber composites with a polymer that degrades faster than the other, thus increasing the porosity for tissue ingrowth. This was shown with the spinning of PCL and gelatin solutions and with the spinning of PCL and PEO. The microporous structure is achieved by nanofibers which can be fast degraded in water.

12.3.3.5 Summary

Design strategies of nanofibrous vascular grafts must consider the needs in vascular tissue regeneration and the capability of nanofiber fabrication technology. Tissue regeneration fundamentally relies on the capability of modulating cell physiology. The essence of nanotechnology is the ability to fabricate and engineer materials where the manipulation of the properties and functionalities is a result of the control of the materials' nanoscale building blocks. In addition to nanotopography, the regulation mechanisms of cell physiology require a variety of nanoscale building blocks that mimic the functions of ECM. These include but are not limited to the building blocks that enhance elasticity, hydrophilicity/hydrophobicity, cell adhesion, cell differentiation, and cell migration. Additionally, nanostructured materials can be advantageously engineered by the formation and ensemble of building blocks. The advancement of nanotechnology techniques allows one to arrange the hierarchical structure of a nanofibrous scaffold for better cell integration and tissue regeneration. Another advantage of the nanofibrous scaffold is to have biomimetic delivery system that allows site-directed molecules, genes, or drugs to be controlled temporally. It is well known to the biologists that an optimal cell signal should be released at a precise rate and dose to match the tissue regeneration or other therapeutic needs. The intricate complexities of the spatial and temporal environment dynamically influence phenotypic and other cellular behavior by providing indirect and direct informational signaling cues. It is believed that the more closely the *in vivo* environment (i.e., chemical composition, morphology, and surface functional groups) can be recreated, the more likely is the success of the tissue engineering scaffolds.

12.4 Suggestions and Future Direction

The future holds very high promise for novel and sophisticated applications of nanofibrous materials in the vascular implants. Tailor-made nanofibrous materials are likely to have tremendous potential in addressing multiple problems facing the current small-diameter blood vessel substitutes. However, the success of these applications depends on our technology ability to fabricate building blocks with a very high degree of control over their composition, property, and the way they are arranged. Therefore, there is a need for the future development of more sophisticated methods for the engineering of the building blocks and the methods of their assembly. For instance, biofunctionalizations of nanofibrous polymers with hybrid composition, surface, and molecule encapsulation can be further developed for more sophisticated mechanisms that nature presents. Nanofibers with programmable release could be an area of future research and development. Chemical methods may be valuable tools for achieving this. Moreover, methods for arranging the building blocks in certain patterns (e.g., gradient pattern for morphogenesis or chemotaxis) are of equal importance. Further, vascular regeneration in grafting implant is largely dependent on the cells. Thus, the nanofibrous scaffolding design must be appropriate for the targeted cells, for example, vascular EC, SMC, fibroblasts, or progenitor/stem cells. The latter are more attractive cell sources, due to the development in stem cell biology. In addition, engineered scaffolds must satisfy the functional parameters under mechanically active conditions.

Nature appears to be the ultimate specialist in the design and manufacture of novel materials with just the right sizes and properties from the nanoscale to microscale to facilitate tissue regeneration. Future investigation and understanding of nature's mechanisms of nanomaterial formation can in turn provide inspirations for the new design strategies of nanofibrous biomaterials for vascular grafts and tissue engineering. Therefore, innovative designs will need interdisciplinary collaborative efforts from cell biologists, chemists, material scientists, bioengineers, and clinicians.

Besides the development in innovative design and fabrication technology, a promising or probably more important area for the future is the one that translates the new technologies into clinically applicable products and transforms the design theory into clinical reality. In addition to the mechanical function, cell physiological functions, tissue remodeling and long-term performances, the clinical impact of design, the manufacturing process, and regulatory affairs are all important considerations for realizing the transition from technology to product.

Bibliography

Alobaid, N., H.J. Salacinski, K.M. Sales, B. Ramesh, R.Y. Kannan, G. Hamilton, and A.M. Seifalian. 1987. 2006. Nanocomposite containing bioactive peptides promote endothelialisation by circulating progenitor cells: An *in vitro* evaluation. *Eur. J. Vasc. Endovasc. Surg.: The Off. J. Eur. Soc. Vasc. Surg.* 32(1): 76–83.

Arts, C.H., G.J. Heijnen-Snyder, P.P. Joosten, et al. 2001. A novel method for isolating pure microvascular endothelial cells from subcutaneous fat tissue ideal for direct cell seeding. *Lab. Invest.* 81: 1461–5.

Asahara, T. and A. Kawamoto. 2004. Endothelial progenitor cells for postnatal vasculogenesis. *Am. J. Physiol. Cell Physiol.* 287(3): C572–79.

Asahara, T., T. Murohara, A. Sullivan, M. Silver, R. van der Zee, T. Li, B. Witzenbichler, G. Schatteman, and J.M. Isner. 1997. Isolation of putative progenitor endothelial cells for angiogenesis. *Science* 275(5302): 964–66.

Ashammakhi, N., A. Ndreu, Y. Yang, H. Ylikauppila, L. Nikkola, and V. Hasirci. 2007. Tissue engineering: A new take-off using nanofiber-based scaffolds. *J. Cranio Surg.* 18: 3–17.

Ayres, C., G.L. Bowlin, S.C. Henderson, L. Taylor, J. Shultz, J. Alexander, T.A. Telemeco, and D.G. Simpson. 2006. Modulation of anisotropy in electrospun tissue-engineering scaffolds: Analysis of fiber alignment by the fast Fourier transform. *Biomaterials* 27: 5524.

Beachley, V. and X.J. Wen. 2009. Effect of electrospinning parameters on the nanofiber diameter and length. *Mater. Sci. Eng. C-Biomimetic Supramol. Systems* 29(3): 663–68.

Behfar, A., L.V. Zingman, D.M. Hodgson, J. Rauzier, G.C. Kane, A. Terzic, and M. Puceat. 2002. Stem cell differentiation requires a paracrine pathway in the heart. *FASEB J.* 16: 1558–66.

Behonick, D.J. and Z. Werb. 2003. A bit of give and take: The relationship between the extracellular matrix and the developing chondrocyte. *Mech. Dev.* 120: 1327.

Berglund, J.D., M.M. Mohseni, R.M. Nerem, and A. Sambanis. 2003. A biological hybrid model for collagen-based tissue engineered vascular constructs. *Biomaterials* 24: 1241–54.

Berndt, P., G.B. Fields, and M. Tirrell. 1995. Synthetic lipidation of peptides and amino acids: Monolayer structure and properties. *J. Am. Chem. Soc.* 117: 9515–22.

Berndt, P., G.B. Fields, and M. Tirrell. 2002. Synthetic lipidation of peptides and amino acids: Monolayer structure and properties. *J. Am. Chem. Soc.* 117: 9515–22.

Bhat, V.D., B. Klitzman, K. Koger, and G.A. Truskey. 1998. Reichert Wm. Improving endothelial cell adhesion to vascular graft surfaces: Clinical need and strategies. *J. Biomater. Sci. Polym. Ed.* 9: 1117–35.

Bhattacharya, V., P.A. McSweeney, Q. Shi, et al. 2000. Enhanced endothelialization and microvessel formation in polyester grafts seeded with Cd34(+) bone marrow cells. *Blood* 95: 581–5.

Bhattacharya, V., M. Cleanthis, and G. Stansby. 2005. Preventing vascular graft failure: Endothelial cell seeding and tissue engineering. *Vasc. Dis. Prevent.* 2: 21–27.

Boland, E.D., J.A. Matthews, K.J. Pawlowski, D.G. Simpson, G.E. Wnek, and G.L. Bowlin. 2004. Electrospinning collagen and elastin: Preliminary vascular tissue engineering. *Front. Biosci.* 9: 1422.

Bondar, B., S. Fuchs, A. Motta, C. Migliaresi, and C.J. Kirkpatrick. 2008. Functionality of endothelial cells on silk fibroin nets: Comparative study of micro- and nanometric fibre size. *Biomaterials* 29(5): 561–72.

Brewster, L.P., D. Bufallino, A. Ucuzian, and H.P. Greisler. 2007. Growing a living blood vessel: Insights for the second hundred years. *Biomaterials* 28(34): 5028–32.

Budd, J.S., K.E. Allen, P.R. Bell, and R.F. James. 1990. The effect of varying fibronectin concentration on the attachment of endothelial cells to polytetrafluoroethylene vascular grafts. *J. Vasc. Surg.* 12: 126–30.

Buttafoco, L., N.G. Kolkman, P. Engbers-Buijtenhuijs, A.A. Poot, P.J. Dijkstra, I. Vermes, et al. 2006. Electrospinning of collagen and elastin for tissue engineering applications. *Biomaterials* 27: 724–34.

Buttafoco, L., P. Engbers-Buijtenhuijs, A.A. Poot, P.J. Dijkstra, I. Vermes, and J. Feijen. 2006. Physical characterization of vascular grafts cultured in a bioreactor. *Biomaterials* 27: 2380–89.

Buttiglieri, S., D. Pasqui, M. Migliori, H. Johnstone, S. Affrossman, L. Sereni, M.L. Wratten, R. Barbucci, C. Tetta, and G. Camussi. 2003. Endothelization and adherence of leucocytes to nanostructured surfaces. *Biomaterials* 24(16): 2731–8.

Byrne, M.E., E. Oral, J.Z. Hilt, and N.A. Peppas. 2002. Networks for recognition of iomolecules: Molecular imprinting and micropatterning poly(ethylene glycol)-containing films. *Poly. Adv. Technol.* 13: 798–816.

Callow, A.D. 1987. Endothelial cell seeding: Problems and expectations. *J. Vasc. Surg.* 6: 318–9.

Callow, A.D. 1990. The vascular endothelial cell as a vehicle for gene therapy. *J. Vasc. Surg.* 11: 793–8.

Casper, C.L., N. Yamaguchi, K.L. Kiick, and J.F. Rabolt. 2005. Functionalizing electrospun fibers with biologically relevant macromolecules. *Biomacromolecules* 6: 1998.

Chew, S.Y., J. Wen, E.K. Yim, and K.W. Leong. 2005. Sustained release of proteins from electrospun biodegradable fibers. *Biomacromolecules* 6: 2017.

Chuaa, K.-N., W.-S. Lima, P. Zhanga, H. Lua, J. Wend, S. Ramakrishna, K.W. Leonga, and H.-Q. Mao. 2005. Stable immobilization of rat hepatocyte spheroids on galactosylated nanofiber scaffold. *Biomaterials* 26: 2537–47.

Clarke, D.R., R.M. Lust, Y.S. Sun, K.S. Black, and J.D. Ollerenshaw. 2001. Transformation of nonvascular acellular tissue matrices into durable vascular conduits. *Ann. Thoracic Surg.* 71(5): S433–S436.

Clowes, A.W. and M.J. Karnovsky. 1978. Suppression by heparin of injury-induced myointimal thickening. *J. Surg. Res.* 24(3): 161–68.

Conte, M.S., L.K. Birinyi, T. Miyata, et al. 1994. Efficient repopulation of denuded rabbit arteries with autologous genetically modified endothelial cells. *Circulation* 89: 2161–9.

Courtney, T., M.S. Sacks, J. Stankus, J. Guan, and W.R. Wagner. 2006. Design and analysis of tissue engineering scaffolds that mimic soft tissue mechanical anisotropy. *Biomaterials* 27(19): 3631–38.

Curtis, A. and C. Wilkinson. 1997. Topographical control of cells. *Biomaterials* 18(24): 1573–83.

de Mel, A., C. Bolvin, M. Edirisinghe, and A.M. Seifalian. 2008. Development of cardiovascular bypass grafts: Endothelialization and applications of nanotechnology. *Expert Rev. Cardiovas. Ther.* 6: 1259–77.

de Mel, A., G. Jell, M.M. Stevens, and A.M. Seifalian. 2008. Biofunctionalization of biomaterials for accelerated *in situ* endothelialization: A review. *Biomacromolecules* 9(11): 2969–79.

Dichek, D.A., R.F. Neville, J.A. Zwiebel, S.M. Freeman, M.B. Leon, and W.F. Anderson. 1989. Seeding of intravascular stents with genetically engineered endothelial cells. *Circulation* 80: 1347–53.

Doi, K.M.T. 1997. Enhanced vascularization in a microporous polyurethane graft impregnated with basic fibroblast growth factor and heparin. *J. Biomed. Mater. Res.* 34: 361–70.

Falk, J., L.E. Townsend, L.M. Vogel, et al. 1998. Improved adherence of genetically modified endothelial cells to small-diameter expanded polytetrafluoroethylene grafts in a canine model. *J. Vasc. Surg.* 27: 902–8.

Feng, L., S.H. Li, J. Zhai, Y.L. Song, L. Jiang, and D.B. Zhu. 2003. Template based synthesis of aligned polyacrylonitrile nanofibers using a novel extrusion method. *Synthetic Metals* 135–136: 817–18.

Feng, L., S. Li, H. Li, J. Zhai, Y. Song, L. Jiang, and D. Zhu. 2002. Super-hydrophobic surface of aligned polyacrylonitrile nanofibers. *Angewandte Chemie International Edition* 41: 1221–23.

Fields, G.B., J.L. Lauer, Y. Dori, P. Forns, Y. Yu, and M. Tirrell. 1998. Proteinlike molecular architecture: Biomaterial applications for inducing cellular receptor binding and signal transduction. *Peptide Sci.* 47: 143–51.

Flemming, R.G., C.J. Murphy, G.A. Abrams, S.L. Goodman, and P.F. Nealey. 1999. Effects of synthetic micro- and nano-structured surfaces on cell behavior. *Biomaterials* 20(6): 573–88.

Fujita, Y., M.H. Wu, A. Ishida, et al. 1999. Accelerated healing of dacron grafts seeded by preclotting with autologous bone marrow blood. *Ann. Vasc. Surg.* 13: 402–12.

Furchgott, R.F. 1999. Endothelium-derived relaxing factor: Discovery, early studies, and identification as nitric oxide. *Biosci. Rep.* 19: 235–51.

Geng, X., O.H. Kwon, and J. Jang. 2005. Electrospinning of chitosan dissolved in concentrated acetic acid solution. *Biomaterials* 26: 5427–32.

Gimbrone, M. 1976. Culture of vascular endothelium. *Prog. Haemost. Thromb.* 3: 1–28.

Gobin, A.S. and J.L. West. 2003. Val-Ala-Pro-Gly, an elastin-derived non-integrin ligand: Smooth muscle cell adhesion and specificity. *J. Biomed. Mater. Res.* 67: 255–9.

Gosselin, C., D.A. Vorp, V. Warty, et al. 1996. Eptfe coating with fibrin glue, Fgf-1, and heparin: Effect on retention of seeded endothelial cells. *J. Surg. Res.* 60: 327–32.

Graham, L., W. Burkel, J. Ford, D. Vinter, R. Kahn, and J. Stanley. 1982. Expanded polytetrafluoroethylene vascular prostheses seeded with enzymatically derived and cultured canine endothelial cells. *Surgery* 91(5): 550–59.

Graham, L.M., D.W. Vinter, J.W. Ford, R.H. Kahn, W.E. Burkel, and J.C. Stanley. 1979. Cultured autogenous endothelial cell seeding of prosthetic vascular grafts. *Surg. Forum.* 30: 204–6.

Gray, J.L., S.S. Kang, G.C. Zenni, D.U. Kim, P.I. Kim, and W.H. Burgess. 1994. Fgf-1 affixation stimulates Eptfe endothelialization without intimal hyperplasia. *J. Surg. Res.* 57: 596–612.

Greisler, H.P., D.U. Kim, J.D. Garfield, et al. 1992. Enhanced endothelialization of expanded polytetrafluoroethylene grafts by fibroblast growth factor type 1 pretreatment. *Surgery* 112: 244–54.

Griese, D.P., A. Ehsan, L.G. Melo, D. Kong, L. Zhang, M.J. Mann, R.E. Pratt, R. Mulligan, and V.J. Dzau. 2003. Isolation and transplantation of autologous circulating endothelial cells into denuded vessels and prosthetic grafts: Implications for cell-based vascular therapy. *Circulation* 108: 2710–15.

Gupta, B.S. and V.A. Kasyanov. 1997. Biomechanics of human common carotid artery and design of novel hybrid textile compliant vascular grafts. *J. Biomed. Mater. Res.* 34: 341–49.

Hartgerink, J.D., E. Beniash, and S.I. Stupp. 2002. Peptide-amphiphile nanofibers: A versatile scaffold for the preparation of self-assembling materials. *Proc. Natl. Acad. Sci.* 99: 5133–38.

Hashi, C.K., Y. Zhu, G.-Y. Yang, W.L. Young, B.S. Hsiao, K. Wang, B. Chu, and S. Li. 2007. Antithrombogenic property of bone marrow mesenchymal stem cells in nanofibrous vascular grafts. *Proc. Natl. Acad. Sci.* 104: 11915–20.

He, H., T. Shirota, H. Yasui, and T. Matsuda. Canine endothelial progenitor cell-lined hybrid vascular graft with nonthrombogenic potential. *J. Thorac. Cardiovasc. Surg.* 126: 455–464.

He, W., T. Yong, W.E. Teo, Z. Ma, and M. Ramakrishna. 2005. Fabrication and endothelialization of collagen blended biodegradable polymer nanofibers: Potential vascular graft for blood vessel tissue engineering. *Tissue Eng.* 11: 1574–88.

Hench, L.L. and J.M. Polak. 2002. Third-generation biomedical materials. *Science* 295: 1014–17.

Herring, M.D.R., T. Cullison, A. Gardner, and J. Glover. 1980. Seeding endothelium on canine arterial prostheses—The size of the inoculum. *J. Surg. Res.* 28: 35–38.

Herring, M., S. Baughman, J. Glover, K. Kesler, J. Jesseph, J. Campbell, et al. 1984. Endothelial seeding of dacron and polytetrafluoroethylene grafts: The cellular events of healing. *Surgery* 96(4): 745–55.

Herring, M.B. 1991. The use of endothelial seeding of prosthetic arterial bypass grafts. *Surg. Annu.* 23: 157–71.

Herring, M.B. 1991. Endothelial cell seeding. *J. Vasc. Surg.* 13: 731–2.

Hersel, U., C. Dahmen, and H. Kessler. 2003. Rgd modified polymers: Biomaterials for stimulated cell adhesion and beyond. *Biomater. Synth. Biomimetic. Polymers* 24(24): 4385–415.

Heydarkhan-Hagvall, S., K. Schenke-Layland, A.P. Dhanasopon, F. Rofail, H. Smith, B.M. Wu, R. Shemin, R.E. Beygui, and W. Robb MacLellan. 2008. Three-dimensional electrospun Ecm-based hybrid scaffolds for cardiovascular tissue engineering. *Biomaterials* 29: 2907–14.

Hinds, M.T., D.W. Courtman, T. Goodell, M. Kwong, H. Brant-Zawadzki, A. Burke, et al. 2004. Biocompatibility of a xenogenic elastin-based biomaterial in a murine implantation model: The role of aluminum chloride pretreatment. *J. Biomed. Mater. Res.* 69A: 55–64.

Hinrichs, W.L., J. Kuit, H. Feil, C.R. Wildevuur, and J. Feijen. 1992. *In vivo* fragmentation of microporous polyurethane- and copolyesterether elastomer-based vascular prostheses. *Biomaterials* 13(9): 585–93.

Hoerstrup, S.P., G. Zund, R. Sodian, A.M. Schnell, J. Grunenfelder, and M.I. Turina. 2001. Tissue engineering of small caliber vascular grafts. *Eur. J. Cardiothorac. Surg.* 20: 164–69.

Holmes, T.C. 2002. Novel peptide-based biomaterial scaffolds for tissue engineering. *Trends Biotechnol.* 20: 16–21.

Hristov, M., W. Erl, and P.C. Weber. 2003. Endothelial progenitor cells: Mobilization, differentiation, and homing. *Arterioscler Thromb Vasc. Biol.* 23: 1185–89.

Hsu, L., G.L. Cvetanovich, and S.I. Stupp. 2008. Peptide amphiphile nanofibers with conjugated polydiacetylene backbones in their core. *J. Am. Chem. Soc. March 26;* (12): 130: 3892–99.

Huang, H., Y. Nakayama, K. Qin, K. Yamamoto, J. Ando, J. Yamashita, H. Itoh, et al. 2005. Differentiation from embryonic stem cells to vascular wall cells under *in vitro* pulsatile flow loading. *J. Artif. Organ.* 8: 110–18.

Huang, L., K. Nagapudi, R.P. Apkarian, and E.L. Chaikof. 2001. Engineered collagen-peo nanofibers and fabrics. *J. Biomater. Sci. Polym. Ed.* 12.

Huang, L., R. Andrew McMillan, R.P. Apkarian, B. Pourdeyhimi, V.P. Conticello, and E.L. Chaikof. 2000. Generation of synthetic elastin-mimetic small diameter fibers and fiber networks. *Macromolecules* 33(8): 2989–97.

Huang, N.F., R.J. Lee, and S. Li. 2007. Chemical and physical regulation of stem cells and progenitor cells: Potential for cardiovascular tissue engineering. *Tissue Eng.* 13: 1809–23.

Huang, Z.M., C.L. He, A.Z. Yang, Y.Z. Zhang, X.J. Hang, J.L. Yin, and Q.S. Wu. 2006. Encapsulating drugs in biodegradable ultrafine fibers through co-axial electrospinning. *J. Biomed. Mater. Res. Part A* 77A(1): 169–79.

Hubbell, J.A. 1999. Bioactive biomaterials. *Curr. Opin. Biotechnol.* 10: 123–29.

Hubbell, J.A. 2003. Materials as morphogenetic guides in tissue engineering. *Curr. Opin. Biotechnol.* 14: 551–58.

Huynh, T., G. Abraham, J. Murray, K. Brockbank, P.O. Hagen, and S. Sullivan. 1999. Remodeling of an acellular collagen graft into a physiologically responsive neovessel. *Nat. Biotechnol.* 17(11): 1083–86.

In Jeong, S., S.Y. Kim, S.K. Cho, M.S. Chong, K.S. Kim, H. Kim, S.B. Lee, and Y.M. Lee. 2007. Tissue-engineered vascular grafts composed of marine collagen and Plga fibers using pulsatile perfusion bioreactors. *Biomaterials* 28: 1115–22.

Isenberg, B.C., C. Williams, and R.T. Tranquillo. 2006. Endothelialization and flow conditioning of fibrin-based media-equivalents. *Ann. Biomed. Eng.* 34: 971–85.

Isenburg, J.C., D.T. Simionescu, and N.R. Vyavahare. 2004. Elastin stabilization in cardiovascular implants: Improved resistance to enzymatic degradation by treatment with tannic acid. *Biomaterials* 25: 3293–302.

Ishikawa, M. and T. Asahara. 2004. Endothelial progenitor cell culture for vascular regeneration. *Stem Cell Dev.* 13: 344–49.

Jarrell, B.E., S.K. Williams, G. Stokes, et al. 1986. Use of freshly isolated capillary endothelial cells for the immediate establishment of a monolayer on a vascular graft at surgery. *Surgery* 100: 392–9.

Jayasinghe, S., S. Irvine, and J.R. McEwan. 2007. Cell electrospinning highly concentrated cellular suspensions containing primary living organisms into cell-bearing threads and scaffolds. *Nanomedicine* 2: 555–67.

Jiang, H., Y. Hu, Y. Li, P. Zhao, K. Zhu, and W. Chen. 2005. A facile technique to prepare biodegradable coaxial electrospun nanofibers for controlled release of bioactive agents. *J. Control Release* 108: 237.

Kakisis, J.D., C.D. Liapis, C. Breuer, and B.E. Sumpio. 2005. Artificial blood vessel: The holy grail of peripheral vascular surgery. *J. Vasc. Surg.* 41: 349–54.

Kambic, H., S. Murabayashi, R. Yozu, T. Morimoto, M. Furuse, H. Harasaki, et al. 1984. Small vessel replacement with elastomeric protein composite materials: Preliminary studies. *Trans. Am. Soc. Artif. Intern. Organs* 30: 406–10.

Kannan, R.Y., H.J. Salacinski, P.E. Butler, G. Hamilton, and A.M. Seifalian. 2005. Current status of prosthetic bypass grafts: A review. *J. Biomed. Mater. Res.* 74B: 570–81.

Karnik, S.K., B.S. Brooke, A. Bayes-Genis, L. Sorensen, J.D. Wythe, et al. 2003. A critical role for elastin signaling in vascular morphogenesis and disease. *Development* 130: 411–23.

Kaushal, S., G.E. Amiel, K.J. Guleserian, O.M. Shapira, T. Perry, F.W. Sutherland, E. Rabkin, et al. 2001. Functional small-diameter neovessels created using endothelial progenitor cells expanded ex vivo. *Nat. Med.* 7: 1035–40.

Keeley, F.W., C.M. Bellingham, and K.A. Woodhouse. 2002. Elastin as a self-organizing biomaterial: Use of recombinantly expressed human elastin polypeptides as a model for investigations of structure and self-assembly of elastin. *Philos. Trans. R Soc. Lond. B Biol. Sci.* 357: 185–89.

Keller, J.D., J. Falk, H.S. Bjornson, E.B. Silberstein, and R.F. Kempczinski. 1988. Bacterial infectibility of chronically implanted endothelial cell seeded expanded polytetrafluoroethylene vascular grafts. *J. Vasc. Surg.* 7: 524–30.

Kenawy, E., G.L. Bowlin, K. Mansfield, J. Layman, D.G. Simpson, E.H. Sanders, et al. 2002. Release of tetracycline hydrochloride from electrospun poly(ethylene-*co*-vinylacetate), poly(lactic acid), and a blend. *J. Control Rel.* 81: 57–64.

Kidoaki, S., I.K. Kwon, and T. Matsuda. 2005. Mesoscopic spatial designs of nano- and microfiber meshes for tissue-engineering matrix and scaffold based on newly devised multilayering and mixing electrospinning techniques. *Biomaterials* 26: 37.

Kimura, H., Y. Sakata, H. Hamada, et al. 2000. *In vivo* retention of endothelial cells adenovirally transduced with tissue-type plasminogen activator and seeded onto expanded polytetrafluoroethylene. *J. Vasc. Surg.* 32: 353–63.

Kinner, B., J.M. Zaleskas, and M. Spector. 2002. Regulation of smooth muscle actin expression and contraction in adult human mesenchymal stem cells. *Exp. Cell Res.* 278: 72–83.

Koike, N., D. Fukumura, O. Gralla, P. Au, J.S. Schechner, and R.K. Jain. 2004. Creation of long-lasting blood vessels. *Nature* 428: 138–39.

Kotnis, R.A., M.M. Thompson, S.L. Eady, J.S. Budd, R.F. James, and P.R. Bell. 1995. Attachment, replication and thrombogenicity of genetically modified endothelial cells. *Eur. J. Vasc. Endovasc. Surg.* 9: 335–40.

Kowalewski, T.A., S. Blonski, and S. Barral. 2005. Experiments and modelling of electrospinning process. *Bull. Pol. Acad. Sci. Tech. Sci.* 53: 385.

Koyama, M., K. Satoh, H. Yoshida, S. Suzuki, H. Koie, and S. Takamatsu. 1996. Surface coverage of vascular grafts with cultured human endothelial cells from subcutaneous fat tissue obtained with a biopsy needle. *Thromb. Haemost.* 76: 610–4.

Kumbar, S.G., R. James, S.P. Nukavarapu, and C.T. Laurencin. 2008. Electrospun nanofiber scaffolds: Engineering soft tissues. *Biomed. Mater.* 3: 034002.

L'Heureux, N., N. Dusserre, Al. Marini, S. Garrido, L. de la Fuente, and T. McAllister. 2007. Technology insight: The evolution of tissue-engineered vascular grafts—From research to clinical practice. *Nat. Clin. Pract. Cardiovasc. Med.* 4: 389–95.

L'Heureux, N., S. Paquet, R. Labbe, L. Germain, and F.A. Auger. 1998. A completely biological tissue-engineered human blood vessel. *FASEB J.* 12: 47–56.

Laflamme, K., C.J. Roberge, J. Labonte, S. Pouliot, P. Dorleans-Juste, F.A. Auger, and L. Germain. 2005. Tissue-engineered human vascular media with a functional endothelin system. *Circulation* 111: 459.

Laflamme, K., C.J. Roberge, S. Pouliot, P. D'Orleans-Juste, F.A. Auger, and L. Germain. 2006. Tissue-engineered human vascular media produced *in vitro* by the self-assembly approach present functional properties similar to those of their native blood vessels. *Tiss. Eng.* 12: 2275.

Lee, J., C.W. Macosko, and D.W. Urry. 2001. Elastomeric polypentapeptides cross-linked into matrixes and fibers. *Biomacromolecules* 2(1): 170–79.

Levenberg, S., J.S. Golub, M. Amit, J. Itskovitz-Eldor, and R. Langer. 2002. Endothelial cells derived from human embryonic stem cells. *Proc. Natl. Acad. Sci.* 99: 4391–96.

Li, M., M.J. Mondrinos, M.R. Gandhi, F.K. Ko, A.S. Weiss, and P.I. Lelkes. 2005. Electrospun protein fibers as matrices for tissue engineering. *Biomaterials* 26: 5999–6008.

Li, M., M.J. Mondrinos, X. Chen, M.R. Gandhi, F.K. Ko, and P.I. Lelkes. 2006. Co-electrospun poly(lactide-co-glycolide), gelatin, and elastin blends for tissue engineering scaffolds. *J. Biomed. Mater. Res. Part A* 79A(4): 963–73.

Li, W.J., R.L. Mauck, and R.S. Tuan. 2005. Electrospun nanofibrous scaffolds: Production, characterization, and applications for tissue engineering and drug delivery. *J. Biomed. Nanotechnol.* 1(3): 259–75.

Li, W.J., C.T. Laurencin, E.J. Caterson, R.S. Tuan, and F.K. Ko. 2002. Electrospun nanofibrous structure: A novel scaffold for tissue engineering. *J. Biomed. Mater. Res. B* 60: 613.

Li, X.R., H. Zhang, H. Li, G.W. Tang, Y.H. Zhao, and X.Y. Yuan. 2008. Self-accelerated biodegradation of electrospun poly(ethylene glycol)-poly(L-lactide) membranes by loading proteinase k. *Polymer Degrad. Stabil.* 93(3): 618–26.

Lindblad, B., S.W. Wright, R.L. Sell, W.E. Burkel, L.M. Graham, and J.C. Stanley. 1987. Alternative techniques of seeding cultured endothelial cells to Eptfe grafts of different diameters, porosities, and surfaces. *J. Biomed. Mater. Res.* 21: 1013–22.

Liu, S.Q., C. Tieche, and P.K. Alkema. 2004. Neointima formation on vascular elastic laminae and collagen matrices scaffolds implanted in the rat aortae. *Biomaterials* 25: 1869–82.

Long, J.L. and R.T. Tranquillo. 2003. Elastic fiber production in cardiovascular tissue-equivalents. *Matrix Biol.* 22: 339–50.

Lu, Q., K. Ganesan, D.T. Simionescu, and N.R. Vyavahare. 2004. Novel porous aortic elastin and collagen scaffolds for tissue engineering. *Biomaterials* 25: 5227–37.

Luong-Van, E., L. Grondahl, K.N. Chua, K.W. Leong, V. Nurcombe, and S.M. Cool. 2006. Controlled release of heparin from poly(epsilon-caprolactone) electrospun fibers. *Biomaterials* 27(9): 2042–50.

Lutolf, M.P. and J.A. Hubbell. 2005. Synthetic biomaterials as instructive extracellular microenvironments for morphogenesis in tissue engineering. *Nat. Biotechnol.* 23: 47–55.

Ma, P.X. and R. Zhang. 1999. Synthetic nano-scale fibrous extracellular matrix. *J. Biomed. Mat. Res.* 46: 60–72.

Ma, Z., M. Kotaki, R. Inai, and S. Ramakrishna. 2005. Potential of nanofiber matrix as tissue-engineering scaffolds. *Tiss. Eng.* 11: 101–09.

Ma, Z., M. Kotaki, T. Yong, W. He, and S. Ramakrishna. 2005. Surface engineering of electrospun polyethylene terephthalate (Pet) nanofibers towards development of a new material for blood vessel engineering. *Biomaterials* 26: 2527–36.

MacNeill, B.D., I. Pomerantseva, H.C. Lowe, S.N. Oesterle, and J.P. Vacanti. 2002. Toward a new blood vessel. *Vascular Medicine* 7(3): 241–46.

Malkar, N.B., J. Lauer-Fields, D. Juska, and G.B. Fields. 2003. Characterization of peptide amphiphiles possessing cellular activation sequences. *Biomacromolecules.* 518–28.

Malone, J.M., K. Brendel, R.C. Duhamel, and R.L. Reinert. 1984. Detergent-extracted small-diameter vascular prostheses. *J. Vasc. Surg.* 181.

Maretschek, S., A. Greiner, and T. Kissel. 2008. Electrospun biodegradable nanofiber nonwovens for controlled release of proteins. *J. Control. Rel.* 127(2): 180–87.

Martins, A., J.V. Araújo, R.L. Reis, and N.M. Neves. 2007. Electrospun nanostructured scaffolds for tissue engineering applications. *Nanomedicine* 2: 929–42.

Matthews, J.A., G.E. Wnek, D.G. Simpson, and G.L. Bowlin. 2002. Electrospinning of collagen nanofibers. *Biomacromolecules* 3: 232.

McKee, J.A., S.S.R. Banik, M.J. Boyer, N.M. Hamad, J.H. Lawson, L.E. Niklason, et al. 2003. Human arteries engineered *in vitro*. *EMBO Rep.* 4: 633–38.

Miller, D.C., K.M. Haberstroh, and T.J. Webster. 2005. Mechanism(S) of increased vascular cell adhesion on nanostructured poly(lactic-*co*-glycolic) acid films. *J. Biomed. Mater. Res.* 73A: 476–84.

Miller, D.C., K.M. Haberstroh, and T.J. Webster. 2007. Plga nanometer surface features manipulate fibronectin interactions for improved vascular cell adhesion. *J. Biomed. Mater. Res.* 81A(3): 678–84.

Miller, D.C., T.J. Webster, and V. Hasirci. 2004. Technological advances in nanoscale biomaterials: The future of synthetic vascular graft design. *Expert. Rev. Med. Devices* 1: 259–68.

Mironov, V., V. Kasyanovand, and R.R. Markwald. 2008. Nanotechnology in vascular tissue engineering: From nanoscaffolding towards rapid vessel biofabrication. *Trends Biotechnol.* 26(6): 338–44.

Mitchell, S.L. and L.E. Niklason. 2003. Requirements for growing tissue-engineered vascular grafts. *Cardiovasc. Pathol.* 12: 59–64.

Mithieux, S.M., J.E. Rasko, and A.S. Weiss. 2004. Synthetic elastin hydrogels derived from massive elastic assemblies of self-organized human protein monomers. *Biomaterials* 25: 4921–27.

Mo, X.M. and H.J. Weber. 2004. Electrospinning P(Lla-Cl) Nanofiber: A tubular scaffold fabrication with circumferential alignment. *Macromol. Symposia.* 217: 413–16.

Mo, X.M., C.Y. Xu, M. Kotaki, and S. Ramakrishna. 2004. Electrospun P(Lla-Cl) nanofiber: A biomimetic extracellular matrix for smooth muscle cell and endothelial cell proliferation. *Biomaterials* 25(10): 1883–90.

Moeen, A., Y. Tintut, and L.L. Demer. 2004. Mesenchymal stem cells and the artery wall. *Circ. Res.* 95: 671–76.

Moghe, A.K. and B.S. Gupta. 2008. Co-axial electrospinning for nanofiber structures: Preparation and applications. *Polymer Rev.* 48(2): 353–77.

Murabayashi, S., H. Kambic, H. Harasaki, T. Morimoto, R. Yozu, and Y. Nose. 1985. Fabrication and long-term implantation of semi-compliant small vascular prosthesis. *Trans. Am. Soc. Artif. Intern. Organs.* 31: 50–54.

Nagapudi, K., W.T. Brinkman, J.E. Leisen, L. Huang, R.A. McMillan, R.P. Apkarian, et al. 2002. Photomediated solid-state cross-linking of an elastin-mimetic recombinant protein polymer. *Macromolecules* 35: 1730–37.

Nagapudi, K., W.T. Brinkman, B.S. Thomas, J.O. Park, M. Srinivasarao, E. Wright, V.P. Conticello, and E.L. Chaikof. 2005. Viscoelastic and mechanical behavior of recombinant protein elastomers. *Biomaterials* 26(23): 4695–706.

Nain, A.S., C. Amon, and M. Sitti. 2006. Proximal probes based nanorobotic drawing of polymer micro/nanofibers. *Nanotechnology, IEEE Transactions on* 5: 499–510.

Nain, A.S., J.C. Wong, C. Amon, and M. Sitti. 2006. Drawing suspended polymer micro-/nanofibers using glass micropipettes. *Appl. Phys. Lett.* 89: 183105–3.

Nam, Y. and T. Park. 1999. Porous biodegradable polymeric scaffolds prepared by thermally induced phase separation. *J. Biomed. Mater. Res.* 47(1): 8–17.

Niklason, L.E., J. Gao, W.M. Abbott, K.K. Hirschi, S. Houser, R. Marini, and R. Langer. 1999. Functional arteries grown *in vitro*. *Science* 284: 489–93.

Oswald, J., S. Boxberger, B. Jorgensen, S. Feldmann, G. Ehninger, M. Bornhauser, and C. Werner. 2004. Mesenchymal stem cells can be differentiated into endothelial cells *in vitro*. *Stem Cells* 22(3): 377–84.

Pasic, M., W. Muller-Glauser, B. Odermatt, M. Lachat, B. Seifert, and M. Turina. 1995. Seeding with omental cells prevents late neointimal hyperplasia in small-diameter dacron grafts. *Circulation* 92: 2605–16.

Patel, A., B. Fine, M. Sandig, and K. Mequanint. 2006. Elastin biosynthesis: The missing link in tissue-engineered blood vessels. *Cardiovasc. Res.* 71(1): 40–49.

Pearce, W.H., R.B. Rutherford, T.A. Whitehill, et al. 1987. Successful endothelial seeding with omentally derived microvascular endothelial cells. *J. Vasc. Surg.* 5: 203–6.

Pham, Q.P., U. Sharma, and A.G. Mikos. 2006. Electrospinning of polymeric nanofibers for tissue engineering applications: A review. *Tissue Engineering* 12(5): 1197–211.

Pittenger, M.F. and B.J. Martin. 2004. Mesenchymal stem cells and their potential as cardiac therapeutics. *Circ. Res.* 95: 9–20.

Riha, G.M., P.H. Lin, A.B. Lumsden, Q. Yao, and C. Chen. 2005. Application of stem cells for vascular tissue engineering. *Tissue Eng.* 11: 1535.

Rincon, A.C., I.T. Molina-Martinez, H.B. de Las, M. Alonso, C. Bailez, J.C. Rodriguez-Cabello, et al. 2006. Biocompatibility of elastin-like polymer poly(Vpavg) microparticles: *In vitro* and *in vivo* studies. *J. Biomed. Mater. Res. A* 78: 343–51.

Rosenman, J.E., R.F. Kempczinski, Y. Berlatzky, W.H. Pearce, G.R. Ramalanjaona, and H.S. Bjornson. 1985. Bacterial adherence to endothelial-seeded polytetrafluoroethylene grafts. *Surgery* 98: 816–23.

Rosenman, J.E., R.F. Kempczinski, W.H. Pearce, and E.B. Silberstein. 1985. Kinetics of endothelial cell seeding. *J. Vasc. Surg.* 2: 778–84.

Rubens, F.D., R.S. Labow, E. Meek, A.K. Dudani, and P.R. Ganz. 1997. Tissue factor expression by cells used for sodding of prosthetic vascular grafts. *J. Surg. Res.* 72: 22–28.

Rupnick, M.A., F.A. Hubbard, K. Pratt, B.E. Jarrell, and S.K. Williams. 1989. Endothelialization of vascular prosthetic surfaces after seeding or sodding with human microvascular endothelial cells. *J. Vasc. Surg.* 9: 788–95.

Sackman, J.E., M.B. Freeman, M.G. Petersen, Z. Allebban, G.P. Niemeyer, and C.D. Lothrop. 1995. Synthetic vascular grafts seeded with genetically modified endothelium in the dog: Evaluation of the effect of seeding technique and retroviral vector on cell persistence *in vivo*. *Cell Transplant.* 4: 219–35.

Salacinski, H.J., G. Punshon, B. Krijgsman, G. Hamilton, and A.M. Seifalian. 2001. A hybrid compliant vascular graft seeded with microvascular endothelial cells extracted from human omentum. *Artif. Organs.* 25: 974–82.

Salacinski, H.J., A. Tiwari, G. Hamilton, and A.M. Seifalian. 2001. Cellular engineering of vascular bypass grafts: Role of chemical coatings for enhancing endothelial cell attachment. *Med. Biol. Eng. Comput.* 39: 609–18.

Sarkar, S., T. Schmitz-Rixen, G. Hamilton, and A.M. Seifalian. 2007. Achieving the ideal properties for vascular bypass grafts using a tissue engineered approach: A review. *Med. Biol. Eng. Comput.* 45: 327–36.

Sauvage, L., K. Berger, S. Wood, Y. Nakagawa, and P. Mansfield. 1971. An external velour surface for porous arterial prostheses. *Surgery* 70(6): 940–53.

Seeger, J.M. and N. Klingman. 1985. Improved endothelial cell seeding with cultured cells and fibronectin-coated grafts. *J. Surg. Res.* 38: 641–7.

Sekiya, I., B.L. Larson, J.R. Smith, R. Pochampally, J. Cui, and D.J. Prockop. 2002. Expansion of human adult stem cells from bone marrow stroma: Conditions that maximize the yields of early progenitors and evaluate their quality. *Stem Cells* 20: 530–41.

Shi, Q., S. Rafii, M. Wu, E.S. Wijelath, A. Ishida, Y. Fujita, S. Kothari, et al. 1998. Evidence for circulating bone marrow-derived endothelial cells. *Blood* 92: 362–67.

Sill, T.J. and H.A. von Recum. 2008. Electrospinning: Applications in drug delivery and tissue engineering. *Biomaterials* 29(13): 1989–2006.

Silva, G.A., C. Czeisler, K.L. Niece, E. Beniash, D.A. Harrington, J.A. Kessler, and S.I. Stupp. 2004. Selective differentiation of neural progenitor cells by high-epitope density nanofibers *Science* 303(5662): 1352–55.

Smith, L.A. and P.X. Ma. 2004. Nano-fibrous scaffolds for tissue engineering. *Colloids Surf. B Biointerfaces* 39: 125.

Snow, A.D., R.P. Bolender, T.N. Wight, and A.W. Clowes. 1990. Heparin modulates the composition of the extracellular matrix domain surrounding arterial smooth muscle cells. *Am. J. Pathol.* 137(2): 313–30.

Stanley, J.C., W.E. Burkel, L.M. Graham, and B. Lindblad. 1985. Endothelial cell seeding of synthetic vascular prostheses. *Acta. Chir. Scand. Suppl.* 529: 17–27.

Stansby, G., C. Berwanger, N. Shukla, T. Schmitz-Rixen, and G. Hamilton. 1994. Endothelial seeding of compliant polyurethane vascular graft material. *Br. J. Surg.* 81: 1286–9.

Stansby, G., N. Shukla, B. Fuller, and G. Hamilton. 1991. Seeding of human microvascular endothelial cells onto polytetrafluoroethylene graft material. *Br. J. Surg.* 78: 1189–92.

Stansby, G., N. Shukla, B. Fuller, and G. Hamilton. 1991. Seeding of human microvascular endothelial cells onto polytetrafluoroethylene graft, and material. *Br. J. Surg.* 78(10): 1189–92.

Stegemann, J.P., S.N. Kaszuba, and S.L. Rowe. 2007. Review: Advances in vascular tissue engineering using protein-based biomaterials. *Tiss. Eng.* 13: 2601–13.

Stegemann, J.P. and R.M. Nerem. 2003. Phenotype modulation in vascular tissue engineering using biochemical and mechanical stimulation. *Ann. Biomed. Eng.* 31: 391–402.

Sterpetti, A.V., W.J. Hunter, R.D. Schultz, et al. 1988. Seeding with endothelial cells derived from the microvessels of the omentum and from the jugular vein: A comparative study. *J. Vasc. Surg.* 7: 677–84.

Stewart, S.F. and D.J. Lyman. 1992. Effects of a vascular graft/natural artery compliance mismatch on pulsatile flow. *J. Biomech.* 25: 297–310.

Stitzel, J., J. Liu, S.J. Lee, M. Komura, J. Berry, S. Soker, et al. 2006. Controlled fabrication of a biological vascular substitute. *Biomaterials* 27: 1088–94.

Sun, Z., E. Zussman, A. Yarin, et al. 2003. Compound core-shell polymer nanofibers by electrospinning. *Adv. Mater.* 15: 1929.

Tang, Y., Q. Zhao, X. Qin, L. Shen, L. Cheng, J. Ge, and M.I. Phillips. 2005. Paracrine action enhances the effects of autologous mesenchymal stem cell transplantation on vascular regeneration in rat model of myocardial infarction. *Ann. Thorac. Surg.* 80: 229–37.

Tannenbaum, G., T. Ahlborn, A. Benvenisty, K. Reemtsma, and R. Nowygrod. 1987. High-density seeding of cultured endothelial cells leads to rapid coverage of polytetrafluoroethylene grafts. *Curr. Surg.* 44: 318–21.

Tao, S.L. and T.A. Desai. 2007. Aligned arrays of biodegradable poly(epsilon-caprolactone) nanowires and nanofibers by template synthesis. *Nano Letters* 7: 1463–8.

Taylor, P.R., J.H. Wolfe, M.R. Tyrrell, A.O. Mansfield, A.N. Nicolaides, and R.E. Houston. 1990. Graft stenosis: Justification for 1-year surveillance. *Br. J. Surg.* 77(10): 1125–8.

Thie, M., W. Schlumberger, R. Semich, J. Rauterberg, and H. Robenek. 1991. Aortic smooth muscle cells in collagen lattice culture: Effects on ultrastructure, prolifaration and collagen synthesis. *Eur. J. Cell. Biol.* 55: 295–304.

Thomson, J.A., J. Itskovitz-Eldor, S.S. Shapiro, M.A. Waknitz, J.J. Swiergiel, V.S. Marshall, and J.M. Jones. 1998. Embryonic stem cell lines derived from human blastocysts. *Science* 282: 1145–47.

Tiwari, A., A. Kidane, G. Punshon, G. Hamilton, and A.M. Seifalian. 2003. Extraction of cells for single-stage seeding of vascular-bypass grafts. *Biotechnol. Appl. Biochem.* 38: 35–41.

Tiwari, A., A. Kidane, H. Salacinski, G. Punshon, G. Hamilton, and A.M. Seifalian. 2003. Improving endothelial cell retention for single stage seeding of prosthetic grafts: Use of polymer sequences of arginineglycine-aspartate. *Eur. J. Vasc. Endovasc. Surg.* 25: 325–9.

Townsend-Nicholson, A. and S.N. Jayasinghe. 2006. Cell electrospinning: A unique biotechnique for encapsulating living organisms for generating active biological microthreads/scaffolds. *Biomacromolecules* 7: 3364–69.

Uchida, N., H. Kambic, H. Emoto, J.F. Chen, S. Hsu, S. Murabayshi, et al. 1993. Compliance effects on small diameter polyurethane graft patency. *J. Biomed. Mater. Res.* 27(10): 1269–79.

Valgimigli, M., E. Merli, P. Malagutti, O. Soukhomovskaia, G. Cicchitelli, G. Macrà, and R. Ferrari. 2003. Endothelial dysfunction in acute and chronic coronary syndromes: Evidence for a pathogenetic role of oxidative stress. *Arch. Biochem. Biophys.* 420: 255–61.

Van Belle, E., B. Witzenbichler, D. Chen, et al. 1998. Potentiated angiogenic effect of scatter factor/hepatocyte growth factor via induction of vascular endothelial growth factor: The case for paracrine amplification of angiogenesis. *Circulation* 97: 381–90.

van der Lei, B., C. Wildevuur, F. Dijk, E. Blaauw, I. Molenaar, and P. Nieuwenhuis. 1987. Sequential studies of arterial wall regeneration in microporous, compliant, biodegradable small-caliber vascular grafts in rats. *J. Thorac. Cardiovasc. Surg.* 93(5): 695–707.

Vasita, R. and D.S. Katti. 2006. Nanofibers and their applications in tissue engineering. *Int. J. Nanomedicine* 1: 15–30.

Venugopal, J. and S. Ramakrishna. 2005. Applications of polymer nanofibers in biomedicine and biotechnology. *Appl. Biochem. Biotechnol.* 125: 147–58.

Vohra, R.K., G.J. Thompson, H. Sharma, H.M. Carr, and M.G. Walker. 1990. Fibronectin coating of expanded polytetrafluoroethylene (Eptfe) grafts and its role in endothelial seeding. *Artif. Organs.* 14: 41–5.

Walter, D.H., M. Cejna, L. Diaz-Sandoval, S. Willis, L. Kirkwood, P.W. Stratford, et al. 2004. Local gene transfer of Phvegf-2 plasmid by gene-eluting stents: An alternative strategy for inhibition of restenosis. *Circulation* 110: 36–45.

Wang, C.-H., W.-J. Cherng, N.-I. Yang, L.-T. Kuo, C.-M. Hsu, H.-I. Yeh, Y.-J. Lan, C.-H. Yeh, and W.L. Stanford. 2008. Late-outgrowth endothelial cells attenuate intimal hyperplasia contributed by mesenchymal stem cells after vascular injury. *Arterioscler Thromb. Vasc. Biol.* 28: 54–60.

Watanabe, Y.D.H. 1997. Vascular permeability factor/vascular endothelial growth factor inhibits anchorage-disruption-induced apoptosis in microvessel endothelial cells by inducing scaffold formation. *Exp. Cell Res.* 233: 340–9.

Whitesides, G.M. J.P. Mathias, and C.T. Seto. 1991. Molecular self-assembly and nanochemistry: A chemical strategy for the synthesis of nanostructures. *Science* 254: 1312–19.

Whitesides, G.M., and B. Grzybowski. 2002. Self-assembly at all scales. *Science* 295: 2418–21.

Williams, S.K., B.E. Jarrell, D.G. Rose, J. Pontell, B.A. Kapelan, P.K. Park, and T.L. Carter. 1989. Human microvessel endothelial cell isolation and vascular graft sodding in the operating room. *Ann. Vasc. Surg.* 3: 5096.

Williams, S.K., T. Carter, P.K. Park, D.G. Rose, T. Schneider, and B.E. Jarrell. 1992. Formation of a multilayer cellular lining on a polyurethane vascular graft following endothelial cell sodding. *J. Biomed. Mater. Res.* 26(1): 103–17.

Wizeman, W. and P. Kofinas. 2001. Molecularly imprinted polymer hydrogels displaying isomerically resolved glucose binding. *Biomaterials* 22: 1485–91.

Woo, K.M., V.J. Chen, and P.X. Ma. 2003. Nano-fibrous scaffolding architecture selectively enhances protein adsorption contributing to cell attachment. *J. Biomed. Mater. Res.* 67A(2): 531–37.

Xu, C., R. Inai, M. Kotaki, and S. Ramakrishna. 2004. Electrospun nanofiber fabrication as synthetic extracellular matrix and its potential for vascular tissue engineering. *Tiss. Eng.* 10: 1160.

Xu, C.Y., R. Inai, M. Kotaki, and S. Ramakrishna. 2004. Aligned biodegradable nanofibrous structure: A potential scaffold for blood vessel engineering. *Biomaterials* 25(5): 877–86.

Xu, X.L., X.L. Zhuang, X.S. Chen, X.R. Wang, L.X. Yang, and X.B. Jing. 2006. Preparation of core-sheath composite nanofibers by emulsion electrospinning. *Macromol. Rapid Commun.* 27(19): 1637–42.

Yamada, K.M. 1991. Adhesive recognition sequences. *J. Biol. Chem.* 266: 12809.

Yamashita, J., H. Itoh, M. Hirashima, M. Ogawa, S. Nishikawa, T. Yurugi, M. Naito, K. Nakao, and S. Nishikawa. 2000. Flk1-positive cells derived from embryonic stem cells serve as vascular progenitors. *Nature* 408: 92–96.

Yang, Y., X.H. Li, M.B. Qi, S.B. Zhou, and J. Weng. 2008. Release pattern and structural integrity of lysozyme encapsulated in core-sheath structured poly(DL-lactide) ultrafine fibers prepared by emulsion electrospinning. *Eur. J. Pharmaceut. Biopharmaceut.* 69(1): 106–16.

Yarin, A.L., S. Koombhongse, and D.H. Reneker. 2001. Bending instability in electrospinning of nanofibers. *J. Appl. Phys.* 89(5): 3018–26.

Yim, E.K. and K.W. Leong. 2005. Significance of synthetic nanostructures in dictating cellular response. *Nanomedicine* 1: 10–21.

Yu, Y., P. Berndt, M. Tirrell, and G.B. Fields. 1996. Self-assembling amphiphiles for construction of protein molecular architecture. *J. Am. Chem. Soc.* 118: 12515–20.

Yu, Y., V. Roontga, V.A. Daragan, K.H. Mayo, M. Tirrell, and G.B. Fields. 1999. Structure and dynamics of peptide amphiphiles incorporating triple-helical protein-like molecular architecture. *Biochemistry* 38: 1659–68.

Yu, Y., M. Tirrell, and G.B. Fields. 1998. Minimal lipidation stabilizes protein-like molecular architecture. *J. Am. Chem. Soc.* 120: 9979–87.

Zarge, J.I., C. Gosselin, P. Huang, D.A. Vorp, D.A. Severyn, and H.P. Greisler. 1997. Platelet deposition on Eptfe grafts coated with fibrin glue with or without Fgf-1 and heparin. *J. Surg. Res.* 67: 4–8.

Zarge, J.I., P. Huang, V. Husak, et al. 1997. Fibrin glue containing fibroblast growth factor type 1 and heparin with autologous endothelial cells reduces intimal hyperplasia in a canine carotid artery balloon injury model. *J. Vasc. Surg.* 25: 840–8.

Zeng, J., A. Aigner, F. Czubayko, et al. 2005. Poly(vinyl alcohol) nanofibers by electrospinning as a protein delivery system and the retardation of enzyme release by additional polymer coatings. *Biomacromolecules* 6: 1484.

Zeng, J., X. Xu, X. Chen, Q. Liang, X. Bian, L. Yang, and X. Jing. 2003. Biodegradable electrospun fibers for drug delivery. *J. Control. Rel.* 92(3): 227–31.

Zhang, R. and P.X. Ma. 2000. Synthetic nano-fibrillar extracellular matrices with predesigned macroporous architectures. *J. Biomed. Mater. Res.* 52: 430–38.

Zhang, S. 2003. Fabrication of novel biomaterials through molecular self-assembly. *Nat. Biotechnol.* 21: 1171–78.

Zhang, Y., C.T. Lim, M. Ramakrishna, and Z.M. Huang. 2005. Recent development of polymer nanofibers for biomedical and biotechnological application. *J. Mater. Sci: Mater. Med.* 16: 933–46.

Zhang, Y., H. Ouyang, C.T. Lim, S. Ramakrishna, and Z.M. Huang. 2005. Electrospinning of gelatin fibers and gelatin/Pcl composite fibrous scaffolds. *J. Biomed. Mater. Res. B* 72: 156.

Zhang, Y.Z., C.T. Lim, S. Ramakrishna, and Z.M. Huang. 2005. Recent development of polymer nanofibers for biomedical and biotechnological applications. *J. Mater. Sci-Mater. Med.* 16(10): 933–46.

Zhang, Y.Z., X. Wang, Y. Feng, J. Li, C.T. Lim, and S. Ramakrishna. 2006. Coaxial electrospinning of (fluorescein isothiocyanate-conjugated bovine serum albumin)-encapsulated poly(epsilon-caprolactone) nanofibers for sustained release. *Biomacromolecules* 7(4): 1049–57.

Zhang, Y.Z., Y. Feng, et al. 2006. Fabrication of porous electrospun nanofibers. *Nanotechnology, IEEE Trans.* 17: 901–8.

Zhang, Y.Z., B. Su, J. Venugopal, S. Ramakrishna, and C.T. Lim. 2007. Biomimetic and bioactive nanofibrous scaffolds from electrospun composite nanofibers. *Int. J. Nanomed.* 2: 623–38.

Zhang, Z., Z. Wang, S. Liu, and M. Kodama. 2003. Pore size, tissue ingrowth, and endothelialization of small diameter microporous polyurethane vascular prostheses. *Biomaterials* 25: 177–87.

Zilla, P., R. Fasol, M. Grimm, et al. 1991. Growth properties of cultured human endothelial cells on differently coated artificial heart materials. *J. Thorac. Cardiovasc. Surg.* 101: 671–80.

Zilla, P., R. Fasol, P. Preiss, et al. 1989. Use of fibrin glue as a substrate for *in vitro* endothelialization of Ptfe vascular grafts. *Surgery* 105: 515–22.

Zilla, P., D. Bezuidenhout, and P. Human. 2007. Prosthetic vascular grafts: Wrong models, wrong questions and no healing. *Biomaterials* 28(34): 5009–27.

13

Engineering Soft Nanostructures for Guided Cell Response

Matt J. Kipper
Colorado State University

Jorge L. Almodóvar
Colorado State University

13.1 Biological Soft Nanostructures

Tissue engineering involves applying the principles of engineering and life sciences toward the development of biological replacements that restore, maintain, or improve tissue function. Investigators have attempted to engineer many mammalian tissues using a variety of approaches. Broadly, these can be classified as *in vitro* approaches and *in vivo* approaches. In the former approaches, cells are cultured on a scaffold *in vitro*, where they form functional tissue for future transplantation. In the latter approaches, scaffolds are designed such that after implantation they recruit native tissue cells that are guided to create new tissue or enhance wound healing. In both approaches, it has been demonstrated that cells respond to a vast array of cues provided by scaffolds and culture conditions, including chemical, biochemical, electrical, mechanical, and topographical stimuli. Thus, in order to achieve predictable cell responses, materials for tissue engineering are often engineered to mimic the structure and properties of natural tissue, both at their surfaces and in the bulk. Surface properties that dictate the interactions between the material and its environment, where the environment consists of cells and important biomolecules, are by nature nanoscale properties. Bulk properties are also dependent on the nanoscale organization of materials. This is because natural tissues are designed and assembled in controlled ways, at a hierarchy of length scales ranging from the macroscale to the nanoscale.

Cartilage serves as a perfect example to demonstrate the hierarchy of tissue structure across multiple length scales (see Figure 13.1). On the macroscopic scale, articular cartilage can be described as a tissue. On the microscopic scale, one observes the organization of a material sparsely populated with cells (chondrocytes) and a relatively small amount of blood vessels. Here, the extracellular matrix (ECM) is organized to contain fibrous structural components in a fluid phase. At the nanoscale, the molecules which make up the ECM are organized into complex nanoassemblies. The ECM in cartilage mostly consists of collagen, but many other proteins and polysaccharides are present, which form a complex nanoscale matrix that controls both mechanical properties and cell behavior (Figure 13.1). The protein collagen forms a triple helix with nanometer dimensions. Many of these helices assemble to form long

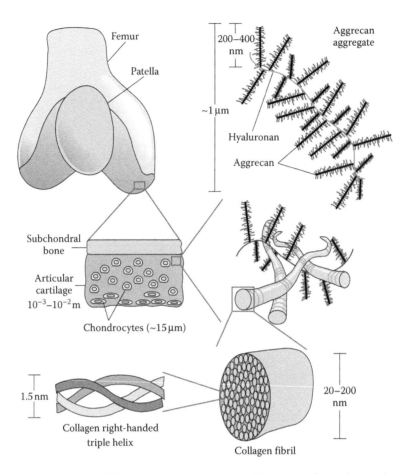

FIGURE 13.1   **(See color insert following page 10-24.)** Structural hierarchy of articular cartilage. In the macroscale, articular cartilage spans about 0.5–15 cm. On the microscale, chondrocytes (around 15 μm in diameter)
are the main components in articular cartilage. On the nanoscale, cartilage is composed of ECM proteoglycan
aggregates embedded within collagen fibers. (Adapted from Mow, V. C., A. Ratcliffe, and A. R. Poole. 1992.
Biomaterials 13(2): 67–97. Copyright 1991, Elsevier. With permission.)

fibrils with diameters ranging from about 20 to 200 nm. These complex nanoassemblies provide tensile
strength to connective tissues. The alignment of fibers can result in anisotropic mechanical properties
appropriate for the particular biomechanics of the tissue in question. Compressive strength and tribo-
logical prosperities are imparted to tissues like cartilage through another soft nanoassembly—the
aggrecan aggregate. Aggrecan is a proteoglycan that carries about 100 highly sulfated polysaccharide
chains (chondroitin sulfate and keratan sulfate). The very high negative charge density results in electrostatic repulsion causing the aggrecan to adopt a rigid bottle-brush conformation in solution, several tens
of nanometers in diameter and 200–400 nm in length. Many aggrecans bind to another polysaccharide,
hyaluronic acid, to form a complex nanoassembly called the aggrecan aggregate in cartilage and other
tissues (Figure 13.1). This dense, rigid nanoassembly with high negative charge density imparts a high
osmotic pressure to the tissues in which it is found providing compressive strength. Polysaccharide
containing assemblies such as the aggrecan aggregate also facilitate the assembly of collagen fibrils and
protect them from biochemical modes of degradation.

    The hierarchical arrangement of materials at multiple length scales illustrated by the cartilage is one
of the hallmarks of what condensed matter physicists refer to as "soft materials." Soft materials generally

have relatively high molecular kinetic energy and relatively low intermolecular bonding energy compared to "hard materials." This combination allows them to explore the configurational space necessary to find local free energy minima that result in self-assembly into hierarchical structures over multiple length scales. These structures are then stabilized by the multiplicity of relatively weak forces whose combined effect holds the structure together, while still allowing local structural changes. As soft materials are characterized by a variety of molecular interactions with different energies and dynamics, their multiscale organization results in physical properties that may vary with the length scales and timescales of experiments. This feature of soft materials is also exhibited by cartilage, as illustrated in Figure 13.2, where its elastic modulus is a function of the loading rate over physiologically relevant ranges.

The relatively weak attractive interactions that stabilize structures in soft materials are often Van der Waals interactions, which arise from the Coulombic forces between permanent and/or inducible dipoles (dipole–dipole, dipole–induced dipole, and induced dipole–induced dipole). In aqueous solutions in particular, hydrogen bonds and electrostatic forces between formally charged groups can also become very important. These typically have higher energies than the Van der Waals interactions. The typical lipid bilayers that compartmentalize cells and intracellular structures and organize membrane-associated proteins exemplify how these forces combine to result in a soft nanoscale assembly. The hydrophobic core of the lipid bilayers is dominated by Van der Waals interactions, while at the surfaces ion–dipole, ion–ion, and hydrogen bond interactions dominate. Differences in the packing density in these two regions tend to frustrate the structure of lipid bilayers, potentially introducing additional fluidity.

The nanoscale organization of the soft materials illustrated by the biological examples discussed above suggests that the design of biomaterials for the repair and/or regeneration of mammalian tissue by mimicking tissue properties require that materials be engineered from the nanoscale up. In many cases, this can be done by judicious manipulation of the noncovalent interactions that govern soft material interactions and assembly. Such approaches can be described as "bottom-up" assembly. In

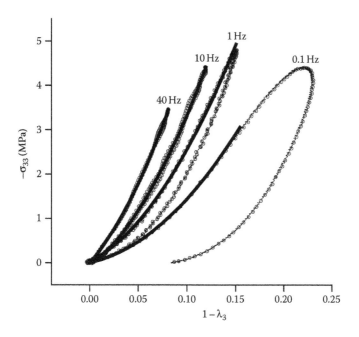

FIGURE 13.2 Stress–strain response for bovine articular cartilage at various loading frequencies. (Reprinted from Park, S., C. T. Hung, and G. A. Ateshian. 2004. *Osteoarthritis and Cartilage* 12(1): 65–73. Copyright 2004, Elsevier. With permission.)

other cases, "top-down" approaches are used to introduce nanoscale features into materials that do not otherwise form nanostructures. This chapter focuses on nanoscale soft materials in mammalian tissues and recent research efforts in manipulating nanoscale properties of soft materials to guide cell and tissue responses. We begin with a brief description of the nanoscale organization of the ECM, followed by a review of the current understanding of cell response to nanoscale features of soft biomaterials, and the techniques used to tailor biomaterials at the nanometer scale.

13.2   Nanoscale Features of the Extracellular Matrix (ECM)

Cells, which are 10–100 μm in diameter, respond differently to topographical features from the macro down to the molecular size. At the very low end of this range (a few nanometers), features such as proteins, polysaccharides, and small protein complexes are found. Proteoglycans, enzymes, cadherins, growth factors, and other proteins have dimensions on the nanometer scale, and are all crucial determinants of cell response to materials. At larger length scales (tens to hundreds of nanometers) these components are organized into more complex assemblies that decorate cell surfaces and form the structural building blocks of the ECM in tissues. Many of these biomolecules can be isolated or produced via biomolecular techniques which can then be used for biomaterials. By tailoring the interactions that govern the organization of these building blocks, biomaterial scientists have the opportunity to explore how the nanoscale structure and organization of these biologically derived materials influences their biochemical and biomechanical functions.

The ECM is the material underlying the epithilia and endothelia, and surrounds all connective tissue cells providing mechanical support and strength to the tissue. The ECM not only provides mechanical support to cells, but also influences their behavior (e.g., adhesion, spreading, migration, and differentiation). The components of the ECM also have important biochemical activity, and can play major roles in growth factor signaling, by sequestering, releasing, and activating growth factors. Thus, the composition of the ECM strongly affects stem cell differentiation and the maintenance of healthy tissue. The ECM is composed of a variety of molecules depending upon the organism and tissue. Connective tissues in mammals have an ECM with fibers composed of mostly the proteins collagen and elastin, and soluble molecules including glycosaminoglycans (GAGs) and proteins (Table 13.1).

Naturally derived polymers found in the ECM, such as proteins and GAGs, are attractive biomaterials, due to their biological, mechanical, and physical properties. Many of these materials are soluble in aqueous solutions, avoiding the need of organic solvents that are often required to process synthetic polymers. Many of these biopolymers also act as polyelectrolytes. Their polyelectrolyte properties can be exploited in the assembly of nanostructured materials by using their water solubility and electrostatic

TABLE 13.1   Components of the ECM along with Their Relative Native Size and Structure

Molecule	Size
Collagen	Fibrillar protein approximately 300 nm in length and 1.4 nm in diameter, organized into larger fibrils and fibers
Aggrecan	Bottlebrush proteoglycan with a length of 400 nm and a radius between 20 and 60 nm
Elastin	Fibrillar protein approximately 10–20 nm in diameter
Fibronectin	Rod-like protein approximately 60 nm long and 2.5 nm wide
Hyaluronic acid	Stiff random coil with radius of gyration about 200 nm
Heparan sulfate	Extended helical structure with 40–160 nm in length
Chondroitin sulfate	Semiflexible coil with intrinsic persistence length in the range of 4.5–5.5 nm
Growth factors (e.g., BMP-2)	BMP-2 is a globular protein $7 \times 3.5 \times 3$ nm in size

interactions to tune nanoscale assembly. As naturally derived polymers have biochemical function, their successful incorporation into engineered ECM provides a bioactive material for the guidance of cell responses.

Proteins are biological polymers composed of amino acids which define their structure and function. Collagen, gelatin (denatured collagen), elastin, and fibrinogen, among others are ECM proteins that form structural networks, and can also be fabricated into biomaterials with nanoscale structure. Collagens are a class of glycoproteins consisting of at least 19 genetically distinct types and are the most abundant protein in mammals, accounting for 20–30% of the total protein content. Collagens type-I, type-II, and type-III are the most abundant fibril-forming molecules in mammalian tissue. They are a primary structural component of the ECM of many tissues, and are an essential building block in the musculoskeletal system. They are synthesized intracellularly as large precursor procollagens forming a continuous triple helix (Figure 13.1). This triple helix is approximately 300 nm in length and 1.5 nm in diameter. This triple helix structure assembles into fibrils tens of nanometers in diameter. In some tissues, these fibrils further assemble into larger fibers. Collagens can be easily isolated for the construction of nanostructured biomaterials. Collagen sponges, nanoparticles, nanofibers, ultra thin films, and hydrogels have been constructed as wound dressings, for the repair of tendon and cartilage, and for studying cell response to nanomaterials. Collagen constructs support mammalian cell growth and are biodegradable. Elastin is a major protein component of lung and vascular tissue responsible for their elastic properties. Elastin is found naturally in the form of fibers approximately 10–20 nm in diameter. It has been used in coatings for vascular grafts, due to its minimal interactions with platelets. Fibrinogen is a fibrous protein that polymerizes to form fibrin–the primary structural component of blood clots. Fibrin forms the structure which supports the early stages of the wound-healing process, and is therefore supportive of key cellular functions during tissue repair. Fibrin is one of the earliest biopolymers used as a biomaterial, due to its biodegradability and injectability. Aside from structural applications, proteins are crucial in modulating cell behavior. Growth factors comprise several protein families, present in every mammalian tissue, and influence cell adhesion, recruitment, proliferation, differentiation, and apoptosis.

Polysaccharides are polymeric carbohydrate structures typically composed of repeating units of mono- or di-saccharides bonded via glycosidic bonds. Polysaccharides widely used as biomaterials include those from nonmammalian sources, such as cellulose, chitosan, chitin, alginate, and dextran. They also include GAGs, often from mammalian tissues, such as heparin, heparan sulfate, hyaluronic acid, chondroitin sulfate, and keratan sulfate. Chitin and chitosan behave as polycations, while alginate and the GAGs behave as polyanions. In fact, heparin, which carries a high number of substituent sulfate groups, has the highest negative charge density of any biological macromolecule. Chitosan is a GAG-like weak polycation derived from the *N*-deacetylation of chitin, the most abundant naturally occurring polysaccharide. Chitosan has been widely used in both the packaging industry and the construction of vascular grafts, due to its antimicrobial activity. Chitosan supports mammalian cell growth and is also an attractive material for wound-healing applications. The GAGs are usually obtained from animal tissues, where their biological functions range from potentiation of enzyme activity in the blood coagulation cascade to influencing the biomechanics of joint tissues. Heparin is used therapeutically as an antithrombotic drug. Heparin and other GAGs also influence the activities of growth factors by binding them in the ECM, sequestering them, stabilizing them with respect to enzymatic degradation, and mediating their binding to growth factor receptors. For example, binding of the transforming growth factor β (TGF-β) proteins by heparin is isoform-specific and has been shown to protect TGF-β1 from proteolytic and chemical inactivation. Binding fibroblast growth factor (FGF) to heparin also increases its half-life almost sixfold. Heparin-bound TGF-β1 and TGF-β3 enhances chondrogenesis, while heparin-bound bone morphogenetic protein (BMP-2) and FGF-2 promote osteogenesis *in vitro* and *in vivo*. Chondroitin sulfate is the major component of aggrecan, a complex ECM nanoassembly (Figure 13.1). Chondroitin sulfate can stimulate metabolic response of cartilage and has anti-inflammatory properties. Hyaluronic acid is the only nonsulfated GAG, making it a weak polyanion of great biological interest. It serves as a lubricant in cartilage, participates in the control of tissue hydration, water transport, and inflammatory response, and organizes the nanostructure of other components of the ECM. It has been used for the construction of polyelectrolyte multilayers (PEM) and hydrogels for mammalian cell culture. Chondroitin sulfate has been used in biomaterials, and it has been shown to support mammalian cell growth when used in hydrogels or polyelectrolyte multilayers. Chondroitin sulfate forms a semiflexible coil in solution with an intrinsic persistence length in the range of 4.5–5.5 nm. All these polysaccharides are biodegradable; degrading into inert products such as disaccharides and monosaccharides (carbohydrates).

Naturally derived polymers are attractive for the construction of tissue engineered constructs, due to their biocompatibility, biodegradability, and ability to bind and stabilize important biomolecules such as growth factors. One of the key features of natural polymers in their native biological environments is their nanoscale assembly, as illustrated by the components of the ECM illustrated in Figure 13.1. This native nanoscale assembly can be exploited to create constructs which mimic the native ECM and control cell response. The next section will review a series of current techniques available to create nanostructured soft materials. It will be divided into three main sections including nanoparticles, surface structures, and nanofibers.

13.3 Engineering Soft Material Nanostructures

There are many techniques currently being investigated for the construction of soft nanostructures. In the following section, a brief review of different nanostructures is presented. We discuss both how the properties of soft materials can be used to engineer their nanostructure and how these nanostructures can be used to tune cell responses. Engineering of these structures can be applied to both naturally derived and synthetic polymers. The nanostructure of synthetic polymers (or combinations of naturally derived and synthetic polymers) has been engineered to tune the biological response to non-natural soft biomaterials. These include, most notably, polyesters such as poly(ε-caprolactone) and poly(L-lactic acid), which have been successfully used for constructs dedicated to the regeneration of bone and cartilage. Natural polymers can also be blended with synthetic polymers to change their chemical, physical, or mechanical properties.

13.3.1 Nanoparticles

Nanoparticles have a wide range of applications in biomedicine, as vehicles for the delivery of therapeutics (via topical, oral, parenteral, and pulmonary administration), as means of introducing topographical features on smooth surfaces, and contrast agents for imaging. Nanoparticles (NP) are very attractive as drug delivery vehicles, because their size alone can be engineered to influence cellular behavior such as cellular uptake. For example, Desai et al., investigated the effect of particle size in gastrointestinal uptake using biodegradable particles made from poly(lactic-*co*-glycolic)acid. The particles were formulated using an emulsion technique, and they investigated the uptake of the particles in the intestinal loop in rat with particles diameter ranging from 100 nm to 10 μm. They discovered that the uptake of the nanoparticles (100 nm in diameter) was from 15-fold to 250-fold higher compared to the larger microparticles (10 μm in diameter). Size differences in the nanometer scale also greatly affect blood circulation time and availability of the particles in the body. Particles with diameters less than 10 nm are quickly removed from the body through renal clearance and extravasation. Particles with diameter between 100 and 200 nm demonstrate the most prolonged blood circulation times, while particles greater than 200 nm are sequestered in the spleen and eventually removed via phagocytosis.

Several methods for creating soft nanoparticles have been investigated which are applicable to both biological and synthetic polymers. In the following two subsections, emulsions and self-assembly methods are discussed.

13.3.1.1 Emulsions

An emulsion is a mixture of two or more immiscible fluids, one making up a dispersed phase, and the other a bulk phase. One technique available to create nanoparticles through emulsions is the oil-in-water method (O/W). O/W emulsions consist of small lipid (oil) droplets dispersed in an aqueous medium. The emulsion is created by the mechanical agitation of the heterogeneous mixture with the addition of a surfactant. The surfactant is added to stabilize the droplets against molecular diffusion, degradation, and against coalescence by collisions. Molecules dissolved in the oil phase can then be precipitated, creating nanoparticles. These molecules could be proteins, polymers, or monomers to induce polymerization (emulsion polymerization), drugs, inorganics, and others. The technique used for mechanical agitation has an effect on particle size. Low-energy techniques (such as stirring) results in large particles with a nonhomogenous size distribution, while high-energy techniques (such as ultrasonication) result in small particles with a homogenous size distribution. Agitation time has also been shown to have an effect on particle size. Surfactants lower the interfacial tension, and improve the stability of smaller particles resulting in reduced particle size. Both the type and amount of surfactant used have a great effect on particle size. Landfester et al., investigated the effect of amount of surfactant (sodium dodecyl sulfate) on latex particles prepared via an O/W emulsion polymerization. They noticed that particle size decreased with an increasing concentration of the sufactant. Mun et al., investigated the effect of using either sodium dodecyl sulfate or Tween-20 as surfactants for O/W droplets coated with chitosan. They found that more stable emulsions were created using Tween 20 for their system. Variations in the amount of the dispersed phase (volume fraction) also affect the size of the emulsion. An increase in diameter was noted on O/W emulsions when the solid content was increased from 5% to 25%. The O/W method creates particles in solvents, which are often toxic. Thus, in order to use the resultant nanoparticles in biological applications the solvent must be removed, usually by drying or solvent extraction. Several factors have been identified which affect the efficiency of these processes including: entrapped particle solubility, internal morphology, solvent type, diffusion rate, temperature, solvent viscosity, solvent vapor pressure, and particulate loading. Many types of nanoparticles have been created through the O/W emulsion and solvent removal method to study cell response; a few of them will be discussed below.

Recently, heparin-conjugated poly(L-lactide-*co*-glycolide) (PLGA) nanospheres were constructed for the delivery of the growth factor FGF-2 through the O/W emulsion and solvent evaporation method. The nanospheres with FGF-2 were loaded on a fibrin gel and the bioactivity of the growth factor was assessed using human umbilical vein endothelial cells (HUVECs). The nanospheres allowed a controlled released of FGF-2, and proliferation of the HUVECs was enhanced when they where in contact with the nanospheres in comparison with the delivery of soluble FGF-2 (Figure 13.3). The nanospheres not only allowed for controlled release of the drugs, but may also have influenced the cell response by the introduction of nanoscale topographical features.

Other investigators have studied similar nanospheres with different cell types yielding similar results. Yilgor et al., created PLGA and poly(3-hydroxybutyrate-*co*-3-hydroxyvalerate) (PHBV) nanocapsules loaded with BMP-2 and BMP-7, respectively. These nanocapsules were incorporated onto a 3-D chitosan fiber mesh and cell response studies were performed using bone marrow-derived rat mesenchymal stem cells (MSCs). The incorporation of the nanocapsules onto the fiber mesh yielded a higher alkaline phosphatase (ALP), a specific marker for osteogenesis activity over the fiber mesh without the nanocapsules (Figure 13.4).

13.3.1.2 Self-Assembled Nanoparticles

Self-assembled nanoparticles are formed when the materials themselves phase separate to form nanoparticles, as opposed to the solvent/nonsolvent-induced phase separation used in emulsion-based techniques described above. Self-assembled nanoparticles can be engineered by controlling the intermolecular forces responsible for their assembly. These forces are tuned by altering the chemistry of the constituent molecules, and by adjusting the assembly conditions, such as temperature and pH of the solution.

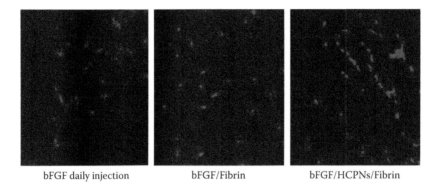

bFGF daily injection   bFGF/Fibrin   bFGF/HCPNs/Fibrin

FIGURE 13.3   (See color insert following page 10-24.) Immunohistochemical analysis of mouse ischemic limbs 4 weeks after treatment with FGF loaded nanoparticles. The specimens were stained with cyanine-conjugated vWF antibodies, which bind specifically to endothelial cells. Note that the delivery of FGF through the heparin modified nanoparticles induces higher growth of endothelial cell when compared to FGF delivered in solution or through a fibrin gel. HCPNs = Heparin-conjugated PLGA nanospheres. (Reprinted from Jeon, O. et al. 2006. *Biomaterials* 27(8): 1598–607. Copyright 2006, Elsevier. With permission.)

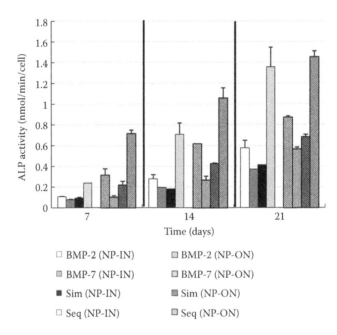

FIGURE 13.4   Specific ALP activity on BMP-loaded particles incorporated chitosan fiber mesh scaffolds. "Sim" denotes simultaneous delivery of BMP-2 and BMP-7, "seq" denotes sequential delivery of BMP-2 and BMP-7, "NP-IN" denotes for nanoparticles that were incorporated into the fibers by allowing them to mix in the chitosan solution before electrospinning, "NP-ON" denotes nanoparticles which were applied on the fibers after electrospinning by a series of vacuum-pressure cycles. (Reprinted from Yilgor, P. et al. 2009. *Biomaterials* 30(21): 3551–59. Copyright 2009, Elsevier. With permission.)

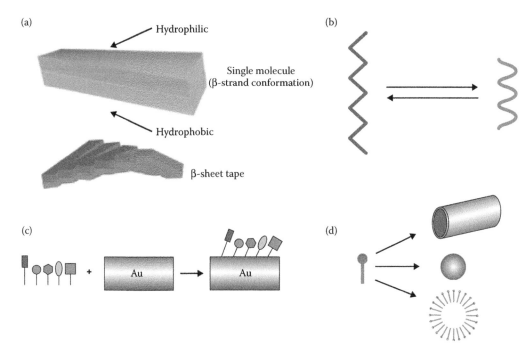

FIGURE 13.5 **(See color insert following page 10-24.)** Various types of self-assembling peptide systems. (a) Amphiphilic peptides in β-strand conformation are chiral objects. As a consequence, they self-assemble into twisted tapes. (b) Helical dipolar peptides can undergo a conformational change between α-helix and β-sheet, much like a molecular switch. (c) Surface-binding peptides can form monolayers covalently bound to a surface. (d) Surfactant-like peptides can form vesicles and nanotubes. (Reprinted from Zhang, S. et al. 2002. *Current Opinion in Chemical Biology* 6(6): 865–71. Copyright 2002, Elsevier. With permission.)

Peptide amphiphiles (PA) are nanometer-sized molecules with a peptide "head group" covalently linked to a hydrophobic "tail." The peptide head group forms a distinct structural element and may introduce some useful biochemical functionality (Figure 13.5). The hydrophobic tail serves to align the peptide strands and induce secondary (α-helices and β-sheets) and tertiary structures (β/α/β motif, hairpin, α-helical-coiled coil, α-helical bundle, Jelly Roll, and the Greek Key). The tail also provides a hydrophobic surface for self-association and/or interaction with other surfaces. Some PA are a promising class of nanoscale biomaterials which can be tuned to promote or inhibit behaviors such as cell proliferation. PA can form nanospheres and nanofibers.

Fields et al., developed PA with a collagen-like structural motif comprised of a dialkyl ester lipid tail with a collagen model peptide head group with a cell-binding sequence that promotes cell spreading. Using human melanoma cells they demonstrated that the PA promotes cell adhesion and spreading. Recently, Aulisa et al. developed a PA which self-assembles into micelles and shows inhibition of pancreatic cancer cells, leukemia cells, and melanoma cells, while noncancerous fibroblasts are less affected. The small size of the PA along with a specific gene added to promote cell uptake of the PA allowed the cancerous cells to absorb the PA to inhibit their proliferation.

The electrostatic interactions of polyelectrolytes can also be exploited to yield different types of assemblies. The complexation of oppositely charged polyelectrolytes to form soluble polyelectrolyte complex nanoparticles (PCNs) has been studied for over 30 years. Nonetheless, the application of this technology to form nanoparticles of soft biomaterials remains an active area of research. The complexation of oppositely charged polyelectrolytes in solution can lead to the formation of colloidally stable nanoparticles by several mechanisms. Generally, one of the charged polymer chains must be in excess.

As the polyelectrolyte in default complexes with the polyelectrolyte in excess, some charge neutralization occurs, forming hydrophobic regions along portions of the polymer chains that are complexed. The hydrophobic regions of these primary complexes tend to aggregate, forming a hydrophobic core, surrounded by a charged, hydrophilic corona. However, some residual surface charge is required to ensure the colloidal stability of the particles. Thus, as the condition of one-to-one charge complexation is approached, the complexes begin to aggregate, forming larger particles and may completely precipitate from the solution.

The size distribution of PCNs tends to be relatively broad. The mean particle size is influenced by a number of factors related to the mechanism of particle formation. Both the complexation between the oppositely charged groups responsible for PCN formation, and the repulsion between the PCN that keeps them from aggregating are due to electrostatic forces. Thus, the same conditions that promote the growth of PCN also tend to stabilize the smaller particles. Thus, any system parameter that promotes the complexation to form larger particles by influencing the electrostatics might also tend to favor the stabilization of smaller ones. For instance, as more of the polyelectrolyte in default is added, the particles may initially collapse to smaller diameters as the magnitude of the charge density in the corona is reduced. However, at higher contents of the excess charged group, the stability of smaller particles is increased, while at lower contents of the excess charged group, the smaller particles tend to be less stable and form aggregates. If the charge density is reduced sufficiently, the smallest particles lose their colloidal stability altogether, and larger particles or aggregates are favored near the one-to-one charge-mixing ratio. Similarly, the solution ionic strength can also influence the sizes of the particles formed by affecting the charge screening length, thereby influencing the electrostatic interactions responsible for the attractive forces and stabilization of PCNs. Solution ionic strength can also influence the osmotic pressure within the complexes. Thus, increasing ionic strengths can lead to both disintegration and aggregation of the particles, depending upon the system. For weak polyelectrolytes, the pH of the solutions in which the PCNs are formed can also be used to tune the electrostatic interactions.

The formation of PCNs using polysaccharides has been studied in our laboratory, as well as by others. In these studies, the tuning of the composition and particle size has been demonstrated by changing the charge-mixing ratios and polymer molecular weights. The complexation between proteins and synthetic polyelectrolytes has also been studied. In one such study, the aggregation of these complexes was shown to depend only on the mixing ratios of the polymer and protein, and not on their concentrations.

PCN can be used to decorate surfaces to induce topographical changes, and for localized delivery of important molecules such as proteins. In fact, chitosan/dextran sulfate polyelectrolyte nanoparticles have been developed for the delivery FGF-10 and vascular endothelial growth factor (VEGF). Hartig et al., recently reported that positively charged PCN containing polysaccharides are rapidly taken up by microvascular endothelial cells, probably by micropinocytosis, suggesting that nanoparticles are an effective means of delivering payloads to the intracellular space. In these studies, the particle size and surface chemistry are key parameters that must be tuned in order to elicit the desired cellular response.

13.3.2 Surface Structures

One of the ongoing challenges in creating biomaterials for tissue repair is their biocompatibility. In particular, many metals and other hard materials are currently being used as biomaterials with limited biocompatibility. To improve the biocompatibility of these materials, researchers have been investigating different surface modifications which could promote or inhibit cell and protein adhesion, ultimately influencing the behaviors of native tissue cells, immune cells, and pathogenic microorganisms such as bacteria and fungi. Soft materials are currently being used to decorate the surfaces of biomaterials with the end of improving wound healing, influencing the inflammation response, preventing thrombosis, and delivering therapeutic proteins and other molecules. The surface techniques discussed in this section include poly-electrolyte multilayers, cell membrane-mimetic thin films, polymer brushes, and soft-lithography.

13.3.2.1 Self-Assembled Polyelectrolyte Multilayers

Layer-by-layer (LBL) assembly of polyelectrolyte multilayers (PEM) was first introduced by Decher and coworkers. This technology has gained attention as an attractive method of surface coating for a broad range of applications, due to its simplicity and the control over coating thickness and composition that can be obtained at the nanometer length scale. The LBL assembly consists of successively adsorbing layers of a polyanion and polycation (or other asymmetrically interacting pair, such as a hydrogen-bond donor/acceptor pair) from solution onto charged substrates (Figure 13.6).

PEMs have been constructed using biomolecules such as DNA, collagen, the polysaccharides chitosan, heparin, hyaluronic acid, chondroitin sulfate, and synthetic polymers such as poly(styrene sulfonate) and poly(allylamine hydrochloride). PEM assemblies can be used to mimic key features of ECM by using biopolymers and embedding important peptides and proteins. The growth factors BMP-2, TGF-β3, and FGF-2 are a few of the many proteins that have been successfully delivered to cells using PEM retaining or enhancing their function. PEMs have been constructed to deliver other types of molecules such as nanoparticles, plasmid vectors, and drugs for cancer treatment.

Engineering of PEM consists in being able to predictively tune their properties that will induce changes in cell behavior. PEM thickness, surface chemistry, stiffness, and surface roughness are just a few of the properties that researchers are investigating. The thickness of PEM can be tuned at the

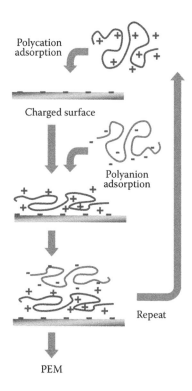

FIGURE 13.6 (See color insert following page 10-24.) Construction of polyelectrolyte multilayers. A charged surface is exposed to a solution of an oppositely charged polyelectrolyte, resulting in polyelectrolyte adsorption and inversion of the surface charge. The charge inversion prevents additional adsorption of the polyelectrolyte, limiting the layer thickness. The surface is then rinsed and exposed to a polyelectrolyte with a charge opposite to that of the first polyelectrolyte. The surface charge is again inverted and the process can be repeated.

nanometer scale by adjusting the number of adsorbed monolayers, and the pH and ionic strength of the polyelectrolyte solution. The effect of pH of the solution on the thickness of PEM has been investigated for weak, strong, synthetic, and natural polyelectrolytes. The thickness of PEM constructed using weak polyelectrolytes can be tuned with great control over a wide range of values on the nanometer scale. The pH dependence on thickness for the polyanion/polycation pair of poly(acrylic acid)/poly(allylamine hydrochloride) was investigated by Shiratori et al. who noted that the thickness of an adsorbed polycation or polyanion layer can be tuned from 0.5 to 8 nm by adjusting the pH of the polymer solution. Boddohi et al., investigated the change in thickness with increasing pH of the solution and ionic strength for the weak polycation/strong polyanion chitosan/heparin pair. They determined that the PEM thickness could be increased from less than 2 nm per bilayer to more than 4 nm per bilayer with increasing pH of the solution and ionic strength. At relatively high values of the solution ionic strength, however, pH had a greatly reduced affect on the layer thickness, presumably because of enhanced electrostatic screening effects. Both the studies show how PEM thickness can increase as charge density on weak polyelectrolytes is decreased (by increasing pH or increasing ionic strength). This could be related to the conformation of the polyelectrolytes in solution, in addition to their interactions at the adsorbing surface. Polyelectrolytes with high charge densities tend to form a more stiff/extended conformation, whereas those with a low charge density adopt a more coiled/globular conformation. Strong polyelectrolytes, such as heparin, tend to be in a stiffer state forming thinner monolayers upon adsorbtion.

Cell behavior as a function of PEM thickness has also been investigated. Li et al., investigated the effect of PEM thickness on smooth muscle cell attachment using poly(allylamine hydrochloride)/poly(sodium 4-styrenesulfonate). They observed that the roundness (and thus attachment) of the cells is greatly affected by the number of monolayers, with cells having a less-rounded, more natural morphology on the thicker films. The interaction of photoreceptor cells and PEM was investigated by Tezcaner et al. The viability of the photoreceptor cells varied with the number of monolayer and terminated layer in the poly(L-lysine)/chondroitin sulfate system. In that system, the 20-monolayer films terminated with chondroitin sulfate were superior to 2-, 21-, and 41-monolayer PEM.

The stiffness of PEM can also be tuned to control cell response. Ren et al., prepared PEM using the weak polycation/weak polyanion poly(L-lysine)/hyaluronan pair with stiffness values ranging between 3 kPa and 400 kPa by cross-linking the films using the 1-ethyl-3-(3-dimethylamino-propyl)carbodiimide (EDC) chemistry to modulate myoblast cell differentiation. Myoblast adhesion, proliferation, and differentiation were strongly affected by PEM stiffness. On soft films, the myotubes exhibited a short and thick morphology, whereas on stiffer films the cells formed elongated and thin striated myotubes.

One of the most active areas of research involving PEMs is their use as coatings to enhance biocompatibility and/or deliver proteins or particles at the surface of metallic implants. Coronary stents, dental screws, and orthopedic implants have all been coated with PEMs to enhance their biocompatibility both *in vitro* and *in vivo*. PEMs have also been used in the coating of soft materials such as microspheres. Coating a smooth surface with a PEM will add nanoscale features which have been shown to enhance cell adhesion and proliferation. Recently, Yan et al., investigated the plasmid uptake response of MSCs for differentiation on titanium films modified with PEMs. They compared smooth unmodified titanium surfaces (with plasmid delivered in solution) with those modified with a chitosan/plasmid DNA PEM. The modified titanium surfaces showed higher cell transfection, which led to a high production of both ALP and osteocalcin, two differentiation markers (Figure 13.7).

A major factor to consider when designing biomaterials is their hemocompatibility. Hemocompatibility of implants can be enhanced by engineering surface coatings from different materials which can be modulated at the nanoscale. Moreover, several groups have engineered biologically inert surfaces which mimic a blood cell membrane using polymeric phospholipds (Figure 13.8). Plasma cell membranes consist of a combination of proteins and glycoproteins embedded on a lipid bilayer. Over 100 different types of lipids are present in the hydrophobic and hydrophilic portion of the lipid bilayer. The hydrophilic

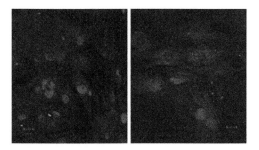

FIGURE 13.7 (See color insert following page 10-24.) Expression of green fluorescence protein (GFP) of cells adhered on titanium surfaces 3 days after culture. (Left) Unmodified titanium surface with GFP plasmid vector delivered in solution with lipofectamine 2000. (Right) Titanium surface modified with chitosan/plasmid LBL assembly. The higher expression of GFP denotes a higher plasmid uptake by the cells. (Reprinted from Hu, Y. et al. 2009. *Biomaterials* 30(21): 3626–35. Copyright 2009, Elsevier. With permission.)

polar head groups are in contact with water, and thus are the main contributors to the interfacial properties of cell surfaces. The major phospholipid head group present in the cell's outer membrane is phosphorylcholine. Thus, researchers are investigating using phosphorylcholine-like molecules to coat surfaces to induce nonthrombogenic characteristics on potential biomedical implants. Gong et al., studied the adhesion of human macrophages to different modified polypropylene surfaces. Different types of plasma-treated polypropylene surfaces (ammonia, nitrogen, and oxygen) were investigated along with a phosphorylcholine-coated surface. The macrophages did not adhere to any of the surfaces except for the phosphorylcholine-coated surface. Their results provide new surfaces on which macrophages can be culture expanded and the interactions between macrophage and cell membrane can be investigated. Wilson et al., coated alginate microcapsules with a phospholipid layer and studied its biocompatibility *in vivo*. The microcapsules were implanted into the peritoneal cavity of mice and removed after 4 weeks of implantation. The phospholipid-coated microcapsules demonstrated an improved biocompatibility, because they were free of cell adhesion and fibrotic overgrowth compared to the noncoated capsule controls.

13.3.2.2 Polymer Brushes

Polymer brushes are an assembly of polymer chains which are closely packed and anchored by one end to a surface. The proximity of the polymer chains forces them to stretch away from the surface with a

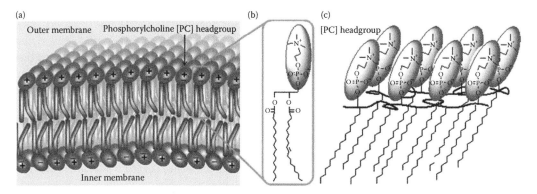

FIGURE 13.8 Schematic structures of the cell membrane and the outer membrane mimetic polymeric assembly: (a) lipid bilayer of cell membrane; (b) phosphatidylcholine; (c) cell membrane mimetic assembly with PC head group and synthetic polymer tails. (Reprinted from Gong, M. et al. 2008. *Applied Surface Science* 255(2): 555–58. Copyright 2008, Elsevier. With permission.)

length significantly higher than the radius of gyration that the molecule would ordinarily adopt in solution. These stretched configurations occur under equilibrium conditions, avoiding the need of a confining geometry or an external field. Polymer brushes can be applied in several systems including polymer micelles, block copolymers at fluid–fluid interfaces, grafted polymers on a solid surface, and diblock copolymers and graft copolymers at fluid–fluid interfaces. In general, there are two ways to create surfaces with polymer brushes, physisorption, and covalent attachment. In physisorption, the polymer chain adsorbs onto a surface with one end interacting strongly with the surface. Covalent attachment can be accomplished using either the "grafting to" or "grafting from" approaches. In the "grafting to" approach, a functionalized end of the chain reacts with an appropriate molecule on the surface to form the brushes. This approach generally yields low grafting densities and low film thickness. In the "grafting from" approach, an initiator is bounded to a surface, and polymer brushes are created through polymerization. The "grafting from" method generally yields high grafting density. The type of initiator used and the method of polymerization are the two important adjustable parameters to control the characteristics of the brushes.

Physisorption is a reversible process achieved by the self-assembly of polymeric surfactants or end-functionalized polymers on a solid surface. The several characteristic dimensions of the brushes, including surface grafting density, are controlled by thermodynamic equilibrium. Physisorption of polymers occurs in the presence of selective solvents or selective surfaces, which gives selective solvation and selective adsorption, respectively. The structure of the brushes depends upon the selectivities of these media and the nature of the polymer (e.g., the architecture of the polymer, the length of the polymer, and the interaction between the polymer end and the surface). Ideal solvents for physisorption are the ones which act like a precipitant for one end of the polymer chain to permit it to anchor to the surface, while acting as a good solvent for the other end to form brushes in solution. Physisorption interactions are in most cases Van der Waals forces or hydrogen bonding. Desorption easily occurs upon exposure to other solvents or other harsh conditions.

Polymer brushes make interesting systems to control cell behavior. Several types of cells have been successfully cultured in polymer brush systems including HUVECs, neurons, osteoblasts, and fibroblasts. Several groups are investigating the effect of brush thickness on cell adhesion using thermo-responsive polymer brushes. Using the "grafting from" technique, Li et al., prepared a poly(*N*-isopropy-lacrylamide) gradient of polymer brushes on a silicon substrate with a linear variation of thickness to study cell attachment and detachment by changes in temperature. The variation in thickness was performed by changing the polymerization time. They used HepG2 cells, and discovered that cells could adhere at 37°C and could be detached at 24°C when the polymer brush thickness was in the range of 20–45 nm. Wischerhoff et al., performed a similar study in which the thickness of the brushes was varied and cell adhesion experiments were performed using thermoresponsive polymers. They tuned the thickness of their polymer brush by using the "grafting from" approach on a PEM. The thickness of the underlying PEM was varied to yield a variation of polymer brush thickness. They studied fibroblast adhesion at 37°C and detachment at 22°C using systems with different thicknesses. They noticed that when the underlying PEM had 4 bilayers, which accounts for a brush thickness between 20 and 40 nm, the cells could attach at 37°C and be detached at 22°C. Mei et al., prepared polymer brush surfaces using poly(2-hydroxyethyl methacrylate) to create a gradient substrate to modulate cell adhesion using fibronectin. The gradient ranged from 2 to 8 nm and from a high graft density to a low graft density region. The substrate was coated with fibronectin, and fibroblasts were allowed to attach. They noticed that protein adsorption and cell adhesion were higher on the low grafting density region. However, the trend was not linear since between 2 and 3 nm of film thickness the amount of protein adsorbed dropped significantly while the cell density remained constant (Figure 13.9).

13.3.2.3 Soft-Lithography

Lithography encompasses a number of techniques which allow modification of the surfaces of materials. These modifications include adding topographical features at the microscale and nanoscale, such as pits,

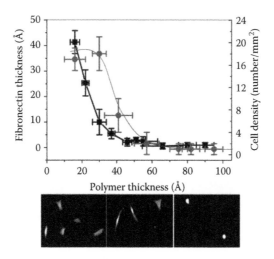

FIGURE 13.9 The effect of polymer brush thickness on the amount of adsorbed fibronectin, cell density, and cell morphology. The black and red lines represent the fibronectin thickness and cell density, respectively. The error bars are the standard from uncertainties from triplicate runs. The lines are to aid the reader's eye. (Reprinted with permission from Mei, Y. et al. 2005. *Langmuir* 21(26): 12309–14. Copyright 2005 American Chemical Society.)

wells, arrays, and chemical and biochemical surface modifications. Lithographic methods are available for both soft and hard surfaces; in this section, we shall discuss several lithographic methods applied on soft surfaces. There are several lithographic methods to create patterns from the micrometer to the nanometer scale. These methods can be divided into several groups including accelerated particle beam lithography, scanning probe lithography, photolithography, and contact printing. Accelerated particle beam lithography involves using charged particles which are accelerated by electric fields and focused into a beam by magnets to strike a surface with high accuracy and nanoscale resolution. One technique which falls in this category is electron beam lithography (EBL) which has a resolution of 10 nm. In scanning probe lithography, a probe, such as an atomic force microscope (AFM) tip, is used to alter surfaces to create features down to 20 nm. Dip-pen lithography uses an AFM tip, which is dipped into a solution of biomolecules or other chemicals, and scans along the surface depositing the inked molecules. In contact printing, a pattern stamp is used to transfer material onto a surface. Microcontact printing uses a flexible stamp to form patterns of self-assembled monolayers onto surfaces with a resolution of 35 nm. In photolithography, a structure is deposited onto a photoresist surface using UV light. It has a resolution of about 250 nm, but depends upon the wavelength of light used. Each technique has a limitation on resolution and price. For example, EBL has an excellent resolution (10 nm), but is an expensive technique and only allows small area printing. Photolithography on the other hand is fairly inexpensive, allows large area printing, but has a resolution of 250 nm and requires specific photoresist surfaces. All these techniques can be used to modify surfaces to study cell responses to nanometer scale features on soft materials.

Recently, EBL was used to create nanopatterned surfaces onto poly(methylmethacrylate) to investigate the effect of symmetric and disordered patterns on MSC differentiation. The behavior of the MSCs greatly differs between highly ordered patterns and random topographies. Indeed, cells on the random topographies exhibited higher cell adhesion and enhancement in cell differentiation (Figure 13.10). Figure 13.10 demonstrates that not only can cell behavior be controlled by topographical features, but also by the spatial arrangement of these features. Lithography may provide efficient tools for studying the interactions between cells and soft nanostructured materials.

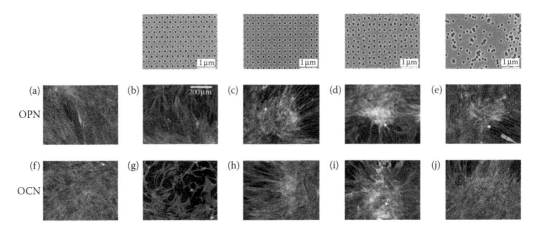

FIGURE 13.10 **(See color insert following page 10-24.)** Osteopontin (OPN) and osteocalcin (OCN) staining of osteoprogenitor cells after 21 days of culture. The top row shows images of nanotopographies fabricated by EBL. All have 120 nm-diameter pits (100 nm deep, absolute or average 300 nm center-center spacing) with hexagonal, square, displaced square 50 (±50 nm from true center) and random placements. a–j, Osteoprogenitors cultured on the control (a,f), note the lack of positive OPN and OCN stain; HEX (b,g), note the loss of cell adhesion; SQ (c,h), note reduced cell numbers compared with the control, but some OPN and OCN positive cells; DSQ50 (d,i), note bone nodule formation (arrows); RAND (e,j), note good cell populations with cells expressing OPN and OCN. Actin = red, OPN/OCN = green. (Reprinted by permission from Macmillan Publishers LTD: Dalby, M. J. et al. 2007. *Nature Materials* 6(12): 997–1003. Copyright 2007.)

13.3.3 Nanofibers

Soft nanofibers are a very attractive class of biomaterials, due to their simple preparation methods, which can provide an environment with features similar to those found in the native ECM. Indeed, nanofibers can be constructed form both biological and synthetic polymers to mimic the ECM of different hard and soft tissues.

13.3.3.1 Electrospun

Electrospinning is a simple and inexpensive method to create fiber meshes with diameters varying from 3 nm to more than 5 μm. Electrospun nanofibers are formed when a polymer solution is drawn into a thin jet by a strong (~1 kV cm^{-1}) electrostatic field, concurrent with evaporation of the solvent and precipitation of the polymer. This is done in practice by slowly pumping a polymer solution through a needle set at a controlled distance from a collector, with a voltage applied between the needle and the collector. Although the apparatus is relatively simple to assemble and use, the process is very complex. There are many adjustable experimental parameters and multiple kinetic processes occurring simultaneously. The flow of the polymer jet occurs along with both conduction and advection of electrical current. Elongation of the jet occurs along with alignment of the polymer chains and evaporation of the solvent. Mechanical and electrical forces acting on the polymer solution jet result in a whipping instability that leads to further elongation of the jet as the solution approaches the collector. The simple spinning geometry uses a stationary flat plate as the collection electrode and results in a nonwoven mat of fibers that have a random orientation of their axes in the plane of the collection electrode surface. Alignment of nanofibers can be achieved by altering the geometry of the electric field, and/or the grounded collector. This can permit axial alignment of fibers, and materials with anisotropic mechanical properties.

Several different biological and synthetic polymers have been successfully electrospun including gelatin, hyaluronic acid, chitosan, PCL, PLLA, and others. The electrospinning process can be manipulated by a number of variables yielding fibers with different diameters. These variables include: solution viscosity, solution charge density, solution surface tension, polymer molecular weight, dipole moment and dielectric constants, flow-rate, electric field strength, distance between tip and collector, needle tip design and placement, collector composition and geometry, and ambient parameters such as temperature and humidity. While complete descriptions of the electrospinning process would be quite complex, several theoretical approaches have enabled successful engineering of the electrospinning process. For example by assuming that the fiber forms as a purely viscous fluid jet, Fridrikh et al., derived a model for the terminal fiber diameter, which predicts that the fiber diameter should scale as the 2/3 power of the ratio of the solution flow-rate to the electric current. This model, although simplified, is parameterized by measurable properties of the polymer solution and correctly predicts the trend in fiber diameter for electrospun poly(ε-caprolactone) from a few hundred nanometers to several microns.

Various researchers have investigated the effect of fiber diameter in cell behavior using several cell types. Cell morphology and proliferation of fibroblasts may not be sensitive to the PLGA fiber diameter. However, many other cell types have been demonstrated to exhibit significant functional responses to nanofiber size. Osteoprogenitor cells cultured on PLLA fibers had an increase of cell density with increasing fiber diameter. However, decreasing the nanofiber diameter has been demonstrated to enhance matrix production by chondrocytes, cell spreading of rat marrow stromal cells, and cell adhesion and proliferation of both HUVECs and neural stem/progenitor cells (NSCs). Reducing the fiber diameter also results in a positive effect on cell differentiation of NSC into oligodendrocytes (Figure 13.11). Adding particles to electrospun fibers is another modification which researchers have used to enhance bioactivity. Electrospun PLLA nanofibers grafted with hydroxyapatite have been evaluated in response to human MSCs and osteoblasts. Cell adhesion and growth was enhanced for osteoblasts (Figure 13.12), while differentiation of human MSCs into chondrocytes was enhanced with the presence of hydroxyapatite nanoparticles in the fiber. The enhanced bioactivity with the presence of nanoparticles is most likely due to the topographical changes induced in the fibers making them structurally similar to native ECM.

13.3.3.2 Molecular Self-Assembly

Molecular self-assembly is controlled by weak noncovalent bonds (hydrogen bonds, electrostatic interactions, hydrophobic interactions, Van der Waals, water-mediated hydrogen bonds, etc.), which may be relatively small in isolation, but when combined together they govern the structure of all biological macromolecules. Self-assembling peptide-based nanofiber scaffolds are a class of self-assembled nanostructures that are attractive for regenerative medicine. These nanofibers are created using the "bottom-up" approach beginning with an alternating sequence of amino acids that contains charged residues. Due to hydrophilic and hydrophobic interactions, these peptides form β-sheets structure spontaneously.

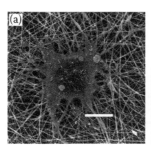
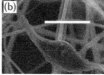

FIGURE 13.11 SEM images of rat NSCs cultured on polyethersulfone fiber meshes of varying fiber diameter. (a) Cells cultured on fiber mesh of 283 nm in diameter. (b) Cells cultured on fiber mesh of 746 nm in diameter. Note the improvement on cell spreading with the lower diameter meshes. Scale bar is 10 μm. (Reprinted from Christopherson, G. T., H. Song, and H. Q. Mao. 2009. *Biomaterials* 30(4): 556–64. Copyright 2009, Elsevier. With permission.)

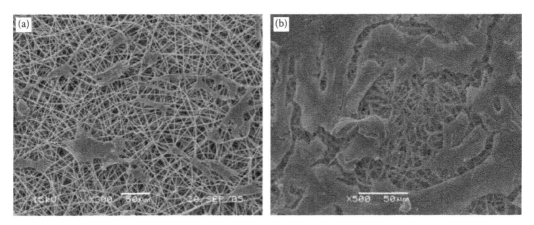

FIGURE 13.12 SEM images of osteoblast cell adhesion and growth on (a) PLLA and (b) PLLA/HA hybrid membranes. (Reprinted from Sui, G. et al. 2007. *Journal of Biomedical Materials Research Part A* 82A(2): 445–54. Copyright 2007, Wiley. With permission.)

Finally, these β-sheet structures are ion screened, by varying the pH of the solution, to form 3-D scaffolds of nanofibers of ~10 nm in diameter. Self-assembled peptides are very attractive, because they can be designed at the single amino acid level, which can be tailored to specific amino acid sequences that change cell behavior. Also, they can be formed in the presence of cells to encapsulate cells in a 3-D environment. Indeed, Horii et al., prepared peptide nanofibers designed specifically for osteoblasts. Their peptide scaffolds contained osteoblast-specific motifs including: osteogenic growth peptides, bone-cell secreted-signal peptides, osteopontin cell adhesion motifs, and arginine-glycine-aspartic acid (RGD) binding sequences. They seeded preosteoblast cells on the specific osteogenic peptide scaffold and on a nonspecific peptide scaffold. The osteogenic specific scaffold demonstrated significant improvement in cell proliferation (Figure 13.13) and osteogenic differentiation. Others have developed peptide self-assembled scaffolds to tune the adhesion and spreading of fibroblasts using the RGD sequence. Peptide nanofibers have also been used as delivery vehicles for important growth factors. Stendahl et al., conducted an *in vivo* study using heparin-binding PA nanofibers to deliver VEGF and FGF-2. They implanted their scaffolds in the omentum of mice with induced diabetes. Their scaffolds induced significant increases in blood vessel density over the control scaffold with no growth factor. Their results pave the way for new therapies for controlling diabetes.

13.4 The Future of Engineering Soft Nanostructures for Guided Cell Responses

In the past two decades, there has been an explosion in the development of nanostructured soft materials for biomedical technologies, fueled in no small part by advances in techniques for synthesizing and characterizing materials with features at the nanometer length scale. These advances have enabled us to begin understanding how biochemical and biomechanical properties emerge from the organization of organs and tissues at multiple length scales. Our ability to control and engineer these soft nanostructures is maturing to the point where dimensions can be tuned with subnanometer, indeed, molecular resolution in some cases. Nanostructures of varying geometries can be reproducibly created, including ultra-thin films, fibers, and spherical particles, using a variety of materials that range from those with potent biochemical activity to the biologically inert. With this repertoire of building blocks at our disposal, we are now exploring the construction of more complex nanoassemblies, and one can begin to imagine the reconstruction of at least some features of the exquisite hierarchy found in natural tissues.

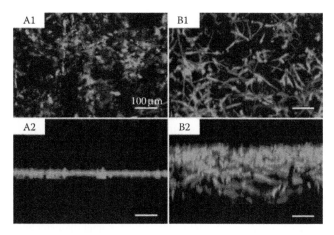

FIGURE 13.13   (See color insert following page 10-24.) Reconstructed image of 3-D confocal micrographs of culturing on the different scaffolds consisting of different mix ratio of RADA16 1% (w/v) and PRG 1% (w/v) using calcein-AM staining. The bar represents 100 μm. A1 and A2: 10% of the 2-unit RGD binding sequence PRG and B1&B2: PRG 70%. A1 and B1 are vertical view and A2 and B2 are horizontal view. In the case of 10% PRG scaffold, the cells were attached on the surface of the scaffold, whereas the cells were migrated into the scaffold in the case of 70% PRG scaffold. There is a drastic cell migration into the scaffold with higher concentration of PRG motif. (Reprinted from Horii, A. et al. 2007. *PLoS ONE* 2(2): e190. doi:10.1371/journal.pone.0000190.)

Transformative advancements in this field will be realized when we move from describing cell behavior, to developing predictive theories of the mechanisms by which cells respond to the myriad stimuli provided by soft nanostructures. To begin with, well-defined and validated nanostructures can be used as platforms to catalog the influence of nanoscale features on cell adhesion, cell proliferation, cell migration, protein transcription, and cell-cell communication. In many cases, the current observations of cell response to nanostructures produce as many or more questions as they have answered. While the questions that have been answered are often, "What will the response be?" the questions that are left unanswered are often of a more mechanistic nature, such as "Why do the cells respond this way?" and "What if this parameter is varied?" These are the types of questions that can be answered by predictive models of cell-nanomaterial interactions. Engineered nanostructures will then provide the realm in which to test and refine these theories.

From predictive theories describing the cell responses to biomaterials, engineering design principles can be developed whereby biomaterials scientists can design novel nanostructures for new biomedical applications. Furthermore, theoretical limits defining the upper and lower bounds of cell response functions can be defined, which can guide the development solutions to new problems. This exciting field offers the opportunity for biomaterials scientists to also make contributions to the biological sciences, by providing new tools and theories to study cellular and molecular biology. The application of materials science to biological materials has already revealed much about the behavior of biomolecules, cells, and tissues, by viewing them as soft nanostructures. Future developments along the lines of predictive theories of cell-nanomaterial interactions will enable realization of the great promise of engineered soft nanostructures for biomaterials.

Bibliography

Aigner, T. and J. Stove. 2003. Collagens—major component of the physiological cartilage matrix, major target of cartilage degeneration, major tool in cartilage repair. *Advanced Drug Delivery Reviews* 55(12): 1569–93.

Antonietti, M. and K. Landfester. 2002. Polyreactions in miniemulsions. *Progress in Polymer Science* 27(4): 689–757.

Atkins, P. W. 1990. *Physical Chemistry*. 4th ed. New York: W.H. Freeman and Company.

Aulisa, L., N. Forraz, C. McGuckin, and J. D. Hartgerink. 2009. Inhibition of cancer cell proliferation by designed peptide amphiphiles. *Acta Biomaterialia* 5(3): 842–53.

Ayad, S., R. P. Boot-Handford, M. J. Humphries, K. E. Kadler, and C. A. Shuttleworth. 1998. *The Extracellular Matrix Factsbook*, 2nd ed., San Diego: Academic Press.

Badami, A. S., M. R. Kreke, M. S. Thompson, J. S. Riffle, and A. S. Goldstein. 2006. Effect of fiber diameter on spreading, proliferation, and differentiation of osteoblastic cells on electrospun poly(lactic acid) substrates. *Biomaterials* 27(4): 596–606.

Ball, V., M. Winterhalter, P. Schwinte, P. Lavalle, J. C. Voegel, and P. Schaaf. 2002. Complexation mechanism of bovine serum albumin and poly(allylamine hydrochloride). *Journal of Physical Chemistry B* 106(9): 2357–64.

Bashur, C. A., L. A. Dahlgren, and A. S. Goldstein. 2006. Effect of fiber diameter and orientation on fibroblast morphology and proliferation on electrospun poly(D,L-lactic-*co*-glycolic acid) meshes. *Biomaterials* 27(33): 5681–88.

Boddohi, S., C. E. Killingsworth, and M. J. Kipper. 2008. Polyelectrolyte multilayer assembly as a function of Ph and ionic strength using the polysaccharides chitosan and heparin. *Biomacromolecules* 9(6):2021–28.

Boddohi, S., N. Moore, P. A. Johnson, and M. J. Kipper. 2009. Polysaccharide-based polyelectrolyte complex nanoparticles from chitosan, heparin, and hyaluronan. *Biomacromolecules* 10(6): 1402–09.

Boddohi, S., J. Almodovar, H. Zhang, P. A. Johnson, and M. J. Kipper. 2010. Layer-by-layer assembly of polysaccharide-based nanostructured surfaces containing polyelectrolyte complex nanoparticles. *Colloids and Surfaces B: Biointerfaces* 77(1): 60–68.

Boddohi, S., N. Moore, P. Johnson, and M. Kipper. 2009. Polysaccharide-based polyelectrolyte complex nanoparticles from chitosan, heparin, and hyaluronan. *Biomacromolecules* 10(6): 1402–09.

Brannigan, G. and F. L. H. 2004. Brown. Solvent-free simulations of fluid membrane bilayers. *Journal of Chemical Physics* 120(2): 1059–71.

Chang, B.-J., O. Prucker, E. Groh, A. Wallrath, M. Dahm, and J. Rühe. 2002. Surface-attached polymer monolayers for the control of endothelial cell adhesion. *Colloids and Surfaces A: Physicochemical and Engineering Aspects* 198, SI: 519-26.

Choi, J. and M. F. Rubner. 2005. Influence of the degree of ionization on weak polyelectrolyte multilayer assembly. *Macromolecules* 38(1): 116–24.

Christenson, E. M., K. S. Anseth, J. J. J. P. van den Beucken, C. K. Chan, B. Ercan, J. A. Jansen, C. T. Laurencin, et al. 2007. Nanobiomaterial applications in orthopedics. *Journal of Orthopaedic Research* 25: 11–22.

Christopherson, G. T., H. Song, and H. Q. Mao. 2009. The influence of fiber diameter of electrospun substrates on neural stem cell differentiation and proliferation. *Biomaterials* 30(4): 556–64.

Crouzier, T., K. Ren, C. Nicolas, C. Roy, and C. Picart. 2009. Layer-by-layer films as a biomimetic reservoir for Rhbmp-2 delivery: Controlled differentiation of myoblasts to osteoblasts. *Small* 5(5): 598–608.

Dalby, M. J., N. Gadegaard, R. Tare, A. Andar, M. O. Riehle, P. Herzyk, C. D. W. Wilkinson, and R. O. C. Oreffo. 2007. The control of human mesenchymal cell differentiation using nanoscale symmetry and disorder. *Nature Materials* 6(12): 997–1003.

Damon, D. H., R. R. Lobb, P. A. Damore, and J. A. Wagner. 1989. Heparin potentiates the action of acidic fibroblast growth-factor by prolonging its biological half-life. *Journal of Cellular Physiology* 138(2): 221–26.

Dautzenberg, H. and W. Jaeger. 2002. Effect of charge density on the formation and salt stability of polyelectrolyte complexes. *Macromolecular Chemistry and Physics* 203(14): 2095–102.

Decher, G. 1997. Fuzzy nanoassemblies: Toward layered polymeric multicomposites. *Science* 277(5330): 1232–37.

Desai, M. P., V. Labhasetwar, G. L. Amidon, and R. J. Levy. 1996. Gastrointestinal uptake of biodegradable microparticles: Effect of particle size. *Pharmaceutical Research* 13(12): 1838–45.

Dubas, S. T., and J. B. Schlenoff. 1999. Factors controlling the growth of polyelectrolyte multilayers. *Macromolecules* 32(24): 8153–60.

Dudhia, J. Aggrecan. 2005. Aging and assembly in articular cartilage. *Cellular and Molecular Life Sciences* 62(19–20): 2241–56.

Durango, A. M., N. F. F. Soares, S. Benevides, J. Teixeira, M. Carvalho, C. Wobeto, and N. J. Andrade. 2006. Development and evaluation of an edible antimicrobial film based on yam starch and chitosan. *Packaging Technology and Science* 19(1): 55–59.

Dutcher, J. R. and A. G. Marangoni, eds. 2005. *Soft Materials: Structure and Dynamics*. New York: Marcel Dekker.

El-Aasser, M. S. and E. D. Sudol. 2004. Miniemulsions: Overview of Research and Applications. *Journal of Coatings Technology and Research* 1(1): 21–31.

Elliott, J. T., M. Halter, A. L. Plant, J. T. Woodward, K. J. Langenbach, and A. Tona. 2008. Evaluating the performance of fibrillar collagen films formed at polystyrene surfaces as cell culture substrates. *Biointerphases* 3(2): 19–28.

Fields, G. B., J. L. Lauer, Y. Dori, P. Forns, Y. C. Yu, and M. Tirrell. 1998. Proteinlike molecular architecture: Biomaterial applications for inducing cellular receptor binding and signal transduction. *Biopolymers* 47(2): 143–51.

Fridrikh, S. V., J. H. Yu, M. P. Brenner, and G. C. Rutledge. 2003. Controlling the fiber diameter during electrospinning. *Physical Review Letters* 90(14): 144502-1–144502-4.

Fujita, M., M. Kinoshita, M. Ishihara, Y. Kanatani, Y. Morimoto, M. Simizu, T. Ishizuka, et al. 2004. Inhibition of vascular prosthetic graft infection using a photocrosslinkable chitosan hydrogel. *Journal of Surgical Research* 121(1): 135–40.

Gelain, F., A. Horii, and S. G. Zhang. 2007. Designer self-assembling peptide scaffolds for 3-D tissue cell cultures and regenerative medicine. *Macromolecular Bioscience* 7(5): 544–51.

Goldberg, M., R. Langer, and X. Q. Jia. 2007. Nanostructured materials for applications in drug delivery and tissue engineering. *Journal of Biomaterials Science-Polymer Edition* 18(3): 241–68.

Gong, M., S. Yang, J. N. Ma, S. P. Zhang, F. M. Winnik, and Y. K. Gong. 2008. Tunable cell membrane mimetic surfaces prepared with a novel phospholipid polymer. *Applied Surface Science* 255(2): 555–58.

Gong, Y.-K., F. Mwale, M. R. Wertheimer, and F. K. Winnik. 2004. Promotion of U937 cell adhesion on polypropylene surfaces bearing phosphorylcholine functionalities. *Journal of Biomaterials Science: Polymer Edition* 15(11): 1423–34.

Halperin, A., M. Tirrell, and T. P. Lodge. 1992. Tethered chains in polymer microstructures. *Advances in Polymer Science* 100: 31–71.

Hamley, I. W. 2007. *Introduction to Soft Matter: Synthetic and Biological Self-Assembling Materials*. Chichester: Wiley.

Hanshaw, R. G., R. V. Stahelin, and B. D. Smith. 2008. Noncovalent keystone interactions controlling biomembrane structure. *Chemistry-A European Journal* 14(6): 1690–97.

Hartig, S. M., G. Carlesso, J. M. 2007. Davidson, and A. Prokop. Development of improved nanoparticulate polyelectrolyte complex physicochemistry by nonstoichiometric mixing of polyions with similar molecular weights. *Biomacromolecules* 8(1): 265–72.

Hartig, S. M., R. R. Greene, G. Carlesso, J. N. Higginbotham, W. N. Khan, A. Prokop, and J. M. Davidson. 2007. Kinetic analysis of nanoparticulate polyelectrolyte complex interactions with endothelial cells. *Biomaterials* 28(26): 3843–55.

Hayward, J. A. and D. Chapman. 1984. Biomembrane surfaces as models for polymer design—the potential for hemocompatibility. *Biomaterials* 5(3): 135–42.

Horii A., X. Wang, F. Gelain, and S. Zhang. 2007. Biological designer self-assembling peptide nanofiber scaffolds significantly enhance osteoblast proliferation, differentiation and 3-D migration. *PLoS ONE* 2(2): e190. doi:10.1371/journal.pone.0000190.

Horkay, F., P. J. Basser, A. M. Hecht, and E. Geissler. 2008. Gel-like behavior in aggrecan assemblies. *Journal of Chemical Physics* 128(13): 7.

Howard, D., L. D. 2008. Buttery, K. M. Shakesheff, and S. J. Roberts. Tissue engineering: Strategies, stem cells and scaffolds. *Journal of Anatomy* 213(1): 66–72.

Hu, S. G., C. H. Jou, and M. C. Yang. 2002. Surface grafting of polyester fiber with chitosan and the antibacterial activity of pathogenic bacteria. *Journal of Applied Polymer Science* 86(12): 2977–83.

Hu, Y., K. Cai, Z. Luo, R. Zhang, L. Yang, L. Deng, and K. D. Jandt. 2009. Surface mediated *in situ* differentiation of mesenchymal stem cells on gene-functionalized titanium films fabricated by layer-by-layer technique. *Biomaterials* 30(21): 3626–35.

Huang, M. and C. Berkland. 2009. Controlled release of Repifermin from polyelectrolyte complexes stimulates endothelial cell proliferation. *Journal of Pharmaceutical Sciences* 98(1): 268–80.

Huang, M., S. N. Vitharana, L. J. Peek, T. Coop, and C. Berkland. 2007. Polyelectrolyte complexes stabilize and controllably release vascular endothelial growth factor. *Biomacromolecules* 8(5): 1607–14.

Ishida, O., K. Maruyama, K. Sasaki, and M. Iwatsuru. 1999. Size-dependent extravasation and interstitial localization of polyethyleneglycol liposomes in solid tumor-bearing mice. *International Journal of Pharmaceutics* 190(1): 49–56.

Ishii, Y., H. Sakai, and H. Murata. 2008. A new electrospinning method to control the number and a diameter of uniaxially aligned polymer fibers. *Materials Letters* 62(19): 3370–72.

Jeon, O., S. W. Kang, H. W. Lim, J. H. Chung, and B. S. Kim. 2006. Long-term and zero-order release of basic fibroblast growth factor from heparin-conjugated poly(L-lactide-*co*-glycolide) nanospheres and fibrin gel. *Biomaterials* 27(8): 1598–607.

Jia, Y. T., J. Gong, X. H. Gu, H. Y. Kim, J. Dong, and X. Y. Shen. 2007. Fabrication and characterization of poly (vinyl alcohol)/chitosan blend nanofibers produced by electrospinning method. *Carbohydrate Polymers* 67(3): 403–09.

Kanai, A. and H. E. Kaufman. 1972. Electron-microscopic studies of elastic fiber in human sclera. *Investigative Ophthalmology* 11(10): 816–21.

Kim, S. E., O. Jeon, J. B. Lee, M. S. Bae, H. J. Chun, S. H. Moon, and I. K. Kwon. 2008. Enhancement of ectopic bone formation by bone morphogenetic protein-2 delivery using heparin-conjugated Plga nanoparticles with transplantation of bone marrow-derived mesenchymal stem cells. *Journal of Biomedical Science* 15(6): 771–77.

Kim, T. G., H. Lee, Y. Jang, and T. G. Park. 2009. Controlled release of paclitaxel from heparinized metal stent fabricated by layer-by-layer assembly of polylysine and hyaluronic acid-G-poly(lactic-*co*-glycolic acid) micelles encapsulating paclitaxel. *Biomacromolecules* 10(6): 1532–39.

Kwon, I. K., S. Kidoaki, and T. Matsuda. 2005. Electrospun nano- to microfiber fabrics made of biodegradable copolyesters: Structural characteristics, mechanical properties and cell adhesion potential. *Biomaterials* 26(18): 3929–39.

Landfester, K., N. Bechthold, F. Tiarks, and M. Antonietti. 1999. Formulation and stability mechanisms of polymerizable miniemulsions. *Macromolecules* 32(16): 5222–28.

Langer, R. and J. P. Vacanti. 1993. Tissue engineering. *Science* 260(5110): 920–26.

Lapcik, L., L. Lapcik, S. De Smedt, J. Demeester, and P. Chabrecek. 1998. Hyaluronan: Preparation, structure, properties, and applications. *Chemical Reviews* 98(8): 2663–84.

Laurencin, Cato T., and Lakshmi S. Nair, eds. 2008. *Nanotechnology and Tissue Engineering: The Scaffold.* Boca Raton, FL: Taylor & Francis.

Laurent, T. C. and J. R. E. Fraser. 1992. Hyaluronan. *FASEB Journal* 6(7): 2397–404.

Lee, C. H., D. S. An, H. F. Park, and D. S. Lee. 2003. Wide-spectrum antimicrobial packaging materials incorporating nisin and chitosan in the coating. *Packaging Technology and Science* 16(3): 99–106.

Lee, C. H., A. Singla, and Y. Lee. 2001. Biomedical applications of collagen. *International Journal of Pharmaceutics* 221(1–2): 1–22.

Lee, J. Y., J. E. Choo, Y. S. Choi, K. Y. Lee, D. S. Min, S. H. Pi, Y. J. Seol, et al. 2007. Characterization of the surface immobilized synthetic heparin binding domain derived from human fibroblast growth factor-2 and its effect on osteoblast differentiation. *Journal of Biomedical Materials Research Part A* 83A(4): 970–79.

Lee, S. H. and H. Shin. 2007. Matrices and scaffolds for delivery of bioactive molecules in bone and carti-lage tissue engineering. *Advanced Drug Delivery Reviews* 59(4–5): 339–59.

Li, J. L., J. L. Pan, L. G. Zhang, X. J. Guo, and Y. T. Yu. 2003. Culture of primary rat hepatocytes within porous chitosan scaffolds. *Journal of Biomedical Materials Research Part A* 67A(3): 938–43.

Li, J. X., A. H. He, J. F. Zheng, and C. C. Han. 2006. Gelatin and gelatin-hyaluronic acid nanofibrous membranes produced by electrospinning of their aqueous solutions. *Biomacromolecules* 7(7): 2243–47.

Li, L. H., Y. Zhu, B. Li, and C. Y. Gao. 2008. Fabrication of thermoresponsive polymer gradients for study of cell adhesion and detachment. *Langmuir* 24(23): 13632–39.

Li, M. Y., D. K. Mills, T. H. Cui, and M. J. McShane. 2005. Cellular response to gelatin- and fibronectin-coated multilayer polyelectrolyte nanofilms. *IEEE Transactions on Nanobioscience* 4(2): 170–79.

Li, Wan-Ju, Yi Jen Jiang, and Rocky S. Tuan. 2006. Chondrocyte phenotype in engineered fibrous matrix is regulated by fiber size. *Tissue Engineering* 12(7): 1775–7285.

Lyon, M., G. Rushton, and J. T. Gallagher. 1997. The interaction of the transforming growth factor-beta S with heparin heparan sulfate is isoform-specific. *Journal of Biological Chemistry* 272(29): 18000–06.

Mathew, G., J. P. Hong, J. M. Rhee, D. J. Leo, and C. Nah. 2006. Preparation and anisotropic mechanical behavior of highly-oriented electrospun poly(butylene terephthalate) fibers. *Journal of Applied Polymer Science* 101(3): 2017–21.

Mccaffrey, T. A., D. J. Falcone, and B. H. Du. 1992. Transforming growth factor-beta-1 is a heparin-bind-ing protein—identification of putative heparin-binding regions and isolation of heparins with vary-ing affinity for Tgf-Beta-1. *Journal of Cellular Physiology* 152(2): 430–40.

Mei, Y., T. Wu, C. Xu, K. J. Langenbach, J. T. Elliott, B. D. Vogt, K. L. Beers, E. J. Amis, and N. R. Washburn. 2005. Tuning cell adhesion on gradient poly(2-hydroxyethyl methacrylate)-grafted surfaces. *Langmuir* 21(26): 12309–14.

Meinel, L., S. Hofmann, O. Betz, R. Fajardo, H. P. Merkle, R. Langer, C. H. Evans, G. Vunjak-Novakovic, and D. L. Kaplan. 2006. Osteogenesis by human mesenchymal stem cells cultured on silk biomateri-als: Comparison of adenovirus mediated gene transfer and protein delivery of Bmp-2. *Biomaterials* 27(28): 4993–5002.

Morgan, S. E., P. Jones, A. S. 2007. Lamont, A. Heidenreich, and C. L. McCormick. Layer-by-layer assem-bly of Ph-responsive, compositionally controlled (Co)polyelectrolytes synthesized via raft. *Langmuir* 23(1): 230–40.

Mow, V. C., A. Ratcliffe, and A. R. Poole. 1992. Cartilage and diarthrodial joints as paradigms for hierar-chical materials and structures. *Biomaterials* 13(2): 67–97.

Nakabayashi, N. and D. F. Williams. 2003. Preparation of non-thrombogenic materials using 2-methacry-loyloxyethyl phosphorylcholine. *Biomaterials* 24(13): 2431–35.

Navarro, M., E. M. Benetti, S. Zapotoczny, J. A. Planell, and G. J. Vancso. 2008. Buried, covalently attached Rgd peptide motifs in poly(methacrylic acid) brush layers: The effect of brush structure on cell adhesion. *Langmuir* 24(19): 10996–1002.

Odonnell, P. B. and J. W. McGinity. 1997. Preparation of microspheres by the solvent evaporation tech-nique. *Advanced Drug Delivery Reviews* 28(1): 25–42.

Papagiannopoulos, A., T. A. Waigh, T. Hardingham, and M. Heinrich. 2006. Solution structure and dynamics of cartilage aggrecan. *Biomacromolecules* 7(7): 2162–72.

Park, J. S., K. Park, D. G. Woo, H. N. Yang, H. M. Chung, and K. H. Park. 2008. Plga microsphere construct coated with Tgf-Beta 3 loaded nanoparticles for neocartilage formation. *Biomacromolecules* 9(8): 2162–69.

Park, J. S., D. G. Woo, H. N. Yang, H. J. Lim, H. M. Chung, and K. H. Park. 2008. Heparin-bound trans-forming growth factor-beta 3 enhances neocartilage formation by rabbit mesenchymal stem cells. *Transplantation* 85(4): 589–96.

Park, S., C. T. Hung, and G. A. Ateshian. 2004. Mechanical response of bovine articular cartilage under dynamic unconfined compression loading at physiological stress levels. *Osteoarthritis and Cartilage* 12(1): 65–73.

Peterson, S., A. Frick, and J. Liu. 2009. Design of biologically active heparan sulfate and heparin using an enzyme-based approach. *Natural Product Reports* 26(5): 610–27.

Pham, Q. P., U. Sharma, and A. G. Mikos. 2006. Electrospinning of polymeric nanofibers for tissue engineering applications: A review. *Tissue Engineering* 12(5): 1197–211.

Pham, Q. P., U. Sharma, and A. G. Mikos. 2006. Electrospun poly(epsilon-caprolactone) microfiber and multilayer nanofiber/microfiber scaffolds: Characterization of scaffolds and measurement of cellular infiltration. *Biomacromolecules* 7(10): 2796–805.

Pileni, M. P. 1997. Nanosized particles made in colloidal assemblies. *Langmuir* 13(13): 3266–76.

Plant, A. L., K. Bhadriraju, T. A. Spurlin, and J. T. Elliott. 2009. Cell response to matrix mechanics: Focus on collagen. *Biochimica Et Biophysica Acta-Molecular Cell Research* 1793(5): 893–902.

Prankerd, R. J. and V. J. Stella. 1990. The use of oil-in-water emulsions as a vehicle for parenteral drug administration. *Journal of Parenteral Science and Technology* 44(3): 139–49.

Pratta, M. A., W. Q. Yao, C. Decicco, M. D. Tortorella, R. Q. Liu, R. A. Copeland, R. Magolda, R. C. Newton, J. M. Trzaskos, and E. C. Arner. 2003. Aggrecan protects cartilage collagen from proteolytic cleavage. *Journal of Biological Chemistry* 278(46): 45539–45.

Pusateri, A. E., S. J. McCarthy, K. W. Gregory, R. A. Harris, L. Cardenas, A. T. McManus, and C. W. Goodwin. 2003. Effect of a chitosan-based hemostatic dressing on blood loss and survival in a model of severe venous hemorrhage and hepatic injury in swine. *Journal of Trauma-Injury Infection and Critical Care* 54(1): 177–82.

Rabenstein, D. L. 2002. Heparin and heparan sulfate: Structure and function. *Natural Product Reports* 19(3): 312–31.

Raghunath, J., J. Rollo, K. M. Sales, P. E. Butler, and A. M. Seifalian. 2007. Biomaterials and scaffold design: Key to tissue-engineering cartilage. *Biotechnology and Applied Biochemistry* 46: 73–84.

Reneker, D. H. and A. L. Yarin. 2008. Electrospinning jets and polymer nanofibers. *Polymer* 49(10): 2387–425.

Richert, L., P. Lavalle, E. Payan, X. Z. Shu, G. D. Prestwich, J. F. Stoltz, P. Schaaf, J. C. Voegel, and C. Picart. 2004. Layer by layer buildup of polysaccharide films: Physical chemistry and cellular adhesion aspects. *Langmuir* 20(2): 448–58.

Rodriguez-Carvajal, M. A., A. Imberty, and S. Perez. 2003. Conformational behavior of chondroitin and chondroitin sulfate in relation to their physical properties as inferred by molecular modeling. *Biopolymers* 69(1): 15–28.

Roughley, P. J., L. I. Melching, T. F. Heathfield, R. H. Pearce, and J. S. Mort. 2006. The structure and degradation of aggrecan in human intervertebral disc. *European Spine Journal* 15: S326–S332.

Ruhe, J., R. Yano, J. S. Lee, P. Koberle, W. Knoll, and A. Offenhausser. 1999. Tailoring of surfaces with ultrathin polymer films for survival and growth of neurons in culture. *Journal of Biomaterials Science-Polymer Edition* 10(8): 859–74.

Saehun, Mun, Decker Eric A., and McClements D. Julian. 2005. Effect of molecular weight and degree of deacetylation of chitosan on the formation of oil-in-water emulsions stabilized by surfactant–chitosan membranes. *Journal of Colloid and Interface Science* 296(2).

Salmivirta, M., K. Lidholt, and U. Lindahl. 1996. Heparan sulfate: A piece of information. *FASEB Journal* 10(11): 1270–79.

Sato, M., M. Ishihara, N. Kaneshiro, G. Mitani, T. Nagai, T. Kutsuna, T. Asazuma, M. Kikuchi, and J. Mochidal. 2007. Effects of growth factors on heparin-carrying polystyrene-coated atelocollagen scaffold for articular cartilage tissue engineering. *Journal of Biomedical Materials Research Part B-Applied Biomaterials* 83B(1): 181–88.

Schatz, C., A. Domard, C. Viton, C. Pichot, and T. Delair. 2004. Versatile and efficient formation of colloids of biopolymer-based polyelectrolyte complexes. *Biomacromolecules* 5(5): 1882–92.

Schatz, C., J. M. Lucas, C. Viton, A. Domard, C. Pichot, and T. Delair. 2004. Formation and properties of positively charged colloids based on polyelectrolyte complexes of biopolymers. *Langmuir* 20(18): 7766–78.

Scheufler, C., W. Sebald, and M. Hulsmeyer. 1999. Crystal structure of human bone morphogenetic protein-2 at 2.7 angstrom resolution. *Journal of Molecular Biology* 287(1): 103–15.

Schneider, A., C. Vodouhe, L. Richert, G. Francius, E. Le Guen, P. Schaaf, J. C. Voegel, B. Frisch, and C. Picart. 2007. Multifunctional polyelectrolyte multilayer films: Combining mechanical resistance, biodegradability, and bioactivity. *Biomacromolecules* 8(1): 139–45.

Schwinte, P., V. Ball, B. Szalontai, Y. Haikel, J. C. Voegel, and P. Schaaf. 2002. Secondary structure of proteins adsorbed onto or embedded in polyelectrolyte multilayers. *Biomacromolecules* 3(6): 1135–43.

Sechriest, V. F., Y. J. Miao, C. Niyibizi, A. Westerhausen-Larson, H. W. Matthew, C. H. Evans, F. H. Fu, and J. K. Suh. 2000. Gag-augmented polysaccharide hydrogel: A novel biocompatible and biodegradable material to support chondrogenesis. *Journal of Biomedical Materials Research* 49(4): 534–41.

Senaratne, W., L. Andruzzi, and C. K. Ober. 2005. Self-assembled monolayers and polymer brushes in biotechnology: Current applications and future perspectives. *Biomacromolecules* 6(5): 2427–48.

Shiratori, S. S. and M. F. Rubner. 2000. Ph-dependent thickness behavior of sequentially adsorbed layers of weak polyelectrolytes. *Macromolecules* 33(11): 4213–19.

Sill, T. J. and H. A. von Recum. 2008. Electro spinning: Applications in drug delivery and tissue engineering. *Biomaterials* 29(13): 1989–2006.

Solans, C., P. Izquierdo, J. Nolla, N. Azemar, and M. J. Garcia-Celma. 2005. Nano-emulsions. *Current Opinion in Colloid & Interface Science* 10(3–4): 102–10.

Stendahl, J. C., L. J. Wang, L. W. Chow, D. B. Kaufman, and S. I. Stupp. 2008. Growth factor delivery from self-assembling nanofibers to facilitate islet transplantation. *Transplantation* 86(3): 478–81.

Stevens, M. M. and J. H. George. 2005. Exploring and engineering the cell surface interface. *Science* 310(5751): 1135–38.

Stolnik, S., L. Illum, and S. S. Davis. 1995. Long circulating microparticulate drug carriers. *Advanced Drug Delivery Reviews* 16(2–3): 195–214.

Suh, J. K. F. and H. W. T. Matthew. 2000. Application of chitosan-based polysaccharide biomaterials in cartilage tissue engineering: A review. *Biomaterials* 21(24): 2589–98.

Sui, G., X. P. Yang, F. Mei, X. Y. Hu, G. Q. Chen, X. L. Deng, and S. Ryu. 2007. Poly-L-lactic acid/hydroxyapatite hybrid membrane for bone tissue regeneration. *Journal of Biomedical Materials Research Part A* 82A(2): 445–54.

Tadros, T., P. Izquierdo, J. Esquena, and C. Solans. 2004. Formation and stability of nano-emulsions. *Advances in Colloid and Interface Science* 108-109: 303-18.

Tezcaner, A., D. Hicks, F. Boulmedais, J. Sahel, P. Schaaf, J. C. Voegel, and P. Lavalle. 2006. Polyelectrolyte multilayer films as substrates for photoreceptor cells. *Biomacromolecules* 7(1): 86–94.

Thierry, B., F. M. Winnik, Y. Merhi, J. Silver, and M. Tabrizian. 2003. Bioactive coatings of endovascular stents based on polyelectrolyte multilayers. *Biomacromolecules* 4(6): 1564–71.

Tsuchida, E. 1994. Formation of polyelectrolyte complexes and their structures. *Journal of Macromolecular Science-Pure and Applied Chemistry* A31(1): 1–15.

Tsuchida, E., Y. Osada, and K. Sanada. 1972. Interaction of poly(styrene sulfonate) with polycations carrying charges in the chain backbone. *Journal of Polymer Science: Polymer Chemistry Edition* 10: 3397–404.

van den Beucken, J. J. J. P., X. F. Walboomers, O. C. Boerman, M. R. J. Vos, Najm Sommerdijk, T. Hayakawa, T. Fukushima, Y. Okahata, R. J. M. Nolte, and J. A. Jansen. 2006. Functionalization of multilayered DNA-coatings with bone morphogenetic protein 2. *Journal of Controlled Release* 113(1): 63–72.

Vinogradov, S. V., T. K. Bronich, and A. V. Kabanov. 2002. Nanosized cationic hydrogels for drug delivery: Preparation, properties and interactions with cells. *Advanced Drug Delivery Reviews* 54(1): 135–47.

Whitesides, G. M., E. Ostuni, S. Takayama, X. Y. Jiang, and D. E. Ingber. 2001. Soft lithography in biology and biochemistry. *Annual Review of Biomedical Engineering* 3: 335–73.

Wilson, J. T., W. X. Cui, X. L. Sun, C. Tucker-Burden, C. J. Weber, and E. L. Chaikof. 2007. *In vivo* biocompatibility and stability of a substrate-supported polymerizable membrane-mimetic film. *Biomaterials* 28(4): 609–17.

Wischerhoff, E., S. Glatzel, K. Uhlig, A. Lankenau, J. F. Lutz, and A. Laschewsky. 2009. Tuning the thickness of polymer brushes grafted from nonlinearly growing multilayer assemblies. *Langmuir* 25(10): 5949–56.

Xia, Y. N. and G. M. Whitesides. 1998. Soft lithography. *Annual Review of Materials Science* 28: 153–84.

Yilgor, P., K. Tuzlakoglu, R. L. Reis, N. Hasirci, and V. Hasirci. 2009. Incorporation of a sequential Bmp-2/Bmp-7 delivery system into chitosan-based scaffolds for bone tissue engineering. *Biomaterials* 30(21): 3551–59.

Yu, Y. C., P. Berndt, M. Tirrell, and G. B. Fields. 1996. Self-assembling amphiphiles for construction of protein molecular architecture. *Journal of the American Chemical Society* 118(50): 12515–20.

Zhang, S. G., D. M. Marini, W. Hwang, and S. Santoso. 2002. Design of nanostructured biological materials through self-assembly of peptides and proteins. *Current Opinion in Chemical Biology* 6(6): 865–71.

Zhang, Y. Z., B. Su, S. Ramakrishna, and C. T. Lim. 2008. Chitosan nanofibers from an easily electrospinnable Uhmwpeo-doped chitosan solution system. *Biomacromolecules* 9(1): 136–41.

Zhao, B. and W. J. Brittain. 2000. Polymer brushes: Surface-immobilized macromolecules. *Progress in Polymer Science* 25(5): 677–710.

Zhao, B. H., T. Katagiri, H. Toyoda, T. Takada, T. Yanai, T. Fukuda, U. I. Chung, T. Koike, K. Takaoka, and R. Kamijo. 2006. Heparin potentiates the *in vivo* ectopic bone formation induced by bone morphogenetic protein-2. *Journal of Biological Chemistry* 281(32): 23246–53.

Zhou, M., A. M. Smith, A. K. Das, N. W. Hodson, R. F. Collins, R. V. Ulijn, and J. E. Gough. 2009. Self-assembled peptide-based hydrogels as scaffolds for anchorage-dependent cells. *Biomaterials* 30(13): 2523–30.

14

Nanoparticles-Incorporated Scaffolds for Tissue Engineering Applications

Hao Xu
University of Texas at Arlington

Zarna Ashwin Bhavsar
University of Texas at Arlington

Kytai Truong Nguyen
University of Texas at Arlington

14.1 Introduction

In tissue engineering, scaffolds are often used to support the cell attachment and growth, thereby repairing and regenerating the diseased tissue or body organ. With the development of modern nanotechnology, scaffolds possessing nanometer-scaled features are attracting increased attention for their application in tissue engineering. It is well known now that cells naturally live within the extracellullar matrix (ECM) complex which has complicated nanometer-scaled three-dimensional structures, including pores, ridges, and fibers (Dufrene, 2001; Flemming et al., 1999). This nanometer-scaled ECM structure interacts with cells and give cells guidance for a number of cell and tissue functions such as cell migration (Wolf et al., 2003) and organelle formation (Dent and Gertler, 2003). It has also been shown that synthetically nanofabricated topography can also influence cell adhesion, proliferation, morphology, alignment, cytoskeleton organization, and migration (Kriparamanan et al., 2006). In addition, the substrate surface properties, including surface energy, chemical compositions, and mechanical properties, also have influences on the tissue–material interactions and determine the fate of medical devices. In the following sections of this chapter, we will discuss the techniques of creating nanotopography using nanoparticles as a surface-modification technique for tissue engineered scaffolds and the effects of this nanotopography to cells and tissues.

In addition to coating on material surfaces to produce surface nanotopography, nanoparticles are also embedded in the bulk material to make nanocomposites which provide the scaffold with special functions for their interactions with cells. These special functions include the following: (1) the nanoparticles provide nanostructure inside the scaffold and nanotopography on top of the scaffold that can change the interaction between the cells with the scaffold; (2) the nanoparticles can be loaded with therapeutic reagents such as drugs, growth factors, and cytokines for time-controlled release; (3) these active factors can be released into the scaffold in a timely manner synchronized with cell and tissue development; (4) nanoparticles embedded in scaffolds can also change the scaffold's mechanical properties and nutrient transport properties, thus making the scaffold better for cell growth. Scaffolds embedded with nanoparticles and their applications in tissue engineering will also be discussed in the next section. The overall schematics of creating nanotopography or nanocomposites are shown in Figure 14.1.

14.2 Nanotopography on Scaffold Surfaces Using Nanoparticles

A number of techniques have been used to make nanoscaled surfaces with either regularly or randomly organized patterns. Techniques to create ordered topography structures include soft lithography, electron-beam or ion-beam lithography, microtransfer molding, replica molding, micromolding in capillaries, solvent-assisted micromolding, and microcontact printing. On the other hand, nanoparticle self-assembly and lithography or chemical etching are the common methods used to make surfaces with randomly organized patterns. In this chapter, only commonly used techniques, surface assembly of nanoparticles, and layer-by-layer (LBL) coating of nanoparticles are reviewed.

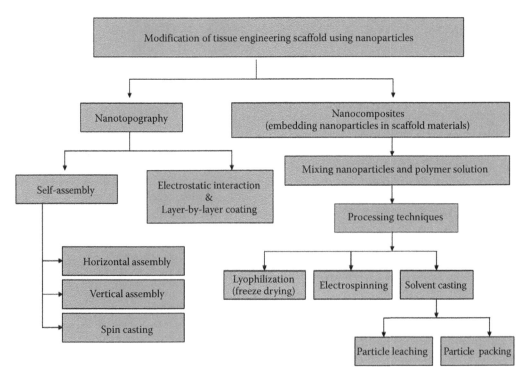

FIGURE 14.1   Schematics of creating nanotopography and nanocomposites using nanoparticles.

14.2.1 Surface Assembly of Nanoparticles

Self-assembly or self-organization, means the spontaneous organization of molecular units into ordered structures. In real life, self-assembly accounts for many key processes, such as nucleic acid synthesis, protein synthesis, and cytoskeleton assembly. Today's definition of self-assembly came from the formation of close-packed amphiphilic molecules, a work of Langmuir and Boldgett in early twentieth century [Blodgett, 1935; Langmuir, 1920]. The binding force of the building units is normally noncovalent interactions (e.g., hydrogen bonds, Van Der Waals, capillary force), which makes the self-assembly process reversible. Three distinctive features of self-assembly include the ordered building unit, the weak interactions (e.g., hydrogen bonds, Van Der Waals, capillary force), and nanoscaled building blocks. Gold (Au) nanoparticles with alkyl disulfide surfaces are among the earliest of colloidal assembly, first produced by Allara and Nuzzo (Nuzzo and Allara, 1983). Au nanoparticles have certain properties, such as high stability, easiness of preparation, and good biocompatibility. Self-assembly of Au nanoparticles with thiol groups has been widely studied and used for DNA delivery. Au nanoparticles are also easy to be conjugated with biofunctional groups, which have wide applications in tissue engineering. In addition to Au, nanoparticles made of other materials such as metal (e.g., copper and silver) (Yu et al., 2007) inorganic materials (e.g., silica) (Wang et al., 2009) and polymers (e.g., polystyrene, poly(lactic-*co*-glycolic acid) (PLGA)) (Miller et al., 2004; Thapa et al., 2003) have also been used by surface self-assembly to create nanotopographies on material surfaces. Three common methods for colloidal particle self-assembly are horizontal deposition, vertical deposition (Kitaev and Ozin, 2003; Wang and Zhao, 2007; Wang et al., 2008) and spin-casting (Mihi et al., 2006). Though these methods were initially invented for other purposes, there are growing interests to use them to create nanotopographic material surfaces for tissue engineering applications.

One common method of particle self-assembly onto the material surface is horizontal deposition where colloidal particles are cast on the substrate horizontally. After the particle suspension spreads on the substrate surface, it is heated to evaporate solvents. A highly ordered colloidal particle layer will form on top of the surface after further heating. This self-assembled nanoparticle layer often has a uniform thickness. Zeng et al., used this method to produce the colloidal polystyrene nanoparticle film (Zeng et al., 2002). Three stages, including evaporation of solvent and particle ordering, particle deformation, and polymer interdiffusion, occur during the nanoparticle layer formation. Mechanisms for particle deformation include dry sintering (driven by the reduction of the polymer/air interfacial energy), wet sintering (driven by the reduction of the polymer/water (serum) interfacial energy), and capillary deformation (driven by the capillary pressure generated across the water/air menisci) (Alexander and William, 1999). The uniformity of the particle layer highly depends on the particle size and dispersity. Other factors that affect the colloidal assembly include particle concentration, electrolyte concentration of the suspending solution, and temperature (Zeng et al., 2002). Horizontal deposition is a fast and flexible method; however, it is usually difficult to create a film more than a few square centimeters without defects. Thus, uniform coating of nanoparticles on a large surface is very hard to achieve.

Different from horizontal deposition, in vertical deposition, the substrate to be coated by nanoparticles is held vertically. After dipping in a colloidal dispersion, the substrate is then lifted away. After drying, a well-ordered nanoparticle mono- or multilayer will form on the substrate surface (Jiang et al., 1999). Alternatively, the substrate can also be dipped in the nanoparticle solution and then held at a tilted angle in a stationary position while the solvent evaporates (Cong and Gao, 2003). The solvent is allowed to evaporate at either the natural ambient rate or at an accelerated rate to create colloidal layers. Factors including temperature and humidity of the surrounding atmosphere can all affect the evaporation rate (Shimmin et al., 2006). Vertical deposition is highly effective when the solvent evaporation rate exceeds the particle sedimentation rate. Two parameters (the particle size and particle/solution volume fraction) control the film thickness; smaller particles yield fewer layers, and higher concentration of the particle solution yields thicker films (Jiang et al., 1999). The tilted angle of the substrate can also affect the thickness of colloidal crystals. In contrast to horizontal deposition, vertical deposition produces superior quality colloidal films with smoother surfaces. Compared to horizontal deposition, vertical deposition takes less time (only a few minutes) to fabricate a colloidal particle film of several square centimeters (Wang et al., 2009). The limitation of vertical deposition is that there is a limited range of particle sizes and densities able to be used in this technique due to the tendency of particle sedimentation, which is also affected by the aqueous phase viscosity. It should be also noted that both sides of the substrate will be coated with the nanoparticle film in vertical deposition.

Spin-casting is another method to make nanoparticle coating on the material surface. In spin-casting, the colloidal particle solution is either dispersed onto the substrate then subjected to spinning or onto the rotating substrate directly. Within seconds, the shear forces will induce the formation of the two- or three-dimensional particle films in nanometer thicknesses (Wang and Möhwald, 2004). In the spin-casting process, the evaporation rate of the continuous medium, spinning velocity, particle dispersion concentration, and medium viscosity are all key parameters to control the particle packing and film thickness. Unlike horizontal or vertical deposition, which usually result in close-packed colloidal particles, spin-casting can fabricate either close-packed or isolated particle arrays depending on the process conditions (Venkatesh and Jiang, 2007; Wang and Möhwald, 2004).

14.2.2 Electrostatic Interaction and Layer-by-Layer Coating of Nanoparticles

Electrostatic interactions are also often used for incorporating nanoparticles on material surfaces. To make this interaction stronger, modifications can be used to intensify or reverse the electrical charges of nanoparticles. For examples, Lo et al., modified PLGA nanoparticle surface charges from negative to high positive by varying the surfactants, and the positively charged nanoparticles resulted in a high percentage of surface coating on the negatively charged material surface (Lo et al., 2009). Though nanoparticles can be self-assembled or electrostatically assembled on material surfaces, their bonding is weak, making the particles unstable on the material surface.

To get a stronger attachment of the particle on the materials surface, LBL coating of the nanoparticles is often used. In LBL coating, polyelectrolytes carrying positive charges (polycation) and polyelectrolytes carrying negative charges (polyanion) are coated on the material surface alternatively, resulting in reversal of the surface charges. Some commonly used polycations include poly(allylamine hydrochloride) (PAH) and polylysine. Poly(acrylic acid) and poly(sodium 4-styrenesulfonate) (PSS) are often used as polyanions. In this process, nanoparticles which carry electrical charges can be deposited on the electrolyte layer carrying the opposite charges to form the LBL coating. For nanoparticles without strong electrical charges, they can also be doped in one of the two polyelectrolytes and spread on top of the substrates to create a nanotopographic surface. The traditional LBL dip-coating process involves multiple deposition and rinsing steps, which extends the processing time and thereby limits its use. To overcome this limitation, other techniques have been employed. Spinning is used with LBL coating, so called the spin-assisted LBL coating. For example, inorganic cadmium sulfide (CdS) nanoparticles or silicon oxide nanoparticles are spin-coated on silicone surface LBL to create multiple nanoparticle layers (Chao and Char, 2001; Yang and Zhang, 2009). Compared with dip-coating, spinning creates better ordered internal structures (Zeng et al., 2002). In addition to spinning, nanoparticles doped in polyelectrolytes can also be sprayed on the surface of the substrates to avoid the rinsing steps (Izquierdo et al., 2005; Krogman et al., 2007). Krogman et al., showed a surface coating of polycation/TiO_2 nanoparticles with nylon fibers using this spray-LBL technique (Krogman et al., 2009). The shortcoming of the spray coating is decreased control over three-dimensional or porous objects with less covering in shadow regions.

To control the pattern of nanoparticles on the surfaces, colloidal particle assembly has also been applied together with surface patterning. Topographical patterns such as various arrays of grooves, holes, or chemical/physical surface patterns on the substrate can guide the colloidal assembly process of particles on these patterns through a variety of mechanisms including electrostatic forces or charges (Lee et al., 2004; Xia et al., 2003). For example, electropositive particles will attach to negative regions or hydrophobic particles will preferentially adsorb onto hydrophobic regions of the substrate. Other mechanisms include capillary force and gravitational forces.

14.2.3 Cell Responses to Nanoparticle-Coated Surfaces

Alterations in material surface topography, particularly nanotopography, elicit diverse cell responses, including cell adhesion, proliferation, morphology, orientation, motility, cytoskeletal condensation, and intracellular signaling pathways (Abrams et al., 2000; Gong, 2002). The development of functional tissue-engineered scaffolds requires the understanding of cellular responses to the nanotopographies. Though great challenges still exist in duplicating the three-dimensional ECM mimicking scaffolds (e.g., scaffolds that mimic the basement tissue membrane which possess a complex network of pores, ridges, and fibers in the nanometer size), the development of nanotechnology allows the creation of some relatively simple nanoscale patterns such as nanochannel, nanoposts (including nanoparticles and nanoislands), and nanopores to study cell and tissue responses. Nanochannels are extensively studied and cells are found to align with the nanochannels. However, cell response to nanoposts and nanopores are found to be uncertain with many conflicts among the researchers due to the disparities in scale features, cell types, and different experimental protocols, as shown on Table 14.1. Since we are more interested in material surface modification with nanoparticles, in this section we intend to compile and analyze the relevant existing information about the cell or tissue behaviors on the material surface modified with nanoparticles and their applications in tissue engineering.

Cell responses to nanotopography generated by nanoparticles are found to be largely dependent on the material properties, particle size, particle density, and cell types. Of those factors, particle size is one of the key factors affecting the cell responses. Large particles are found to inhibit cell adhesion and proliferation compared to smaller particles or flat surfaces. For example, Miura and Fujimoto, found that human umbilical vein endothelial cells seeded on a 527-nm diameter poly(styrene-*co*-acrylamide) particle monolayer had slower cell growth than on flat tissue culture plates. On the 1270 nm-diameter particle monolayer, the amount of cells decreased even more after 24 h growth (Miura and Fujimoto, 2006). Dalby et al., also found that fibroblasts grown on 27-nm- or 95-nm high poly(4-bromostyrene) nanoislands showed slower cell growth compared to cells grown on a smooth surface (Dalby et al., 2003; Dalby et al., 2004). In addition, cell adhesion/proliferation was found to be related to nanoparticle density. Kunzler et al. found that rat calvarial osteoblasts seeded on polylysine-RGD-treated silica nanoparticles (73 nm in diameter) demonstrated a continuously reduced cell proliferation rate with the increasing particle densities (Kunzler et al., 2007). In addition, the particle shape has also been found to affect cell functions. Spherical HA nanoparticles are found to better support L929 fibroblast proliferation than needle-shaped HA nanoparticles (Fu and Li, 2008).

In addition to cell proliferation, cell morphology can also be affected by the nanoparticle coating on material surfaces. Human endothelial cells grown on poly(styrene-*co*-acrylamide) nanoparticle films demonstrated stretched, narrow stalk-like shapes (Miura and Fujimoto, 2006). An established human endothelial cell line (HGTFN) showed better cell spreading with more accurate cells when grown on polystyrene and poly(4-bromostyrene) nanoislands of 13, 35, and 95 nm heights (Dalby et al., 2002). The cells also showed stronger interaction with the nanoparticles with more filopodias "grasping" the nanoparticles, as well as less cytoskeleton stress fibers compared to the cells grown on a flat surface (Miura and Fujimoto, 2006). Similar hindered actin network was found in rat calvarial osteoblast cells grown on dense nanoparticle layers (Kunzler et al., 2007). Though the mechanisms of how nanotopographies affect cell behaviors are not yet understood, it is likely that nanotopography modulates the interfacial forces that guide cytoskeletal formation and membrane receptor organization in the cells, which in turn can modify intracellular signaling (Curtis et al., 2004; Curtis et al., 2006). It is also suspected

TABLE 14.1   Cellular Responses to Nanopost Topography

Materials	Dimensions	Cell Types	Cell Responses
Poly(styrene-*co*-acrylamide) nanoparticles	527 nm, 1270 nm diameter	Human umbilical vein endothelial cells	Cell growth was slower than on flat TCPS, cell numbers even decreased on 1270 nm particle layer (Miura and Fujimoto, 2006)
Polylysine-RGD treated silica nanoparticles	73 nm in diameter	Rat calvarial osteoblasts	Reduced cell proliferation rate with the increasing particle densities (Kunzler et al., 2007)
Polystyrene nanoislands	27 and 95 nm high	Human fibroblasts	Inhibited cell growth with large pseudopodial processes compared to the cells grown on smooth surface (Dalby et al., 2004)
Polystyrene nanoislands	13, 35, and 95 nm high	Human endothelial cell type HGTFN	Cells spread bigger with more filopodia interacting with the nanoislands (Dalby et al., 2002)
Polystyrene nanoislands	11, 38, and 85 nm high	Human fetal osteoblastic cell	Cells cultured on 11 nm high islands displayed significantly enhanced cell spreading and larger cell dimensions than cells on larger nanoislands or flat PS control (Lim et al., 2005)
PEG nanopillars	300–500 nm	Mouse P19EC stem cells	Increased cell adhesion (Kim et al., 2005)
PLA nanopillars	400–700 nm	Human fibroblasts	Lower cell proliferation, smaller cell size, enhanced cell elongation (Choi et al., 2007)
Silver nanoparticles	7–30 nm	Human platelets	Resist platelet adhesion and human plasma fibrinogen adsorption, antibacterial activity against MRSA (Yu et al., 2007)
Titanium nanopyramids	23–80 nm	Human fibroblasts Human astrocytoma-derived glial cells	Reduced cell proliferation, more elongated cell morphology, less mature cytoskeleton (Pennisi et al., 2009)
Polystyrene nanopillars	160–1000 nm	HeLA cells	Decreased cell spreading (Nomura et al., 2006)
Polyethylene glycol (PEG) nanopillars	400 nm high 150 nm width	Human cardiomyocytes	Enhanced cell adhesion, guided filopodial growth (Kim et al., 2005)
Silica nanoparticles	20 or 50 nm in diameter	Human fibroblasts	Increased cell adhesion, earlier cell–cell interaction (Wood et al., 2006)
PMMA nanocolumns	160 nm high, 100 nm wide	Immortalized Human fibroblasts	Less cell speading, punctuate actin organization, many filopodia (Dalby et al., 2005)

that the availability of an integrin binding site, which can further affect the downstream signaling pathways, might be responsible for the nanotopographical affects.

Though the mechanism of cell–nanotopography interaction is still yet to be elucidated, nanotopography cues have been used in tissue engineering applications. For example, nanosized hydroxyapatite particles were coated on the PLLA fiber surfaces to increase mouse fibroblast adhesion while reducing inflammation when subcutaneously implanted compared to untreated PLLA fibers (Spadaccio et al., 2009; Yanagida et al., 2009). It not only increased mouse fibroblasts adhesion but induced less inflammation when subcutaneously implanted than untreated PLLA fibers (Yanagida et al., 2009). Better induction of human mesenchymal stem cells (MSCs) to chondrocyte-like cells was also found on the HAp nanoparticle-coated PLLA fibers, which is favorable for cartilage regeneration (Spadaccio et al., 2009). Particularly, soluble drugs or growth factors can be incorporated in the nanoparticles and released into the surrounding environment. When nanoparticles are used to create the nanotopographical surfaces, the nanotopography can work synergistically with the controlled release of therapeutic agents to affect cellular behaviors.

14.3 Embedment of Nanoparticles to Make Nanocomposites for Tissue Engineering Applications

The tissue engineering approach investigates various techniques to form 3-D scaffolds which can guide the growth of mammalian cells by providing an artificial ECM or a scaffold and mimic the local environment of the natural tissue (Yang et al., 2001). For mimicking the ECM in structures and properties and thereby enhancing the cell growth, nanoparticles can be embedded in the scaffold to provide the cells with favorable properties for adhesion, differentiation, and growth. In addition, scaffolds formed by polymeric matrix and inorganic nanoparticles would provide materials with optical, electronic, or magnetic properties for various applications while maintaining the processing ease of polymers. These nanoparticle-embedded scaffolds are sometimes called nanocomposites. The method for formation of the nanocomposite scaffold is chosen based on the application, size, and characteristics of the required scaffold. In general, conventional techniques such as solvent casting, freeze-drying, and electro-spinning used to make tissue engineering scaffolds can be applied to form scaffolds embedded with nanoparticles. However, the ability to control the dispersion and distribution of nanoparticles within the polymeric matrix when forming the scaffolds can be difficult. Clumping and sedimentation of nanoparticles are often occurred when nanoparticles are introduced into the scaffolds. In the next sections, several methods to form scaffolds from polymeric matrix and nanoparticles will be discussed.

14.3.1 Techniques to Form Scaffolds with Embedded Nanoparticles

Scaffolds with embedded inorganic and organic nanoparticles can be made by several techniques such as plastic processing technologies, solvent solution, melt processing, *in situ* polymerization and emulsion polymerization (Šupová, 2009). Plastic processing methods include compounding, milling, and compression or injection molding. Ceramic nanoparticles have been mixed with polymer pellets before compression molding step to form composite scaffolds. Mixing ceramic powders with polymer pellets led to a ceramic nanoparticle network around the polymer pellets. Yet these techniques might cause formation of air bubbles and thermal degradation of matrix polymers during the process. Solvent solution technique is based on the dispersion of nanoparticles into a polymer–solvent solution. This method can produce a homogeneous dispersion of nanoparticles depending on polymers, solvent, and viscosity of the materials; however, the main drawback is the potential toxicity that results from organic solvent residues. Unlike plastic processing and solvent solution techniques, melt extrusion method has been shown to produce homogenous distribution of inorganic nanoparticles within the polymer matrix. In this technique, nanoparticles are mixed with the polymer in the molten state, thus no organic toxic solvent is required. Similar to plastic processing techniques, melt processing might also cause the thermal degradation of materials.

In addition to traditional composite methods such as plastic processing, solvent solution, and melt extrusion, several techniques and modifications have been made to produce homogenous distribution of nanoparticles within the polymeric matrix while avoiding several drawbacks such as toxicity and thermal degradation. One of them is the *in situ* polymerization. In this method, nanoparticles are dispersed in the polymeric monomers and formed into scaffolds after exposure to UV, which is used to initiate the photopolymerization to produce a crosslinking network. Another method is *in situ* formation of nanocomposites by forming nanoparticles in the presence of polymers using the co-solution and coprecipitation. This technique is more attractive as it avoids particle aggregations that are often produced by a mechanical mixing process. For example, Kato et al. (1997), have investigated various hydroxyapatite (HA) nanoparticles/polymer composites via *in situ* synthesis. They have found that crystallization of HA was reduced when the ionized polymers were introduced and that the crystallization was concentration-dependent. This method has been successfully used to form nano-HA/polyamide, HA/chitosan, and HA/collagen nanocomposites.

Recently, Zhao et al. developed a new, interesting technique that can control the spatial distribution of nanoparticles within the polymer matrix without the use of chemical modification of the original nanoparticles. They used a small-molecule-directed nanoparticle assembly approach by binding a surfactant to one of the polymer blocks through hydrogen bonding. This induces a favorable interact of the alkyl-chain covered nanoparticles to the surfactant-modified block in a noncovalent manner. Interestingly, the noncovalent binding of nanoparticles and polymer matrix can be strengthened or decoupled by external stimuli via the use of functional, stimuli-responsive small molecules. This responsiveness to external stimuli would open up new perspectives for tissue engineering applications. For example, it is possible to design stimuli-responsive scaffolds that control and release the encapsulated nanoparticles toward the surrounding via an external stimulation. Noncovalent control of nanoparticle assembly in hierarchically organized block copolymer/surfactant complexes can also provide more novel particle arrangements within the polymeric matrix. This method provides the advantages of flexibility, ease of implementation, spatial control of nanoparticle distribution, and reversibility while avoiding the tedious modification of nanoparticles. The authors have provided the success in controlling spatial distribution of various nanoparticles with different shapes and sizes such as Au, CdSe, and PbS. The authors also demonstrate the thermo- and light-responsive behaviors to control the temperature-dependent partitioning of nanoparticles within the scaffolds. This approach seems very simple, robust, versatile, and applicable to a wide range of nanoparticles. If successful with various materials, it will open new routes for scaffold and device fabrication using nanoparticles and polymeric matrix.

To form scaffolds embedded with organic nanoparticles, the nanocomposite synthesis procedure basically involves mixing nanoparticles at certain concentrations in the bulk polymeric materials. The mixture of nanoparticles and polymer solution is then processed by various methods to form a 3-D scaffold. Freeze drying or lyophilization is the most widely used method in the scaffold formulation process to produce a porous nanocomposite scaffold. This process removes all the aqueous parts from the scaffold resulting in a porous, dry scaffold (Tan et al., 2009). Another scaffold formation technique is the solvent casting method in which the nanoparticle–polymer solution is casted into a 3-D mold similar to standard casting methods. In addition, the electrospinning technique can also be used to spin the polymer–nanoparticle solution into mesh-like scaffolds (Li et al., 2006). Combinations of different techniques like solvent casting, particle leaching, and particle packing can also be used. After casting the polymer–nanoparticle solution in the mold, the porogen can be leached to produce a porous nanocomposite scaffold (Chen et al., 2008). Other new technologies to form 3D polymer scaffolds such as 3D printing, selective laser sintering, multiphase jet solidification, and fused deposition modeling can also be applied to the nanoparticle-polymer solution to form the 3D scaffolds with embedded nanoparticles (Stevens et al., 2008). Various types of nanoparticles have been used to embed in the materials for many tissue engineering applications as shown in Table 14.2. In the next section, commonly used nanoparticles will be discussed.

14.3.2 Scaffolds Embedded with Inorganic Nanoparticles

Magnetic nanoparticles: Hydrogel-based nanocomposite scaffolds embedded with magnetic nanoparticles have been shown to give rise to a unique approach, that is, tissue engineering aided by drug-delivery using magnetic nanoparticles. The magnetically sensitive hydrogel was fabricated by *in situ* coprecipitation of magnetic nanoparticles deposited in biodegradable gelatin by sol–gel method (Hu et al., 2007). Vitamin B12 was used as a model growth factor loaded in the gelatin scaffold and its release was dependent on the application of an external magnetic field. On application of the external magnetic field, the authors found that the release of Vitamin B12 was evidently lower as compared to release in the absence of the external magnetic field. The magnetic field blocked the drug molecules from freely diffusing through the scaffold, and removal of the magnetic field allowed a generous release of drug into the surroundings of the scaffold (Hu et al., 2007). This type of controlled release of growth factor in the scaffold would allow the slow release of growth factors, and thereby leading to better cell growth and production

TABLE 14.2 Applications of Nanocomposites in Tissue Engineering

Tissue Engineering Applications	Scaffold Materials	Nanoparticles		Results
		Materials	Size	
Bone tissue engineering	Poly(ester urethane)	Nano-HA	10–15 nm	Increased tensile properties, osteoconductivity (Boissard et al., 2009)
	Chitosan-Polylactic acid	Nano-HA	Diameter 50 nm, length 300 nm	Significant improvements in elastic modulus and compressive strength (Cai et al., 2009)
	Poly(propylene fumarate)	Nano-HA	100 nm	Enhanced cell attachment, spreading, and proliferation (Lee et al., 2008)
	Collagen I	nHA	12–15 nm	Enhanced mechanical properties, strong interaction between organic and inorganic phases (Tampieri et al., 2003; Du et al., 1999; Soichiro et al., 2004)
	Collagen I-Alginate	nHA	12–15 nm	Increased compressive yield strength and compressive modulus as compared to collagen-nHA composite (Zhang et al., 2003)
	Gelatin	HAp		Gelatin is readily available as compared to collagen, increased chemical bonding between the two phases (Chang et al., 2003)
	Poly(2-hydroxyethyl methacrylate) (pHEMA) hydrogel	HAp		Increased mineral-hydrogel interfacial adhesion strength (Song et al., 2003)
	Poly(L-lactic acid) (PLLA)	Bioactive glass ceramic	20–40 nm	Increased compressive strength, bioactivity, and hydrophilicity of the composite (Hong et al., 2008)
	Chitin	Nano-silica		Increased bioactivity (Yang et al., 2001)
	Poly(propylene fumarate)/ propylene fumarate-diacrylate	Surface modified alumoxane nanoparticles		Enhanced bone ingrowth, bone contact, and degradability (Mistry et al., 2009)
	Collagen-polylactic acid (PLA)	nHA		Composition and hierarchy similar to natural bone, bioactive, high mechanical strength (Liao et al., 2004)
Cartilage tissue engineering	Poly-L-lactic acid (PLLA)	Nano-HA	<200 nm	Increased chondrogenic differentiation of human MSCs (Spadaccio et al., 2009)
	Collagen	Gold (Au)	5 nm	Increased mechanical properties, antioxidative effect (Chen et al., 2008)
	Chitosan	Chitosan	0.2–1.5 µm (for microspheres loaded with growth factors)	Rapid proliferation of chondrocytes on chitosan scaffold by release of growth factor (Kim et al., 2003)
	Gelatin/chitosan/ hyaluronan	PLGA	<50 µm	Increased compressive strength while maintaining excellent biocompatibility (Tan et al., 2009)

TABLE 14.2 (continued) Applications of Nanocomposites in Tissue Engineering

Tissue Engineering Applications	Scaffold Materials	Nanoparticles		Results
		Materials	Size	
Neural tissue engineering	Chitosan	Gold (Au)	5 nm	Improved mechanical strength and cellular responses (Lin et al., 2008)
	Polyurethane	Zinc oxide(ZnO)	60 nm	Increased electrical, mechanical, and antibacterial properties (Chen et al., 2008)
Cardiac and vascular tissue engineering	Polyvinyl alcohol	Bacterial cellulose	<100 nm	Enhanced mechanical properties similar to aortic heart valve (Millon and Wan, 2006)
	Polycaprolactone (PCL)	PLGA	$0.437 \pm 0.29\ \mu m$	Highly interconnected porous scaffold, increased diffusion of media through the porous scaffold (Sarkar et al., 2006)
Wound healing	Chitin	Nanosilver	5 nm	Bactericidal property and enhanced blood clotting ability (Madhumathi et al., 2009)
	Gelatin	PLGA	1–$15\ \mu m$	Decreased swelling properties, increased degradation rate, enhanced mechanical properties (Banerjee et al., 2009)
	Collagen	Gelatin	60–$120\ \mu m$	Improved environment for wound healing and controlled release of drug (Adhirajan et al., 2009)

of the ECM to increase tissue regeneration. Magnetic nanoparticles have also a great potential for tissue engineering applications like enhancing cell seeding, cell invasion, and tissue engineering-based drug delivery.

Ceramic Nanoparticle: Ceramic nanoparticles are often used to embed into various biomaterial scaffolds for bone and cartilage tissue engineering applications as ceramic nanoparticles are known to increase the mechanical properties of the scaffold (Spadaccio et al., 2009; Yang et al., 2001; Ma et al., 2006). Many types of ceramic materials like HA, bioactive glass, silica nanoparticles, and zinc oxide (ZnO) have been investigated as embedding materials in the scaffolds. Some of these materials are inorganic parts of the natural bone, thus they possess properties like biocompatibility, bioactivity, and osteoconductivity which gives the scaffold characteristics of natural bone (Murugan and Ramakrishna, 2005). Nano-HA has been incorporated into different polymeric matrices for different applications. For example, nano-HA particles were added to the polyelectrolyte complex (PEC) of natural cationic polymer chitosan and anionic polygalacturonic acid to increase cell adhesion and proliferation on the scaffolds and to induce mechanical properties. The property of the scaffold was enhanced because of the interaction of the scaffold and nanoparticles which mimicked the ECM of the natural bone (Verma et al., 2009). Another example is nano-HA particles embedded in a highly elastic and biocompatible polymer, poly(ester urethane) with polycaprolactone (PCL) segments, to increase the osteoconductivity property and protein adhesion on the scaffold as well as maintain the elastic properties. Enhanced bone invasion and surface properties was found on this nanocomposite along with a good bonding with the native tissue. Along with the enhanced properties by the nano-HA particle incorporation, the poly(urethane) soft segments were responsible for the extensibility and the hard segments for the stiffness and strength of the polymer resulting in a suitable nanocomposite for bone tissue engineering (Boissard et al., 2009; Cai et al., 2009).

In addition to nano-HA, glass ceramic nanoparticles embedded in materials have also shown superior results. For instance, bioactive glass ceramics have been reported to influence osteoblast and bone marrow stromal cell proliferation and differentiation (Bosetti and Cannas, 2005; Hench et al., 1991). Bioactive glass ceramic nanoparticles were embedded into a poly(L-lactic acid) (PLLA) matrix and the nanocomposite matrix exhibited higher mechanical properties and mineralization compared to the PLLA scaffold without any bioglass nanoparticles (Hong et al., 2008). Another important concept is the use of bioactive glass ceramic nanoparticles embedded in synthetic polymers from the family of polylactide to overcome a local acidic environment generated by the polymer degradation (Bosetti et al., 2005). When these biodegradable polymers are degraded, their acidic degraded products accumulate in the vicinity of the scaffold which tends to trigger inflammatory reactions. This can be overcome by the basic degradation of the glass ceramic-based particles as it will buffer the acidic environment. These significant developments have led researchers to divert their attention towards the use of newly developed, bioactive glass ceramic nanoparticles for tissue engineering applications.

Silica is another class of ceramic materials which can be synthesized in the form of nanosilica and added to the polymeric scaffolds to increase the bioactivity of the scaffold. Silica is a component of bioactive glasses which form an apatite layer *in vitro* and *in vivo*. This material has been found to produce apetite formation in simulated body fluid (SBF). Silica particles were successfully embedded into the chitin matrix to increase the swelling and biocompatibility properties of the scaffold (Madhumathi et al., 2009). The formation of apetite layer on the scaffold also makes this silica embedding scaffold a good candidate for bone tissue engineering.

Nanoparticles made of ZnO, a piezoelectric material, were chosen to embed in scaffolds for neural tissue engineering. Piezoelectric ZnO nanoparticles of diameter 60 nm were synthesized and embedded in polyurethane scaffolds to closely mimic the scale of the building blocks that form natural neural support tissues. Additionally, the piezoelectric characteristics of ZnO allowed for a transient electrical charge across the guidance channel upon mechanical deformation of the material. Moreover, nanoscale ZnO showed reduced adhesion and density of bacteria found naturally on the skin providing the nanocomposite with antibacterial properties. The combination of these characteristics into one nanostructured scaffold could produce the necessary electrical and structural cues (along with a desirable antibacterial property) for axonal guidance and nervous system tissue regeneration (Seil et al., 2008).

Gold nanoparticles: Au nanoparticles have been embedded into natural as well as synthetic polymers to provide the composite structure with many favorable properties for tissue growth. Au nanoparticles of size 5 nm were embedded into collagen II scaffolds seeded with chondrocytes for cartilage tissue regeneration. These scaffolds exhibited better interaction of the filipodia of the cells with the anionic Au nanoparticles and resulted in better anchoring and attachment of the cells. The incorporation of the Au nanoparticles also made the scaffolds less elastic and stiff which decreased the epithelial cell apoptosis by degradation of the polymer. The addition of Au nanoparticles also made the nanocomposite antioxidative, avoiding problems caused by oxidative reactions. Although a small amount of Au nanoparticles were released from the collagen scaffold resulting in the uptake of Au nanoparticles by chondrocytes, no cytotoxicity was seen to occur in the scaffold while using the optimum amount of Au nanoparticles (Hsu et al., 2007). Au nanocomposites with poly(ether urethane) and poly(ester urethane) have also been previously studied. Addition of Au nanoparticles to the polymeric scaffolds resulted in increased biocompatibility, thermal, mechanical, and free radical scavenging properties of the composite (Hsu et al., 2008). For sciatic nerve repair, micropatterned Chitosan-Gold conduits were synthesized. The addition of Au nanoparticles to the scaffold increased the mechanical properties by changes in the temperature. Also, specific amounts of Au nanoparticles had a stimulating effect on cell proliferation capacity and gene expression (Lin et al., 2008).

14.3.3 Scaffolds Embedded with Organic (Degradable) Nanoparticles

Degradable polymers are of much interest in the fields of both tissue engineering and drug delivery. These materials can be used to synthesize the polymeric scaffolds as well as the micro/nanoparticles to be used as embedding materials in the scaffold, and this combination aids the regenerative medicine based on following features. First, it acts as a mechanical scaffold for the transplanted cells by providing the growing cells with temporary support and bearing of the mechanical loads. Biodegradable materials can also be used to synthesize carriers (nanoparticles) which can be used to load and release therapeutic agents such as drugs, growth factors, and differentiating factors upon the degradation of the polymer (Martina and Hutmacher, 2007). In addition, embedded degradable nanoparticles can act as porogens in synthesizing the porous scaffolds for vascularization and transport of nutrients, ions, and waste materials to and from the cells. Currently many exciting studies are being done to investigate the changes in the behavior of the scaffolds and resulting tissue regeneration by using scaffolds embedded with degradable nanoparticles. Natural as well as synthetic polymers have been investigated for formation of nanocomposites. Natural polymers like gelatin, fibrin, alginate, and collagen are used to synthesize nanoparticles to be embedded in the polymeric scaffolds mainly to mimic the ECM of the natural tissue to be regenerated. Another role of synthetic polymeric nanoparticles is for delivery of growth factors, cytokines to aid cell growth, attachment, and proliferation.

Natural degradable nanoparticles: Nanoparticles made of natural materials including collagen, which is a component of natural cartilage, bone, skin, and connective tissue and is also found in abundance in the ECM, have been incorporated into the scaffolds for tissue regeneration purposes. For instance, collagen nanoparticles embedded into polymeric scaffolds made of chitosan promoted the attachment of dermal fibroblast cells on the scaffold. Results from animal studies also showed that there was minimal inflammation caused by the nanocomposite scaffold of collagen nanoparticles embedded in chitosan membrane crosslinked by genipin crosslinker as compared to conventional wound healing methods. In addition, the composite scaffold allowed drainage of the wound exudates, proliferation of the fibroblast cells, and formation of the epithelial tissue which makes this nanocomposite a suitable matrix typically for wound healing and skin regeneration applications (Chen et al., 2009).

Synthetic degradable polymer particles: Nanoparticles made of synthetic degradable polymers have been widely developed and used to embed in the scaffolds for tissue engineering applications. PLGA can carry various hydrophilic/hydrophobic drugs, growth factors, and chemicals for chemical and physical stimulation of growth and differentiation of seeded cells on the scaffold. Using stem cells to differentiate into a particular cell lineage is a growing concept in the modern tissue engineering field which requires stimulating factors for differentiation of the cells. In one of the approaches using stem cells for articular cartilage tissue regeneration, sustained release of transforming growth factor $TGF-\beta_1$ from PLGA nanoparticles embedded within the scaffolds was used to promote differentiation of chondroblasts and MSCs. The nanocomposite system used for this application consisted of heparin-functionalized $TGF-\beta_1$-loaded PLGA nanoparticles and fibrin gels which further helped the differentiated cells to maintain their phenotype and produce cartilage ECM (Jung et al., 2009).

14.4   Conclusion and Future Outlook

Employing nanoparticles for the creation of nanotopography or nanocomposites has been attracting increasing interest in tissue engineering applications. Nanoparticles made of various inorganic and organic materials have been used to either modify the scaffold surfaces or embed into the scaffold materials to create nanotopography and nanostructure as well as to encapsulate and control release of therapeutic reagents to enhance cell adhesion, growth, and other functions within the scaffolds for tissue engineering applications. Although ample evidence demonstrates the efficacy of these nanostructures in improving the biocompatibility of the scaffold and enhancing tissue regeneration, the mechanism is yet to be elucidated. Some studies are still qualitative and many conflicting results still exist. In-depth studies with strictly regulated protocols and large number of repeats are needed to fully understand the effects of nanotopography and nanocomposites on cellular and tissue responses. Better particle incorporation techniques are needed to be developed in order to control the uniform distribution of nanoparticles throughout the surfaces or within the structures of tissue-engineering scaffolds for more reliable studies and results in tissue engineering applications. Nevertheless, advances in this field will reap significant rewards of achieving desired cell and tissue responses to create a future generation of biomaterials.

References

Abrams, G. A., S. L. Goodman, P. F. Nealey, M. Franco, and C. J. Murphy. 2000. Nanoscale topography of the basement membrane underlying the corneal epithelium of the rhesus macaque. *Cell Tissue Res.* 299(1): 39–46.

Adhirajan, N., N. Shanmugasundaram, S. Shanmuganathan, and M. Babu. 2009. Functionally modified gelatin microspheres impregnated collagen scaffold as novel wound dressing to attenuate the proteases and bacterial growth. *Eur. J. Pharm. Sci.* 36(2–3): 235–45.

Alexander, F. R. and B. R. William. 1999. A process model for latex film formation: Limiting regimes for individual driving forces. *Langmuir* 15(22): 7762–33.

Banerjee, I., D. Mishra, and T. K. Maiti. 2009. PLGA microspheres incorporated gelatin scaffold: Microspheres modulate scaffold properties. *Int J Biomater.* 2009: Article ID 143659.

Blodgett, K. B. 1935. Films built by depositing succesive monomolecular layers on a solid surface. *J. Am. Chem. Soc.* 57: 1007–22.

Boissard, C. I. R., P. E. Bourban, A. E. Tami, M. Alini, and D. Eglin, 2009. Nanohydroxyapatite/poly(ester urethane) scaffold for bone tissue engineering. *Acta Biomater.* 5(9): 3316–27.

Bosetti, M., and M. Cannas. 2005. The effect of bioactive glasses on bone marrow stromal cells differentiation. *Biomaterials* 26: 3873–79.

Cai, X., H. Tong, X. Shen, W. Chen, J. Yan, and J. Hu. 2009. Preparation and characterization of homogeneous chitosan-polylactic acid/hydroxyapatite nanocomposite for bone tissue engineering and evaluation of its mechanical properties. *Acta Biomater.* 5(7): 2693–703.

Chang, M. C., C.-C. Ko, and W. H. Douglas. 2003. Preparation of hydroxyapatite-gelatin nanocomposite. *Biomaterials* 24(17): 2853–62.

Chao, J. and K. Char. 2001. Fabrication of highly ordered multilayers films using a spin self-assembly method. *Adv. Mater.* 13(14): 1076–78.

Chen, K.-Y., W.-J. Liao, S.-M. Kuo, F.-J. Tsai, Y.-S. Chen, C.-Y. Huang, and C.-H. Yao. 2009. Asymmetric chitosan membrane containing collagen I nanospheres for skin tissue engineering. *Biomacromolecules* 10(6): 1642–49.

Chen, Q., J. A. Roether, and A. R. Boccaccini. 2008. Tissue engineering scaffolds from bioactive glass and composite materials. *Top. Tissue Eng.* 4. N.A.

Choi, C. H., S. H. Hagvall, B. M. Wu, J. C. Y. Dunn, R. E. Beygui, and C. J. Kim. 2007. Cell interaction with three-dimensional sharp-tip nanotopography. *Biomaterials* 28(9): 1672–79.

Cong, H. L. and W. X. Gao. 2003. Colloidal crystallization induced by capillary force. *Langmuir* 19(20): 8177–81.

Curtis, A. S., M. Dalby, and N. Gadegaard. 2006. Cell signaling arising from nanotopography: Implications for nanomedical devices. *Nanomedicine* 1(1): 67–72.

Curtis, A. S., N. Gadegaard, M. J. Dalby, M. O. Riehle, C. D. Wilkinson, and G. Aitchison. 2004. Cells react to nanoscale order and symmetry in their surroundings. *IEEE Trans. Nanobiosci.* 3(1): 61–5.

Dalby, M. J., S. Childs, M. O. Riehle, H. J. Johnstone, S. Affrossman, and A. S. Curtis. 2003. Fibroblast reaction to island topography: Changes in cytoskeleton and morphology with time. *Biomaterials* 24(6): 927–35.

Dalby, M. J., D. Giannaras, M. O. Riehle, N. Gadegaard, S. Affrossman, and A. S. Curtis. 2004. Rapid fibroblast adhesion to 27 nm high polymer demixed nano-topography. *Biomaterials* 25(1): 77–83.

Dalby, M. J., M. O. Riehle, H. Johnstone, S. Affrossman, and A. S. Curtis. 2002. *In vitro* reaction of endothelial cells to polymer demixed nanotopography. *Biomaterials* 23(14): 2945–54.

Dalby, M. J., M. O. Riehle, D. S. Sutherland, H. Agheli, and A. S. Curtis. 2004. Changes in fibroblast morphology in response to nano-columns produced by colloidal lithography. *Biomaterials* 25(23): 5415–22.

Dalby, M. J., M. O. Riehle, D. S. Sutherland, H. Agheli, and A. S. Curtis. 2005. Morphological and microarray analysis of human fibroblasts cultured on nanocolumns produced by colloidal lithography. *Eur. Cell Mater.* 9: 1–8; discussion 8.

Dent, E. W. and F. B. Gertler. 2003. Cytoskeletal dynamics and transport in growth cone motility and axon guidance. *Neuron* 40(2): 209–27.

Du, C., F. Z. Cui, X. D. Zhu, and K. de Groot. 1999. Three-dimensional nano-hap/collagen matrix loading with osteogenic cells in organ culture. *J. Biomed. Mater. Res.* 44(4): 407–15.

Dufrene, Y. F. 2001. Application of atomic force microscopy to microbial surfaces: From reconstituted cell surface layers to living cells. *Micron* 32(2): 153–65.

Flemming, R. G., C. J. Murphy, G. A. Abrams, S. L. Goodman, and P. F. Nealey. 1999. Effects of synthetic micro- and nano-structured surfaces on cell behavior. *Biomaterials* 20(6): 573–88.

Fu, Q. and H. F. Li. 2008. *In vitro* study on different cell responses to spherical hydroxyapatite nanoparticles. *J. Biomater. Appl.* 23(1): 37–50.

Gong, H. 2002. A new view of human trabecular meshwork using quick-greeze, deep-etch electron microscopy. *Exp. Eye Res.* 75: 347.

Hench, L. L. 1991. Bioceramics: From concept to clinic. *J. Am. Ceramic Soc.* 74: 1487–510.

Hong, Z., R. L. Reis, and J. F. Mano. 2008. Preparation and *in vitro* characterization of scaffolds of poly(L-lactic acid) containing bioactive glass ceramic nanoparticles. *Acta Biomater.* 4(5): 1297–306.

Hsu, S.-h., H.-J. Yen, and C.-L. Tsai. 2007. The response of articular chondrocytes to type Ii Collagen Au nanocomposites. *Artif. Organs* 31(12): 854–68.

Hsu, S.-h., C.-M. Tang, and H.-J. Tseng. 2008. Biostability and biocompatibility of poly(ester urethane)-gold nanocomposites. *Acta Biomater.* 4: 1797–808.

Hu, S.-H., T.-Y. Liu, C.-H. Tsai, and S.-Y. Chen. 2007. Preparation and characterization of magnetic ferroscaffolds for tissue engineering. *J. Magn. Magn. Mater.* 310(2), Part 3: 2871–73.

Itoh, S., K. Masanori, K. Yoshihisa, T. Kazuo, S. Kenichi, and T. Junzo. 2004. Development of a hydroxyapatitecollagen nanocomposite as a medical device. *Cell Transpl.* 13: 451–61.

Izquierdo, A., S. S. Ono, J. C. Voegel, P. Schaaf, and G. Decher. 2005. Dipping versus spraying: Exploring the deposition conditions for speeding up layer-by-layer assembly. *Langmuir* 21(16): 7558–67.

Jiang, P., J. F. Bertone, and V. L. Colvin. 1999. Single-crystal colloidal multilayers of controlled thickness. *Chem. Mater.* 11(8): 2132–40.

Jung, Y., Y.-Il Chung, S. H. Kim, G. Tae, Y. H. Kim, J. W. Rhie, S.-H. Kim, and S. H. Kim. 2009. *In Situ* chondrogenic differentiation of human adipose tissue-derived stem cells in a Tgf-B$_1$ loaded fibrin-poly(lactide-caprolactone) nanoparticulate complex. *Biomaterials* 30: 4657–64.

Justin, T. S. and T. J. Webster. 2008. Decreased astroglial cell adhesion and proliferation on zinc oxide nanoparticle polyurethane composites. *Int. J. Nanomed.* 3(4): 523–31.

Kato, K., Y. Eika, and Y. Ikada. 1997. *In situ* hydroxyapatite crystallization for the formation of hydroxyapatite/polymer composite. *J. Mater. Sci.* 32(20): 5533–43.

Kim, D. H., P. Kim, K. Suh, S. Kyu Choi, S. Ho Lee, and B. Kim. 2005. Modulation of adhesion and growth of cardiac myocytes by surface nanotopography. *Conf. Proc. IEEE Eng. Med. Biol. Soc.* 4: 4091–94.

Kim, P., D. H. Kim, B. Kim, S. K. Choi, S. H. Lee, A. Khademhosseini, R. Langer, and K. Y. Suh. 2005. Fabrication of nanostructures of polyethylene glycol for applications to protein adsorption and cell adhesion. *Nanotechnology* 16(10): 2420–26.

Kim, S. E., J. H. Park, Y. W. Cho, H. C., Seo Y. Jeong, E. B. Lee, and I. C. Kwon. 2003. Porous chitosan scaffold containing microspheres loaded with transforming growth factor-[beta]1: Implications for cartilage tissue engineering. *J. Control. Rel.* 91(3): 365–74.

Kitaev, K., and G. A. Ozin. 2003. Self-assembled surface patterns of binary colloidal crystals. *Adv. Mater.* 15(1): 75–8.

Kriparamanan, R., P. Aswath, A. Zhou, L. Tang, and K. T. Nguyen. 2006. Nanotopography: Cellular responses to nanostructured materials. *J. Nanosci. Nanotechnol.* 6(7): 1905–19.

Krogman, K. C., J. L. Lowery, N. S. Zacharia, G. C. Rutledge, and P. T. Hammond. 2009. Spraying asymmetry into functional membranes layer-by-layer. *Nat. Mater.* 8(6): 512–18.

Krogman, K. C., N. S. Zacharia, S. Schroeder, and P. T. Hammond. 2007. Automated process for improved uniformity and versatility of layer-by-layer deposition. *Langmuir* 23(6): 3137–41.

Kunzler, T. P., C. Huwiler, T. Drobek, J. Voros, and N. D. Spencer. 2007. Systematic study of osteoblast response to nanotopography by means of nanoparticle-density gradients. *Biomaterials* 28(33): 5000–6.

Langmuir, I. 1920. The mechanism of the surface phenomenon of flotation. *Trans. Faraday Soc.* 15: 62–74.

Lee, K.-W., S. Wang, M. J. Yaszemski, and L. Lu. 2008. Physical properties and cellular responses to cross-linkable poly(propylene fumarate)/hydroxyapatite nanocomposites. *Biomaterials* 29(19): 2839–48.

Lee, W., A. Chan, M. A. Bevan, J. A. Lewis, and P. V. Braun. 2004. Nanoparticle-mediated epitaxial assembly of colloidal crystals on patterned substrates. *Langmuir* 20(13): 5262–70.

Li, C., C. Vepari, H.-J. Jin, H. J. Kim, and D. L. Kaplan. 2006. Electrospun silk-Bmp-2 scaffolds for bone tissue engineering. *Biomaterials* 27(16): 3115–24.

Liao, S. S., F. Z. Cui, W. Zhang, and Q. L. Feng. 2004. Hierarchically biomimetic bone scaffold materials: Nano-ha/collagen/pla composite. *J. Biomed. Mater. Res. Part B: Appl. Biomater.* 69B(2): 158–65.

Lim, J. Y., J. C. Hansen, C. A. Siedlecki, J. Runt, and H. J. Donahue. 2005. Human foetal osteoblastic cell response to polymer-demixed nanotopographic interfaces. *J. R. Soc. Interface* 2(2): 97–108.

Lin, Y.-L., J.-C. Jen, S.-h. Hsu, and I.-M. Chiu. 2008. Sciatic nerve repair by microgrooved nerve conduits made of chitosan-gold nanocomposites. *Surg. Neurol.* 70(Suppl. 1): S9–S18.

Lo, C. T., P. R. Van Tassel, and W. M. Saltzman. 2009. Simultaneous release of multiple molecules from poly(lactide-*co*-glycolide) nanoparticles assembled onto medical devices. *Biomaterials* 30(28): 4889–97.

Ma, P. X. and J. Elisseeff. 2006. *Scaffolding in Tissue Engineering*. CRC Press, Boca Raton, FL.

Madhumathi, K., P. Sudheesh Kumar, S. Abhilash, V. Sreeja, H. Tamura, K. Manzoor, S. Nair, and R. Jayakumar. 2009. Development of novel chitin/nanosilver composite scaffolds for wound dressing applications. *J. Mater. Sci.: Mater. Med.* 21(2): 807–13.

Madhumathi, K., S. Kumar, P. T. Kavya, K. C. Furuike, T. Tamura, H. Nair, and S. V. Jayakumar, R. 2009. Novel chitin/nanosilica composite scaffolds for bone tissue engineering applications. *Int. J. Biol. Macromol.* 45(3): 289–92.

Martina, M. and D. W. Hutmacher. 2007. Biodegradable polymers applied in tissue engineering research: A review. *Polymer Int.* 56(2): 145–57.

Mihi, A., M. Ocaña, and H. Míguez. 2006. Oriented colloidal-crystal thin films by spin-coating microspheres dispersed in volatile media. *Adv. Mater.* 18(17): 2244–49.

Miller, D. C., A. Thapa, K. M. Haberstroh, and T. J. Webster. 2004. Endothelial and vascular smooth muscle cell function on poly(lactic-*co*-glycolic acid) with nano-structured surface features. *Biomaterials* 25(1): 53–61.

Millon, L. E. and W. K. Wan. 2006. The polyvinyl alcohol-bacterial cellulose system as a new nanocomposite for biomedical applications. *J. Biomed. Mater. Res. Part B: Appl. Biomater.* 79B(2): 245–53.

Mistry, A. S., Q. P. Pham, C. Schouten, T. Yeh, E. M. Christenson, A. G. Mikos, and J. A. Jansen. 2009. *In vivo* bone biocompatibility and degradation of porous fumarate-based polymer/alumoxane nanocomposites for bone tissue engineering. *J. Biomed. Mater. Res. Part A* 9999(9999): NA.

Miura, M. and K. Fujimoto. 2006. Subcellular topological effect of particle monolayers on cell shapes and functions. *Colloids Surf. B-Biointerfaces* 53(2): 245–53.

Murugan, R. and S. Ramakrishna. 2005. Development of nanocomposites for bone grafting. *Composites Sci. Technol.* 65(15–16): 2385–406.

Nomura, S., H. Kojima, Y. Ohyabu, K. Kuwabara, A. Miyauchi, and T. Uemura. 2006. Nanopillar sheets as a new type of cell culture dish: Detailed study of Hela cells cultured on nanopillar sheets. *J. Artif. Organs* 9(2): 90–6.

Nuzzo, R. G. and D. L. Allara. 1983. Adsorption of bifunctional organic disulfides on gold surfaces. *J. Am. Chem. Soc.* 105: 4481.

Pennisi, C. P., C. Sevcencu, A. Dolatshahi-Pirouz, M. Foss, J. L. Hansen, A. N. Larsen, V. Zachar, F. Besenbacher, and K. Yoshida. 2009. Responses of fibroblasts and glial cells to nanostructured platinum surfaces. *Nanotechnology* 20(38): 385103.

Sarkar, S., G. Y. Lee, J. Y. Wong, and T. A. Desai. 2006. Development and characterization of a porous micro-patterned scaffold for vascular tissue engineering applications. *Biomaterials* 27(27): 4775–82.

Seil, J. T. and T. J. Webster. 2008. Decreased astroglial cell adhesion and proliferation on zinc oxide nano-particle polyurethane composite. *Int J Nanomedicine* 3(4): 523–31.

Shimmin, R. G., A. L. Dimauro, and P. L. Braun. 2006. Slow vertical deposition of colloidal crystals: A Langmuir–Blodgett process? *Langmuir* 22(15): 6507–13.

Soichiro, I., M. Kikuchi, Y. Koyama, K. Takakuda, K. Shinomiya, and J. Tanaka. 2004. Development of a Hydroxyapatite/Collagen Nanocomposte as a Medical Device. *Cell Transplant* 13(4): 451–61.

Song, J., E. Saiz, and C. R. Bertozzi. 2003. A new approach to mineralization of biocompatible hydrogel scaffolds: An efficient process toward 3-dimensional bonelike composites. *J. Am. Chem. Soc.* 125(5): 1236–43.

Spadaccio, C., A. Rainer, M. Trombetta, G. Vadalá, M. Chello, E. Covino, V. Denaro, Y. Toyoda, and J. A. Genovese. 2009. Poly-L-lactic acid/hydroxyapatite electrospun nanocomposites induce chondrogenic differentiation of human msc. *Ann. Biomed. Eng.* 37(7): 1376–89.

Stevens, B., Y. Yang, A. Mohandas, B. Stucker, and K. T. Nguyen. 2008. A review of materials, fabrication methods, and strategies used to enhance bone regeneration in engineered bone tissues. *J. Biomed. Mater. Res. Part B: Appl. Biomater.* 85B(2): 573–82.

Šupová, M. 2009. Problem of hydroxyapatite dispersion in polymer matrices: A review. *J. Mater. Sci.: Mater. Med.* 20(6): 1201–13.

Tampieri, A., G. Celotti, E. Landi, M. Sandri, N. Roveri, and G. Falini. 2003. Biologically inspired synthesis of bone-like composite: Self-assembled collagen fibers/hydroxyapatite nanocrystals. *J. Biomed. Mater. Res. Part A* 67A(2): 618–25.

Tan, H., J. Wu, L. Lao, and C. Gao. 2009. Gelatin/chitosan/hyaluronan scaffold integrated with plga microspheres for cartilage tissue engineering. *Acta Biomater.* 5(1): 328–37.

Thapa, A., D. C. Miller, T. J. Webster, and K. M. Haberstroh. 2003. Nano-structured polymers enhance bladder smooth muscle cell function. *Biomaterials* 24(17): 2915–26.

Venkatesh, S., and P. Jiang. 2007. Generalized fabrication of two-dimensional non-close-packed colloidal crystals. *Langmuir* 2007(23): 8231–35.

Verma, D., K. S. Katti, and D. R. Katti. 2009. Polyelectrolyte-complex nanostructured fibrous scaffolds for tissue engineering. *Mater. Sci. Eng. C* 29(7): 2079–84.

Wang, A. J., S. L. Chen, and P. Dong. 2009. Rapid fabrication of a large-area 3d silica colloidal crystal thin film by a room temperature floating self-assembly method. *Mater. Lett.* 63(18–19): 1586–89.

Wang, D. and H. Möhwald. 2004. Rapid fabrication of binary colloidal crystals by stepwise spin-coating. *Adv. Mater.* 16(3): 244–47.

Wang, J., S. Ahl, and Q. Li. 2008. Structural and optical characterization of 3d binary colloidal crystal and inverse opal films prepared by direct co-deposition. *J. Mater. Chem.* 18(9): 981–88.

Wang, L. K. and X. S. Zhao. 2007. Fabrication of crack-free colloidal crystals using a modified vertical deposition method. *J. Phys. Chem. C* 111(24): 8538–42.

Wolf, K., R. Muller, S. Borgmann, E. B. Brocker, and P. Friedl. 2003. Amoeboid shape change and contact guidance: T-lymphocyte crawling through fibrillar collagen is independent of matrix remodeling by Mmps and other proteases. *Blood* 102(9): 3262–69.

Wood, M. A., C. D. Wilkinson, and A. S. Curtis. 2006. The effects of colloidal nanotopography on initial fibroblast adhesion and morphology. *IEEE Trans. Nanobiosci.* 5(1): 20–31.

Xia, Y., Y. Yin, and J. Mclellan. 2003. Template-assisted self-assembly of spherical colloids into complex and controllable structures. *Adv. Funct. Mater.* 13(12): 907–18.

Yanagida, H., M. Okada, M. Masuda, M. Ueki, I. Narama, S. Kitao, Y. Koyama, T. Furuzono, and K. Takakuda. 2009. Cell adhesion and tissue response to hydroxyapatite nanocrystal-coated poly(L-lactic acid) fabric. *J. Biosci. Bioeng.* 108(3): 235–43.

Yang, G. B. and P. Y. Zhang. 2009. Preparation and characterization of layer-by-layer self-assembled polyelectrolyte multilayer films doped with surface-capped SiO_2 nanoparticles. *J. Colloid Interface Sci.* 333(2): 776–81.

Yang, S., K.-F. Leong, Z. Du, C.-K. Chua. 2001. The design of scaffolds for use in tissue engineering. Part i. traditional factors. *Tissue Eng.* 7(6): 679–89.

Yu, D. G., W. C. Lin, and M. C. Yang. 2007. Surface modification of poly(L-lactic acid) membrane via layer-by-layer assembly of silver nanoparticle-embedded polyelectrolyte multilayer. *Bioconj. Chem.* 18(5): 1521–29.

Zeng, F., Z. W. Sun, and C. Y. Wang. 2002. Fabrication of inverse opal via ordered highly charged colloidal spheres. *Langmuir* 18(24): 9116–20.

Zhang, S. M., F. Z. Cui, S. S. Liao, Y. Zhu, and L. Han. 2003. Synthesis and biocompatibility of porous nano-hydroxyapatite/collagen/alginate composite. *J. Mater. Sci.: Mater. Med.* 14(7): 641–45.

Zhao, Y., K. Thorkelsson, A. J. Mastroianni, T. Schilling, J. M. Luther, B. J. Rancatore, K. Matsunaga, et al. 2009. Small-molecule-directed nanoparticle assembly towards stimuli-responsive nanocomposites. *Nat. Mater.* 8(12): 979–85.

Index

Printed and bound by CPI Group (UK) Ltd, Croydon, CR0 4YY

23/10/2024

01778257-0004